MW01273841

Carnivore Diet Cookbook

Approach to Modern Wholesome Meat Recipes to Healthy Living and Delay Aging

Haile Banister

Contents

The Carnivore Meal Plan Cookbook for Athletes

The Ultimate Electric Smoker Cookbook

Air Fryer Cookbook for Summer

The Healthy Air Fryer Cookbook with Pictures

Air Fryer Cookbook for Summer

Carnivore diet Cookbook

The Carnivore Meal Plan Cookbook for Athletes

The Protein-Based Program You Need to Build Progressive Endurance and Strength like a Pro [Meal Plan Worth: 1.375$]

By

Haile Banister

Contents

Introduction

Nutrition is crucial for athletes at the most fundamental level because it offers an energy source to conduct the task. Our power, preparation, productivity, and training are influenced by the meal we intake. Not only is the kind of food important to sports nutrition, but the times we consume across the day also affect our levels of performance and the ability of our bodies to recover after exercise. It's important to set your goals before you start eating the carnivorous diet method.

Keep in mind this is a change in lifestyle - no carbs, no plants, only products from animals and lots of good fat. You need to know why you are getting into the carnivore diet throughout the first place, whether it's to achieve your intended body weight, fight food allergies, decrease body fat battle with an autoimmune condition, and construct some muscular strength.

The Carnivore Diet arises from the widespread concept that mainly meat and fish were consumed by human ancestor communities and that high-carb diets are responsible for today's high rates of infectious disease.

Meals ingested before and after the workout are the most important thing about sports performance, but you should always be vigilant with all you put into your body. Athletes should eat around two hours before practicing as a general rule, and this diet should be low in fat, high in carbohydrates and high in protein.

The primary source of nutrition that drives your exercise schedule is protein, and carbohydrates are needed to help muscle recovery. You, therefore, need to replace the nutrients you have lost after exercising, and by incorporating protein in your post-workout meal, you need to allow consistent muscle recovery.

Chapter 1: Whatisthe carnivore diet?

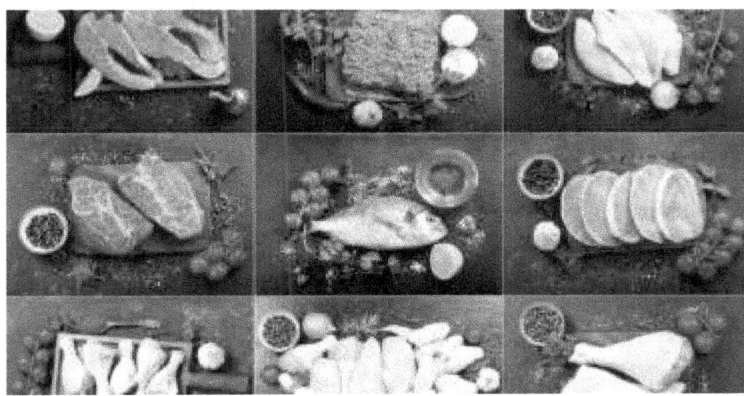

The Carnivore diet consists of foods dependent on animals, including fish, meat, low lactose milk and eggs products. Honey, zero carb seasoning, salt and pepper may also be used by a consumer pursuing the diet.

Certain items are eliminated from the diet, like grains, vegetables and fruits, plant-based oils, high lactose milk and carbohydrates.

The carnivore diet is based on the controversial theory that it was rich in meat eaten by human ancestors long ago. It assumes that when boosted by high protein and fat levels, human bodies operate best.

Figures such as Jordan Peterson (bestselling author and psychologist), Joe Rogan (standup comedian and podcast host), Shawn Baker (retired orthopedic surgeon) have made the diet popular.

On Carnivore Diet, once the appetite is satisfied, you eat fatty cuts of the high-quality meal and avoid all carbs, Sauces, Fruits, Nuts, Plant-based food, and Veggies.

Therefore, a carnivore diet is considered an "elimination diet" that can clarify its effectiveness in supporting others with digestive issues, constipation, and food sensitivities.

1.1 How to organize your meal plan for your Carnivore Diet.

In Carnivore Diet, these tips have enabled us a great deal to remain encouraged and accomplish some auxiliary goals. That's the opportunity to get rid of extra fat, lose weightand attain that little muscular strength without missing the micronutrients needed. So, get into it now.

1. Know Your Why

It's necessary to set your objectives before you start your carnivore diet plan. Note that it is indeed a shift of lifestyle no carbs, no plants, just products from animals and lots of healthy fat. You have to remember why you are going into a carnivore diet from the first place, whether it's to achieve your target body weight, decrease body fat, battle digestive problems, cure an autoimmune condition, or create some lean muscle.

Depending on your needs, you have to assign yourself a clear goal. Perhaps it's about losing 20 lbs. Whether you go out on a summer break and acquire 5 pounds of muscle mass in six months - whatever it is, in the entire process, Stay close to the meat-only diet style.

It would be like a suggestion to help you stay on track to proceed with the carnivore diet. Whatever that is, to inform you of your diet pattern, experienced carnivore dieters may write it all down and upload it somewhere that you can see each day. Based on your losing weight and other fitness objectives, it'll be like a way to remind you to keep you active to proceed with the carnivore diet.

2. Plan for sticking to The Meal Plan

It requires absolute devotion and determination to consume a moderate animal fat, carnivore diet for further than a few days or weeks. On the carnivore diet, the worst thing you can do is start taking it day by day and postpone it until the morning to find out what you're going to eat next. Instead, set specific targets for the week, use a diet planner, and list carnivore diet foods to schedule what animal products to consume in advance.

We also involve items like how many runs and visits to the workout we do, as well as what we'll have with each meal for our regular carnivore diet, in addition to having a carnivore diet food chart.

You may take some further time to discover new kinds of varieties of meat products you may like and methods of preparation to introduce a little more variety to your menu of animal meat. To try more diet choices and taste new tastes, you can also try on eating fresh animal organs (such as heart or cow liver). You can benefit from meal delivery if you are not dependent on cooking your foods while on the diet weight loss diet. It's an efficient method to reignite your Carnivore diet, and most significantly, according to your body's needs, you receive quality meats, pork, or chicken meat.

3.Preparations toward social life

The reality is that, on a carnivore diet, eating at social events seems to be one of the most disturbing situations. If you eat at a dinner party like that and tell people how every day eats lunch at McDonald's, eat Donuts and dinner pizza, you're not going to be judged more by people.

Suppose you tell another person on the table that you are on a carnivore diet meal schedule, though, because it includes eating only animal fat, zero plant foods and red meat because of your favorite diet. In that case, the entire table is now shocking. There's a vegetarian at the table, and Heaven forbid, you won't hear another word of it. Firstly, tell people you are doing so because of multiple problems with food allergies, and determining the underlying reasons, you are sticking with a carnivore diet.

Generally, at the start, we don't like speaking regarding weight loss. You'll only get remarks from several people so with this way, such as: "You're totally crazy not to eat fruit and veg, and it's so stupid." The vegetarian at the table will also have a lot of fruitier nutritional vocabulary and a long discussion about the need to eat fruit and veggies to get more nutrition. In this scenario, we find that asking if they are associated with their fitness or yours is the only solution that helps? It fits us nine times in a row, and if you get yourself sitting beside the vegetarian, then change the topic to another one.

4. Dining Out

The pleasant deal for people upon this carnivore diet is with quality nutrition meats that will suit your needs; there are many places you can eat out. Eating at BBQ and steak restaurants is probably the best decision you can make. But make sure to avoid animal meats that are frozen. In the carnivorous weight loss diet, consuming meat products is not tolerated. Everything you need to do is pay attention to the way the meals are prepared. While on a carnivore diet, the main thing is to avoid consuming something that includes stir-fried vegetables or sauces.

Unfortunately, in many Indian and Chinese restaurants, you'll most likely stop eating out for a carnivore diet because almost all their meals are heavy with sauces and salt. What we usually do when we start our all-meat diet is review the menus online. We'd be likely to eat there as long as we see filet mignon and are steaks accessible.

1.215daysmeal plan for the Carnivore Diet.

Carnivore Diet For 1st week

On Monday

Breakfast 1 or 2 100 percent pure pork sausages (3 ounces) and Five bacon slices (about 4 ounces)

Lunch just 10 ounces of grilled beef patty burger with a slice of cheese.

Dinner four stacks of healthy lamb (12 ounces)

On Tuesday

Breakfast 3 bacon slices (4 ounces) 3 grilled 100 percent pure pork sausages (about 5 ounces)

Lunch Slammed buttery cutlets of salmon upon the bone (about 15 ounces).

Dinner Porterhouse steak (12 ounces) grilled with butter.

On Wednesday

Breakfast Grilled trout fillets with butter (about 10 ounces)

Lunch Grilledbelly ofpork (about 10 ounces)

Dinner Slowbeef roast upper side (about 12 ounces)

On Thursday

Breakfast Roasted ground beef burger patty with cheese (about 8 ounces)

Lunch Roast salmon cutlets with butter on the bone (about 15 ounces)

Dinner Grilled steak porterhouse (about 12 ounces)

On Friday

Breakfast 2 breasts of grilled chicken with skin (about 8 ounces)

Lunchfillets of fried trout (about 16 ounces)

Dinner Slow grilledupper side of beef (about 12 ounces)

On Saturday

Breakfast three100 percent pure pork sausages grilled (about 5 ounces)

Lunch Three slices of bacon (about 4 ounces) Fourhealthy lamb chops (about 12 ounces)

Dinner Grilled steak ribeye (about 12 ounces)

On Sunday

Breakfast two breasts of grilled chicken with skin (about 8 ounces)

Lunch 4 grilled or fried pork chops (about 12 ounces)

Dinner Grilledsteak ribeye (about 12 ounces)

Shopping list for 1st week

- Pork belly about 10 ounces
- Lamb Chops about 24 ounces
- Beef Grounded abouteighteen ounces
- Porterhouse steak about twenty-four ounces
- Topside of beef about twenty-four ounces
- Salmon cutlets about thirty ounces (or other fatty fish)
- Trout about twenty-six ounces
- Butteraround one lb.
- Cheese around half lbs.

- Bacon about twelve ounces
- 100 percent pork sausages around 13 ounces
- Pork chops about twelve ounces
- Chicken breasts
- Ribeye steak about twenty-four ounces
- The topside of beef about twenty-four ounces
- salmon cutlets aboutthirty ounces (or any otherfish with fats)

Carnivore diet meal plan for 2nd week

We will be reducing much of the milk from items on our carnivore diet during the next week. We're still going to allow the butter to be utilized for the food, but dairy foods such as cheese will now be gone.

On Monday

Breakfast Two breasts of grilled chicken with skin (about 8 ounces)

Lunch Slow beef grilledtopside (about 12 ounces)

Dinner fourhealthy lamb pieces (about 12 ounces)

Tuesday

Breakfast roasted ground beef patty burger (about 8 ounces)

Lunchon the bone roasted salmon cutlets (about 15 ounces)

Dinner Grilled steak ribeye (about 8 ounces) and roasted liver of beef (about 4 ounces)

On Wednesday

Breakfast 5 bacon slices (about 4 ounces) and one- or two-100 percent pork sausages (about 3 ounces)

Lunch grilled porterhouse steak with butter (about 12 ounces)

Dinner Slowbeef roast topside (about 12 ounces)

On Thursday

Breakfast Grilled steak with ribeye (about 12 ounces)

Lunch 3 chicken breasts grilled with skin (around 12 ounces)

Dinner barbequed ground beef patty burger (around 12 ounces)

On Friday

Breakfast sirloin steak grilled with butter (about 8 ounces)

Lunch Slowbeef roast topside (about 8 ounces) and roastedliver of beef (4 ounces)

Dinner with fourfried or grilled pork pieces (about 12 ounces)

On Saturday

Breakfast Grilled ground beefpatty burger (about 8 ounces)

Lunch Roast salmon cutlets on the bone with butter (about 15 ounces)

Dinner Grilled steak of sirloin (12 ounces)

On **Sunday**

Breakfast Grilled steak ribeye (about 8 ounces)

Lunch Slow roast beef upside (about 12 ounces)

Dinner 3 grilled with skin chicken breast (about 12 ounces) and roastedliver of beef (about 4 ounces)

Shopping list for 2nd week:

- Salmon cutlets aboutthirty ounces or any other fatty fish
- Ribeye steak abouttwenty-eight ounces
- Pork chops aroundtwelve ounces
- Beef's liver aroundtwelve ounces
- Ribeye steak aroundtwenty-four ounces
- 100 percent pork sausages aboutthree ounces
- Porterhouse steak abouttwelve ounces
- Chicken breasts aboutthirty-two ounces
- Topside of beef around forty-four ounces
- Lamb chops around twelve ounces

1.3 What food is included in the carnivore diet?

The Carnivore Diet falls completely under one category of food: animal products.

Though animal products can break into additional categories, there are various content standards within each category. Now let's look into those classifications.

MEAT

Any type: lamb, beef, poultry, pork etc. Preferably choose grass-fed or organic meats.

ORGANS

Organs are an excellent substitute but are a key element of a well-formulated carnivore diet. Try to include chicken liver, kidneys, beef heart, beef liver, and brains.

EGGS.

Eggs of all kinds from most birds. Where possible, choose organic.

FISH AND SEAFOOD

Choose fatty fish such as sardines, mackerel, salmon herring are great and might even have health privilege due to high amounts of omega-3 fatty acids. Other seafood includes shrimp, squid tilapia, tuna, swordfish, and trout scallops.

DAIRY

Choose full-fat options where possible, like full-fat cream, real butter, sour cream, high-fat cheeses, and Greek yogurt. Try to use skim milk minimum, reduced fat, and regular milk as they contain many sugars.

FATS AND OILS

For cooking, use ghee, butter, tallow, lard, chicken fat, suet and tallow duck fat.

CARNIVORE DRINKS

WATER

Wherever appropriate, water must be your first preference. Try sparkling water if you think you're going to struggle with your water intake.

BONE BROTH

Broth from any animal's bones will make a drink that is warm and comforting.

TEA

Tea would Be OK with a drop of cream or milk. Green tea is best with no milk.

COFFEE

Coffee with milk, Black coffee or coffee with cream is all fine. Remember that the cream provides extra calories that you do not account for when attempting to lose weight.

1.4 What Food items avoided on the Carnivore diet?

The Carnivore Diet prohibits all food that does not come from animals.

Restricted foods include:

Vegetables: green beans, cauliflower, potatoes, broccoli, peppers, etc.

Legumes: lentils, beans, etc.

Nuts and seeds: sunflower seeds, pumpkin seeds, almonds, pistachios, etc.

Grains: quinoa, bread, pasta, rice, wheat, etc.

Alcohol: wine, liquor, beer, etc.

Sugars: maple syrup, brown sugar, table sugar etc.

"Beverages" other than water: coffee, tea, fruit juice, soda etc.

PROCESSED MEATS

Process meats are highly insufficient in diet and moderate in chemical substances.

LOW-FAT MILK.

High sugar usually consists of skimmed milk and low fat. Unless you need to, restrict it to a few drops in your coffee or tea.

Sauces & Seasoning

While seasoning a steak with thyme, salt, or even paprika is not unusual, going too deep on sauces and seasoning can cause stomach issues for those with a weak immune system.

Foods on the Carnivore Diet that might be OK.

Foods that may be permissible include:

Milk

Yogurt

Cheese

1.5 How carnivore diets have beneficial effects?

The carnivore diet has helped thousands of people fix the effects of many health conditions or improve them. Check out some favorable circumstances of the carnivore diet.

Minimize Acid Reflux

As stomach acid rises into the esophagus, acid reflux occurs, causing discomfort that can lead to heartburn symptoms. In the United States, this is relatively a common medical complaint, and many of us live on the belief that there is little we can do to change it. Fortunately, that isn't valid.

Although no food form has yet been shown to cure this disorder entirely, your dietary choices will help minimize or even eradicate symptoms a great deal. That makes a decent amount of sense, provided that in your stomach, this condition begins.

IMPROVED ACNE

Acne, defined by the occurrence of spots mostly on the face, neck and shoulders and is also a sign of hormonal changes that causes inflammation elsewhere in the body. It can be physically and psychologically uncomfortable, depending on your diet, and it's avoidable.

There are several reasons why the carnivore diet helps hold spots at bay. The key theory connects carbohydrate intake and acne. Image Inflammation is a significant cause of acne as well. Incidentally, in those that eat so many carbohydrates, inflammation is identified.

Meat also provides vital nutrients, which have also been observed to affect breakouts, including omega 3s and zinc. Several meat substitutes, such as milk, can also worsen no-ending acne. If you want flawless skin, a carnivore diet could provide an alternative.

Maintain ADD/ADHD

Hyperactivity disorders that affect kids, teenagers, and even adults are called ADD and ADHD. Either syndrome may contribute to hyperactivity, impaired control of impulses, and trouble paying attention.

It is no secret that in problems such as these, diet plays a major role. Although many studies of ADHD and diet effects are still needed, the wrong foods appear to worsen troublesome symptoms.

The advantages of the carnivore diet have been shown to improve the symptoms. Perhaps because of the interaction of plant foods with the gut microbiome.

PREVENT ALZHEIMER'S

Alzheimer's is a steady brain disease that kills memory, cognitive capacity, and comprehension of even basic activities such as brushing teeth. It has a devastating effect on the lives of patients affected and on their loved ones and sometimes results in hospitalization or treatment for the long term.

The good news is that there is evidence to indicate a diet that can help with such a carnivore diet free of plant foods. Although there is no way to reverse the effect of Alzheimer's, modifying diets like this might minimize symptoms. Studies show that consuming a lower diet of plant foods over your life can also minimize the risk of Alzheimer's by up to 44%!

The association between the lectins present in plants and Alzheimer's is the key explanation why plant foods are causing concern. As such, patients who eat large quantities of plant food can intensify their symptoms and put themselves at risk. By contrast, healthy fats such as those present in beef can hold symptoms at bay and, as a result, delay Alzheimer's expansion.

IMPROVE BLOOD PRESSURE

Blood pressure associate with the pressure of circulating blood on the walls of blood vessels. Lifestyle and diet control of blood pressure is essential for ongoing health and the prevention of progressive health problems such as heart disease. While meat gave a bad perspective when it comes to blood pressure, it is not reasonable.

In terms of blood pressure regulation, limiting carbohydrate intake and consuming red meat and fish, turkey, or skinless chicken have shown positive results.

It is mainly due to high levels of protein present in animal foods, according to studies. There is also some evidence that a balanced intake of vitamin D and omega-3 will help maintain an even keel for blood pressure rates. Obviously, with a very well carnivore diet, they are simple enough to come by.

REDUCE CANCER RISK

A disease that no one wishes to obtain is cancer, marked by the uncontrolled division of cancerous cells. It's one of the most serious diseases we struggle with without a cure today, despite medical advances and increased recovery rates.

Our chances of developing cancer will affect our lifestyle. Smoking, for instance, increases the probability of irregular cells. What fewer people know is that cancer and what we eat also have close ties. Although research is underway on exactly what effect food can have, a balanced diet is important to keep this problem at bay.

In particular, studies have shown that diets that are low in carbohydrates and rich in healthy proteins may help keep the body fit and resistant to cancer growth. Red meat and poultry can provide any diet with a great deal of protein while also maintaining gut bacteria as safe for cancer-fighting potential as possible.

DIABETES CONTROL

Diabetes is a chronic disorder that impacts the body's ability to maintain the consumption of sugar.

Type 1 diabetes happens when the body's immune system kills cells that contain insulin.

Type 2 diabetes happens when a person does not, in the first place, generate enough insulin. This disease, as you are probably aware, occurs mainly in people with low, high-sugar diets. In reality, by simply changing what they eat, some individuals with type 2 diabetes might completely turn around. Management of diabetes is a considerable health improvement of carnivore diet, and it is not unbelievable to see that high-quality meat may help minimize sugar intake. That's because the protein found in red meats will hold the level of satiety stable for longer, often without causing blood pressure to increase. Zero carbs, which has been proven to be one of the effective methods of controlling blood glucose levels, is also a carnivore diet.

WEIGHT LOSS

While we're on the topic of losing weight, the carnivore diet has become just another possible health gain. In the U.S. alone, estimates that there are approximately 160 million people above.

It is a set of problems because overweight itself can contribute to many of the issues we have addressed here, including heart diseases, thyroid issues, and diabetes.Fortunately, meat has one of the planet's most weight-loss-friendly ingredients. That's why the carnivore diet is so satisfying for so many.

Thanks to its high nutritional value, lean beef has specifically been found to be useful here. A high-quality steak will keep you energized, manage blood sugar, and also ensure that you don't need to have a snack. Protein was quite good for this; in particular, research has shown that a 25 percent increase in protein can reduce cravings by 60 percent. Even better, to appreciate those all-important advantages, you don't need to compromise on taste.

CONSTIPATION RELIEF

Constipation refers to irregular bodily functions that are hard to get through. What we eat will play a major role in producing symptoms in a condition of this type. And you can guarantee that when you spend all night in the bathroom, you will regret those unhealthy choices.

In contrast, it will help to keep our digestive system normal and flowing by shifting our preference to constipation-friendly menus. That, in turn, if we put the effort in, will hold the C-word at bay for our entire lives for a long period.

Here, the carnivore diet is also helpful as it offers delicious, low fiber meals that ensure that things move for you. No studies support the argument that high in fiber foods are beneficial for digestive health, and zero fiber diets have shown the best improvements in some research.

EPILEPSY MANAGEMENT

Epilepsy disrupts the mechanisms of brain messaging and thus causes frequent seizures. Some patients will only have seizures in their childhood and teenage years, whereas others will continue to fight epilepsy through their lifetime. Epilepsy causes fluctuate and may include head injuries and disorders of the brain. However, you might be surprised to learn that specialists have found proven advantages for patients concentrating on dietary changes, particularly low-carb diets such as the carnivore diet. Eating just meat may have such an effect that certain patients can decrease or eliminate drugs and encounter fewer or no seizures. In situations like this, high-fat products such as hamburgers and bacon also seem to have the best outcomes. Although it is not generally understood why all these foods have such a major effect on seizures (up to a reduction of

90%!), the research suggests that it can make a huge difference to eat more fat and to steer clear of carbohydrates.

Reduce THYROIDs Problems

Thyroid issues come in a variety of forms and often occur due to thyroid hormone production issues. The overproduction of certain hormones is hyperthyroidism. When the thyroid stops producing enough hormones, hypothyroidism occurs. Problems such as these can be dangerous for patients, although they are fully treatable with hormone substitutes or, in several cases, diet.

Evidence indicates that it can go a long way to minimize or even avoid thyroid disorders by consuming a diet rich in unique nutrients. When you look at just what those nutrients are, it's obvious to see that most of them are in meat.

In particular, zinc can stimulate thyroid hormones in hypothyroidism and is not in short supply from a diet rich in beef. All meats are, in truth, recommended for those who need to increase the development of thyroid hormone. It's also worth noting that it has been shown that weight loss on a low-carb diet helps reduce the development of excess thyroid hormones. That implies that increased intake of meat will enhance this situation all around.

1.6 Side Effects of carnivore diet and their Cures?

Without its health consequences, no diet appears that's also part of the carnivore diet. Fortunately, on an animal-based diet, the human body performs exceptionally well, and any harmful side effects are temporary. Here are a few side effects of a carnivorous diet and how to treat them.

DIARRHEA ON CARNIVORE DIET

Your gastrointestinal tract may experience disruptions if you have diarrhea, feel uneasy in the bathroom, or get alarming signals from the digestive system.

What happens?

Diarrhea may happen when food moves too rapidly through your digestive tract. Transit times are typically slower if you've been consuming plant foods to give your body time to cope with the extra fiber and extract nutrients from the food. Transit time can be affected as you move to a zero-fiber diet and diarrhea occurs.

What's the effective cure?

On the carnivore diet, the treatment for diarrhea is:

Give your body time to adjust to a zero-fiber diet - food can move too quickly through the large intestine at first so that the large intestine pulls water from the food.

Minimize the intake of rendered fats - liquid fats such as tallow and cream are commonly rendered fats. These fat types can move too easily through your system.

BAD BREATH ON THE CARNIVORE DIET

One of the side effects of going from a high protein diet using glucose as the primary fuel source to a low carb diet while using ketones as a fuel source is bad breath. "The "keto breath" is often considered to.

What Happens?

Compound acetone is responsible for the change in the scent of your breath. Acetone is the simplest and perhaps most rapidly changing of the various forms of ketones and is formed from acetoacetate, ketone muscle dissolution. Acetone disperses into the lungs during ketosis and leaves the body as you exhale.

What's the effective cure?

Some individuals don't get a keto breath, but with time, it goes away on its own for those who do. If you do have it, during the carnivore diet, there are some things you can do to minimize bad breath.

Wait - if it's not that bad, sitting it out and waiting for it to go on its own is OK.

Drink more - As you urinate, ketones can often leave the body, so drinking more water will also eliminate extra ketones in the urine.

Stay fresh- Keep your teeth, tongue, gums, and mouth clean so the air you breathe does not mix with any other unpleasant odors.

HEART PALPITATIONS ON THE CARNIVORE DIET

The carnivore diet's common symptom is heart palpitations, beating heart, and flutters, but it is generally episodic and nothing to stress about in these situations.

What Happens

It's normal to find that your heart rate increases, or your stroke volume increases when you first adopt a carnivore diet. It is generally due to a lower blood volume, dehydration, and a loss of electrolytes, which can be the product of low blood volume. The heart needs to toughen up to work harder to maintain the blood pressure when you feel those fast heartbeats.

What's the effective cure?

Drinking enough water is the easiest cure and ensuring that you keep the salt your body requires will help fight those palpitations in the heart. Additional options include:

Take some magnesium - the recommended daily amount is up to 400 mg per day and is safe for most individuals.

Get on point with your salt intake - too little or too much can cause palpitations in the chest. It's probably more likely that you have too little rather than too many.

Add in carbs - You will need to add more carbs to raise blood flow if the heart palpitations do not go away within a few weeks.

HIGH CHOLESTEROL ON THE CARNIVORE DIET

What Happens?

The Carnivore Diet is high in sodium, cholesterol and fat, and the elevation of your cholesterol levels may be one of the diet's most important concerns. The rise in saturated fat increases your levels of cholesterol with time. Cholesterol, however, is not bad. The media and recent studies show that low carb and higher fat diets can contribute to an improved lipid profile.

What's the effective cure?

Before you start the carnivore diet, have your cholesterol levels tested first and foremost, so you have a baseline on which to operate. There are a few things you can do if you get a relevant lipid profile on the carnivore diet:

Reduce the consumption of liquid fat. It can also, on its own, boost your lipid profile.

For at least 12 hours a day, try fasting. There is sufficient evidence to suggest that this would lower total cholesterol levels.

Consult the physician. Most doctors are willing to speak with you about your carnivore way of life and give suggestions, particularly younger ones.

LEG CRAMPS ON CARNIVORE DIET

Among those who just started the carnivore diet, leg cramps are a frequent issue, but they typically fade over time. With that said, on the carnivore diet, there are some items you can do to avoid or remove leg cramps completely.

What Happens?

Muscle cramps are caused by the change of nutrients, especially magnesium. Consequently, it is also not unusual to get leg cramps due to low potassium or sodium intake.

What's the effective cure?

On the carnivore diet, leg cramps treatment is to even magnesium, sodium, and potassium levels. It can attain in two ways:

Increase sodium - Maybe the best way to balance your mineral levels is to add additional salt to your diet to avoid mineral loss. As levels of sodium decline, amounts of magnesium and potassium normally follow.

Supplement - consider replacing with magnesium in some situations where more sodium does not help.

Slow down - you might want some more time to adapt and in the worst situation where nothing works. Although pushing through is possible, it's also OK to add more carbs and then slowly decrease them over time to allow your body time to adjust.

Adaption: Nausea, Headaches, Lack of focus, Irritability

Due to your body's normal reaction to carbohydrate limitation and the elimination of unnecessary chemicals and additives, you will notice some unpleasant side effects and side symptoms during adaptation.

Some of the other effects of the adaption process include headache, chills, digestive issues, dizziness, irritability, bad breath/smell, dry mouth, brain fog, nausea, bad taste in the mouth, poor focus, insomnia, decreased physical performance, sore throat cramping, cravings, diarrhea, rapid heart rate, night sweats, poor focus, and muscle soreness.

These effects are the result of significant hormonal and metabolic changes.

What Happens?

Your body will have to re-learn about using fat as a source of energy as the muscle glycogen levels start dropping due to a lack of carbohydrate intake. It takes time for this "switch," and you feel low energy during that time, feel irritable and extreme cravings. How much you suffer will depend on how metabolically active you are.

As if that weren't enough, while your gallbladder and pancreas react to the extra fat intake, you may also notice gastrointestinal problems such as diarrhea.

Finally, the hormones will take a hit as your body re-balances minerals, fluids, and sources of energy. T3 and Cortisol, in particular. T3 is a thyroid hormone that depends on carbohydrates' ingestion to manage metabolism, and Cortisol would be a stress hormone.

What's the effective cure?

Many of the signs of adjusting to the carnivore diet can be minimized or even removed using a couple of easy tricks:

Eat more - the carnivore diet is naturally full of protein and high in fat, ensuring you can feel satisfied for a very long time. It could mean your daily intake of calories is much smaller. Find out how many calories you have to live and then consider when deciding on the amount of food.

Drink more - it's natural to drop a lot of fluids, particularly during the first few days, but if you don't want to experience the symptoms, these fluids need to be replaced.

Electrolytes - you can need more electrolytes if more water and food don't help. First, try to add some extra salt to your diet, but suggest an electrolyte supplement if you need to.

Sweat more - exercise is a perfect way to naturally eliminate excess contaminants and re-equalize the electrolyte levels.

Chapter 2: Breakfast Recipes for the Carnivore Diet

You may not have eaten for up to 10 hours when you wake up after your overnight sleep. Breakfast recharges the body's energy and nutrient reserves. In a brief period, it increases the energy levels and ability to focus and can decrease the risk of type 2 diabetes, long-term heart disease and improved weight management.

1.Carnivore Breakfast Sandwich

It's delicious, easy, and rich in protein, fat, with no plants. This breakfast sandwich is appreciated by those on the carnivore diet or anyone who loves their diet with fat and protein. Although the Carnivore Breakfast Sandwich appears to criticize the mainstream cholesterol-preventing dietary advice, what we enjoy about this breakfast sandwich is how Incredibly delicious it is!

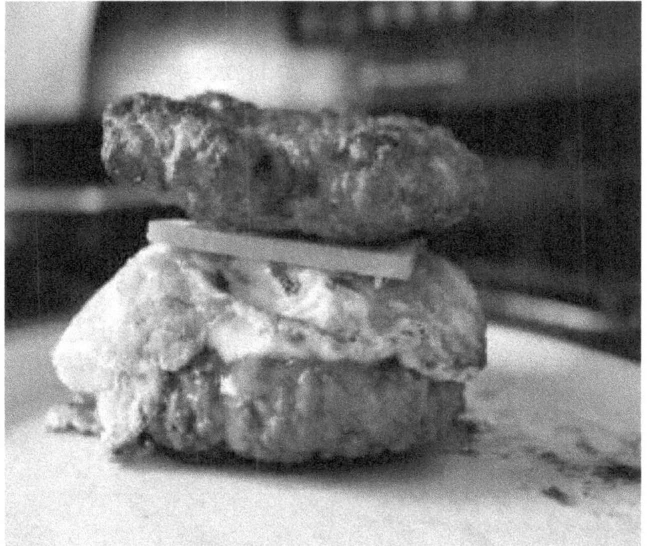

Prep Time: 5 Minutes

Cook Time: 5 Minutes

Total Time: 10 Minutes

Serving: 1

INGREDIENTS

- One egg
- Onetsp bacon grease or butter.
- Two Sausage Patties beef
- 1-ounce cheddar cheese

INSTRUCTIONS

1. Melt butter on moderate temperature in a big skillet.
2. Shape the sausage into thin patties, about 1/2 inch thick but about the length of the palm. On the otherside, cook patties until it turns to brown color, then flip, cook the other side for further 2-3 minutes, till then cooking continuously.
3. Fry an egg in the same pan at the same time. If not, in an additional pan (moderate temperature and take some time until the pan is hot to avoid sticking), use a little more butter and then prepare your carnivore breakfast sandwich. As with your sauce and keep sauce thin withyolk.
4. Set one sausage patty on a tray for preparation, then top it with a slice of cheese egg, another sausage patty, and top with a fried egg.
5. You can add sliced onion, sautéed spinach, or avocado as well. Enjoy the meal.

2.Cheesy 3-Meat Breakfast CasseroleRecipe

There's all in this Cheesy 3-Meat Breakfast Casserole recipe: sausage, plenty of cheese, bacon, and ham. Perfect for a weekend breakfast or even during the holidays for visitors. A breakfast for lovers of meat!

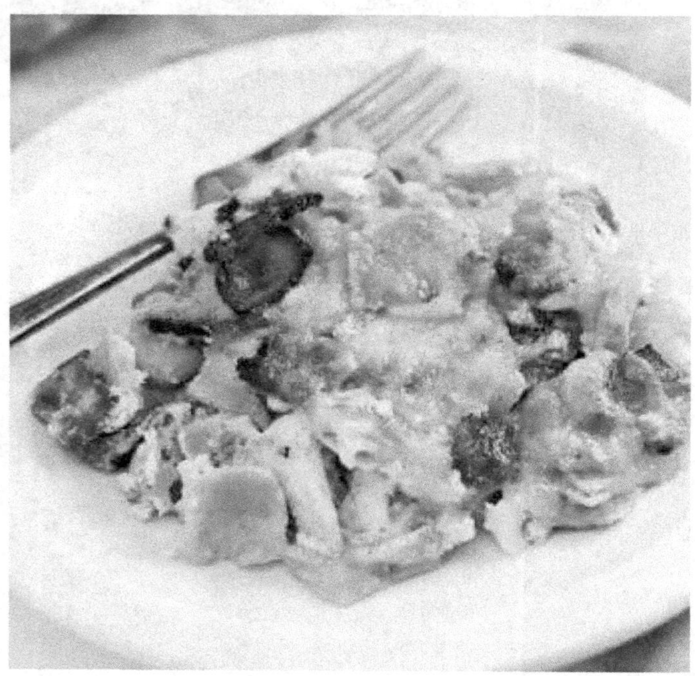

Prep Time: 15 Minutes

Cook Time: 40 Minutes

Total Time: 55 Minutes

Servings: 10

Ingredients

- Seven ounces of ham chopped.
- Potatoes cut into cubes.
- 32 ounces chilled hash brown
- Two cups shreddedcheddar cheese.
- Two cups of milk, eight large eggs,onetspof salt.
- One medium onion (diced)
- Half teaspoon pepper.
- Twelve ounces breakfast sausage
- Twelve ounces bacon (diced into 1" pieces)
- Half tsp. garlic powder

Instructions

1. Spray with cooking spray on a 9x13" baking dish. Preheat oven to 350°F.
2. Cook the bacon pieces in a large non - stick frying pan once cooked thoroughly and become crispy. Don't overcook anymore. Remove the bacon from the bowl with a slotted spoon, leave the grease in the pan. Cook the sausage in the same frying pan over medium-high heat, breaking up the connections so that you have bite-sized bits (or smaller). When the sausage is roughly halfway finished, add the onion, and cook until the sausage is fully cooked. Stir the sausage/onion mixture into a bowl with a slotted spoon and leave the pan's grease.
3. After cooking both the bacon and the sausage and removing them from the pan, add the pan's brown hash potatoes. Cook the potatoes in the remaining grease over medium heat until they are softened and browned slightly. In the lower part of the prepared baking dish, layer the hash browns.
4. Layer the cooked bacon on top of the hash browns, the ham, and the sausage/onion mixture. Then, scatter the cheese equally over the beef.
5. Whisk the eggs with the milk, garlic powder, salt, and pepper together in a big cup. On the upper side of the covered ingredients of the baking dish, add the egg mixture on top.
6. Bake for about 35-40 minutes in the oven or until the egg is fully set and the cheese is soft and bubbly.

3.One-Pan Egg and Turkey Skillet Recipe

You now need to have this One-Pan Egg and Turkey Skillet if you are looking for an easy, nutritious, and delicious meal. You're going to love that. The most important meal of the day is breakfast. So, with this balanced breakfast, start your day right off.

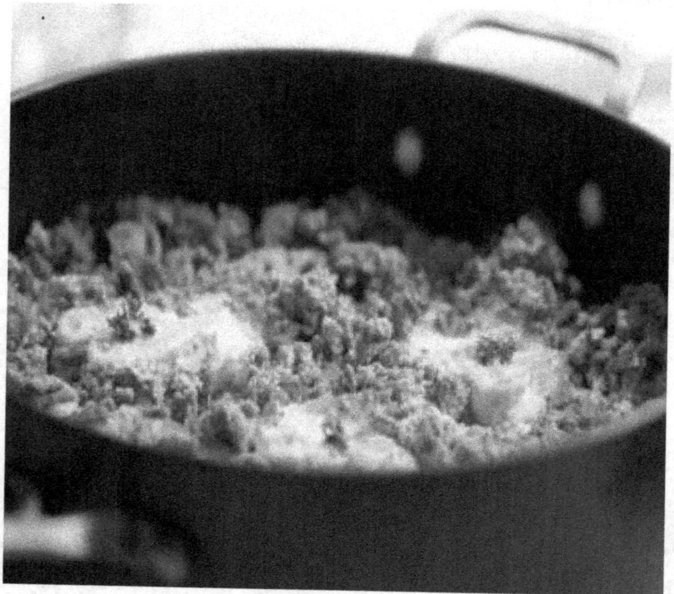

Prep Time: 5 Minutes

Cook Time: 20 Minutes

Total Time: 25 Minutes

Servings: 6

INGREDIENTS

- Six eggs
- One cup salsa
- Pepper and salt according to taste.
- 1 pound ground turkey

INSTRUCTIONS

1. Spray with non-stick cooking spray on the skillet and add in ground turkey.
2. Cook until the turkey is golden brown, over moderate flame. Also, drain all grease.
3. Connect the salsa mixture and blend well. For 2-3 minutes, cook the turkey and salsa.

4. Put the eggs in the skillet and cover them for 7 to 9 minutes or until the eggs are cooked to your taste.

4.Keto and Carnivore Meatloaf Muffin

It's quick to make this amazing Keto and Carnivore Meatloaf Muffin Meal, tasty but without all the fillers and perfect for taking for work or breakfast on-the-go. You can keep them all week long to eat in advance.

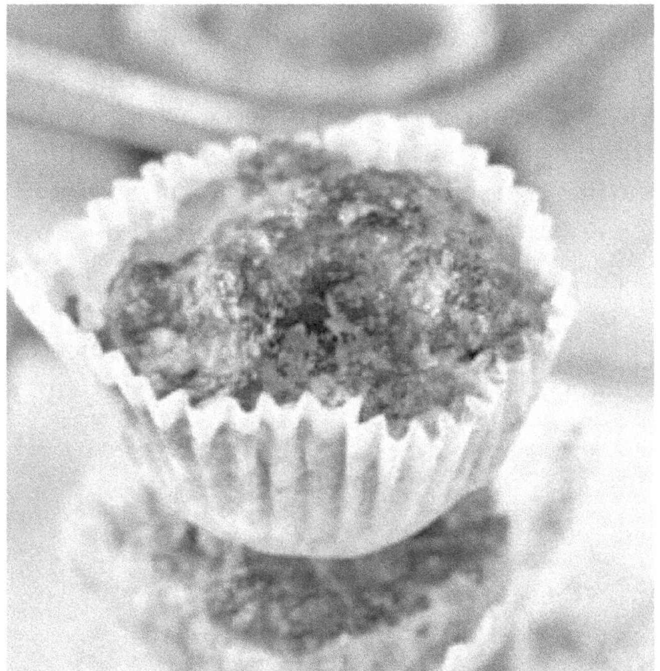

Prep Time: 15 Minutes

Cook Time: 25 Minutes

Servings:2

Ingredients

- Two eggs
- 2 lbs. 85 percent ground beef
- Two tsps. Sea salt.

Optional Ingredients:

- Two tsps. paprika
- No-sugar added ketchup for topping.
- One tbsp. garlic powder

- Half tsp. black powder

Instructions

1. To 350 degrees, set the oven.
2. Mix the eggs, meat, spices, and salt, if used, in a large mixing bowl with both hands until well mixed.
3. Using the liners to prepare the muffin pan.
4. Use meat to fill each cup until it is three times the amount filled.
5. Put the muffins in the oven with the meatloaf and put it in the oven for 25-35 minutes.
6. Muffins can cook quicker or slower, based on your oven.
7. Check a muffin by gently cut the hot muffin in half after about 20 minutes.
8. Take the muffin pan from the oven. If it seems done enough in your taste, present the muffins with tongs, and eat.

5.Carnivore Keto Burgers

If you are considering the Carnivore diet, these burgers will become one of your favorite meals. You get enough calories from this to keep your energy up, so fattier meat cuts are best.

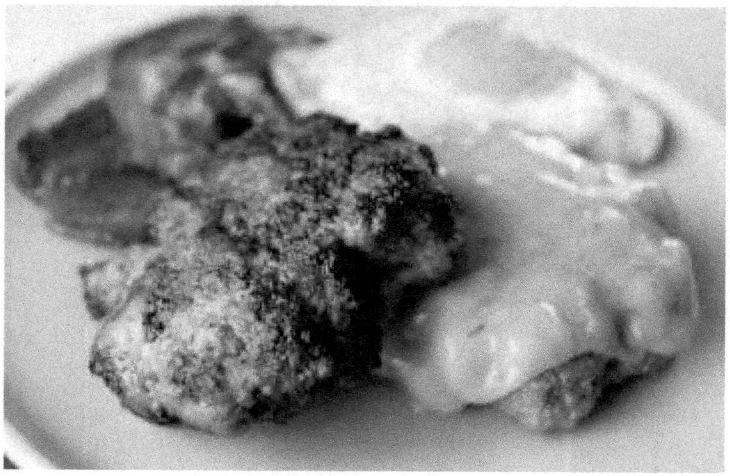

Prep Time:5 Minutes

Cook Time:10 Minutes

Total Time:15 Minutes

Servings: 8

Ingredients

- One teaspoon salt.

- 200 grams Speck or bacon 0.5 pound
- 500 grams Ground Beef (Beef grind) 1 pound
- 500 grams Ground Pork (Pork grind) 1 pound
- Two tablespoons Southwest Seasoning

Instructions

1. Cut the speck to the smallest possible size. If you want everything chopped/ground more equally, you can also use a mincer or food processor.
2. Combine it in a large bowl with all the items.
3. Generally, divide the mixture into eight patties and shape each by hand into a patty style.
4. BBQ on high/heat grill
5. Switch the grill/Barbeque down to low and put patties and straighten with a spatula on the grill/BBQ.
6. Please enable it to cook for 5 minutes on the grill, then flipped and cook for another five min. It is going to make the burgers well done.
7. Add and display your favorite seasonings.

6 Low-carb baked eggs

A great low-carb combination of eggs and beef. Please, yes! At any moment, cook up this delicious gem-lunch, dinner, or breakfast. You will be thanked by your every taste buds!

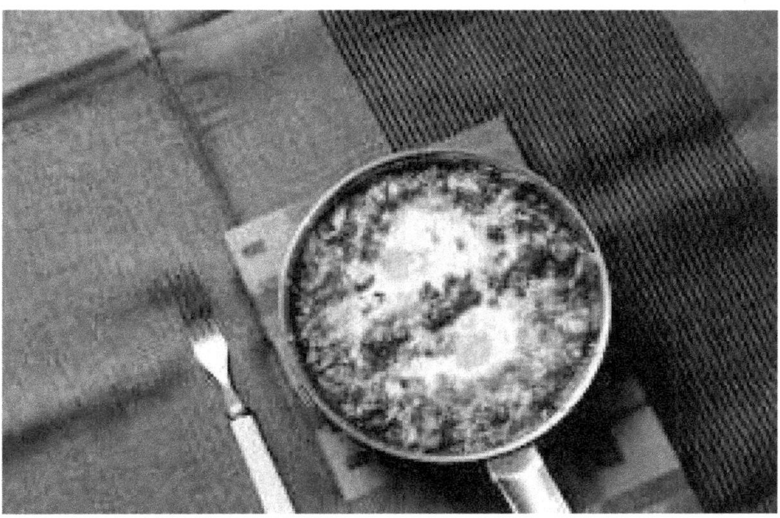

Prep Time: 5 Minutes

Cook Time: 10 Minutes.

Serving: 1

Ingredients

- Two eggs
- Half cup (2 oz.) grated cheese
- Three oz. Ground turkey or ground pork or ground beef cook it any way you like.

Instructions

1. Heat the oven to 200 °C (400 °F).
2. Arrange a cooked mixture of ground beef in a little baking dish. Then, using a spoon, make two holes and crack the eggs into them.
3. Sprinkle the end with shredded cheese.
4. Cook in the oven for around 10-15 minutes, till the eggs are cooked.
5. Allow it to cool for a little while. The ground meat and eggs get very hot.

Tip for the recipe

- It is a great recipe for the remaining hamburger you weren't sure what to do. Accumulate the recipe by the number of people and the entire family; you'll have dinner. Tada!
- Complement this with fresh herbs and avocado with quite a crunchy, crisp salad. Or give this a try with this amazing homemade mayonnaise (made without additives and soybean oil).

7. Spam and Eggs

A delicious recipe eaten for lunch, breakfast, or dinner is this easy Spam and Eggs. These cheesy meat eggs in less than fifteen min make a perfect, fast breakfast!

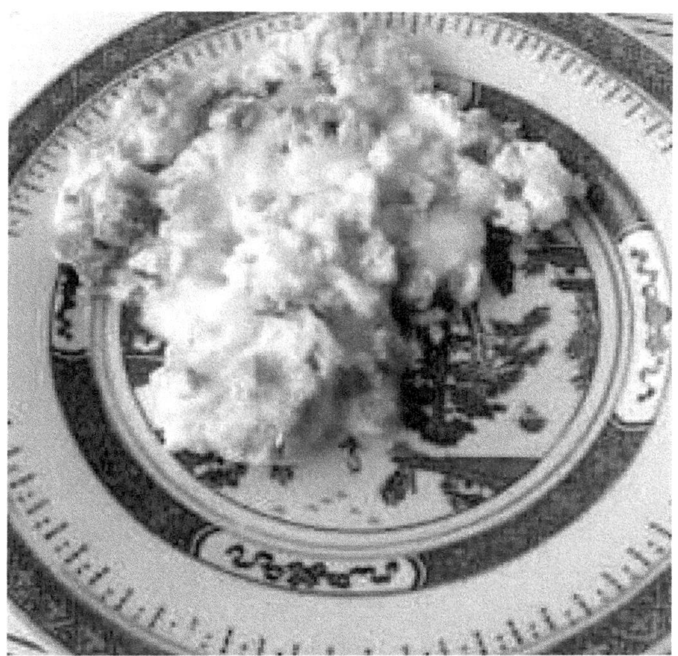

Prep Time: 5Minutes.

Cook Time: 10 Minutes.

Total Time:15 Minutes

Servings: 2

Ingredients

- Two eggsare well beaten.
- Two ounces Cheddar cheese, shredded.
- One (12 ounces) bowl of fully cooked luncheon meat (for example, spam)cut into cubes.

Instructions

Under moderate heat on a non-stick pan, put the eggs in, then spam. Cooked and stir till the eggs are almost ready, then spread over the cheese and mix until it is melted.

Chapter 3: Lunch Recipes for Carnivore Diet

The lunch hour helps your brain to relax, refresh, and remain focused, although it will directly increase your productivity for the rest of the day. Taking some time out during the day, yet if you choose to take some brief breaks, offers your brain an opportunity to recharge. Getting the proper ratio of meals is the secret to a balanced packed lunch to give you the nutrition you have to remain healthy.

1. Carnivore Chicken Nuggets

Everyone enjoys chicken nuggets. This beautiful and tasty recipe is simple and full of nutrients to develop. Appreciate the meals which everyone enjoys in a healthily!

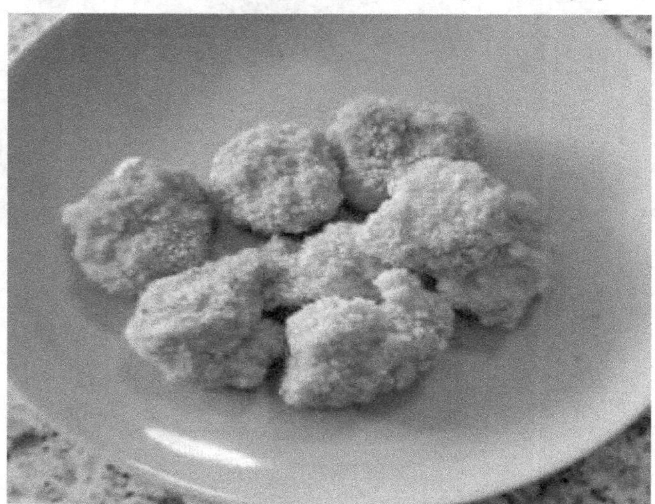

Prep Time: 40 minutes

Cook Time: 20 minutes

Servings: 60 nuggets.

Ingredients

- One large egg
- Mixture of bread
- half teaspoon oregano
- One cup of parmesan cheese is shredded.
- One cup pork rinds ground
- Three lbs. ground chicken or chop your own.
- Chicken Mixture

- half teaspoon pink salt

Instructions

1. Preheat the oven to 400°C.
2. Step cookie sheet with baking paper.
3. In a flat pan, merge the cheese and ground pork.
4. Stir up your egg, spices, and chicken.
5. From the chicken mixture, shape a small patty of the size you want. On the breading, put the mixture.
6. Cover the chicken with the mixture using a fork.
7. Place it on a cookie sheet lined with parchment.
8. Please continue with steps 5 - 7 till you have used all the chicken. If you are out of bread, make more of it.
9. Bake for 20 minutes at 400 degrees.

2. Cheesy Air Fryer Meatballs

You can make tasty, healthy meatballs in even less than thirty min, without any greasy mess! Real easy low carb meal in your air fryer for Cheesy Meatballs made fast and easy. Perfect for those who are on the carnivore diet.

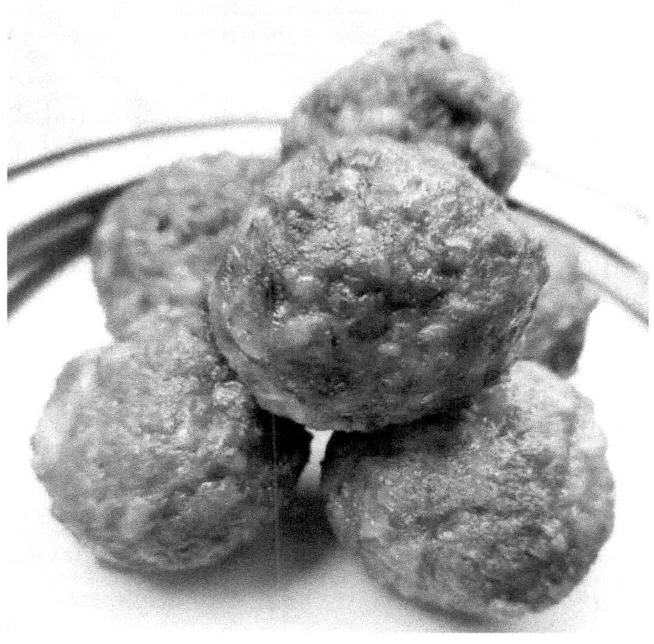

Prep Time: 20 Minutes

Cook Time: 12 Minutes

Resting Time: 8 Minutes

Total Time: 40 Minutes

Servings:6(4 meat-balls servings)

Equipment

Air Fryer

Ingredients

- One tablespoon lard
- 2 ounces pork rinds
- Three ounces shredded Italian cheese blend.
- One teaspoon pink sea salt
- Two pounds grass-fed ground beef
- Two large, well-blended eggs

Instructions

1. In a mixing bowl, add all of the items. Mash the mixture with clean hands till it is fully mixed.
2. Roll around 1 1⁄2 inches in diameter into balls. Twenty-four meatballs will be prepared by this method.
3. You'll cook them in parts, which vary according to the size of your air fryer.
4. If you use them, fill your fryer basket with liners. Otherwise, spray with cooking spray.
5. Put meatballs in the basket, ensuring they do not touch the basket's sides and each other.
6. Cook for 8 minutes at 350 degrees. Bring the basket out and switch over the balls of meat. Return to the frying pan and cook for another 4 minutes at 350 degrees.
7. The core temperature of the meatballs should approach 165 degrees, and then they're cooked!

3. Scallops with Wrapped Bacon

Jumbo scallops covered in a flavorful glaze are the bacon-wrapped scallops and broiled to satisfaction. A quick but tasteful appetizer and the main course choice that will get rave reviews for sure!

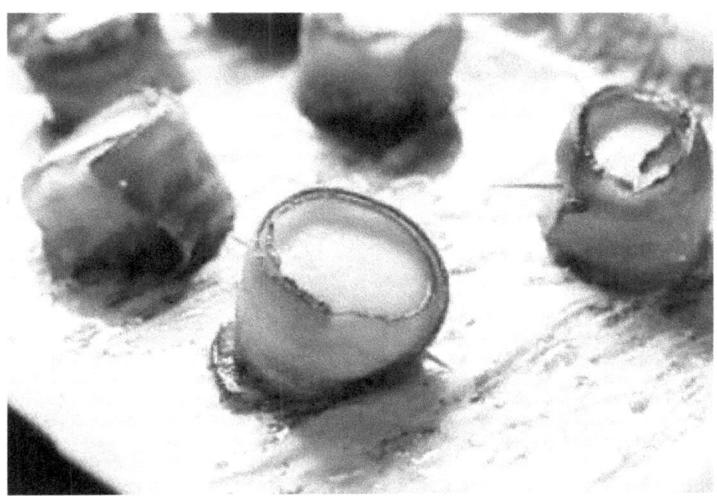

Prep Time: 20 minutes

Cook Time: 15 minutes

Total Time: 35 minutes

Servings:6

INGREDIENTS

- One-pound bacon slices diced in the half crossway.
- Two tablespoons of well-diced parsley.
- Two tablespoons soy sauce
- Pepper and saltaccording to your taste.
- 2 pounds large sea scallops patted dry.
- A cup of quarter fourth maple syrup
- 1/4 teaspoon garlic powder and
- cooking spray

INSTRUCTIONS

1. Preheat your broiler. Utilizing cooking spray to cover a sheet pan.

2. Cover each scallop around a slice of bacon and fix it with a toothpick. Put the scallops on the baking pan in a single layer.
3. Whisk all together soy sauce, pepper, salt, garlic powder and maple syrup in a small cup. Brush from over the top from each of the scallops with half the paste.
4. Broil around 10-15 minutes, just until the bacon becomes crispy and cooked through scallops. Half the way through the cooking process, brush the leftover sauce and over scallops.
5. Sprinkle parsley and serve.

4. Steak Tartare

If you are on the carnivore diet and love healthy, fresh flavors, this homemade Steak Tartare (or Beef Tartare) is something youcan make at home.

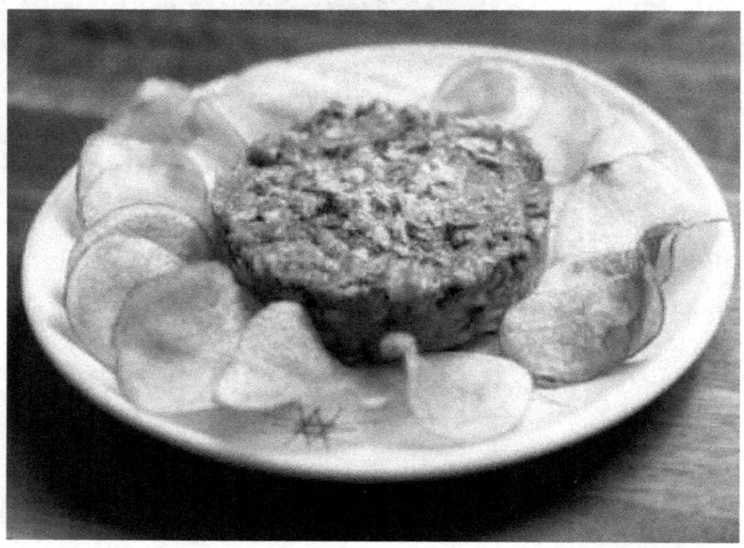

Total Time: 30 minutes (includes freezing time)

Active Time: 25 minutes

Servings: 4

Ingredients:

- Two large egg yolks
- Sixtbsps. finely diced shallots
- One tsp. kosher salt

- Half tsp. dry mustard
- Two tsps. sherry vinegar
- Sixteen ounces top sirloin cleaned and trimmed.
- 2 tbsps.Fresh parsley isfinely diced and divided.
- One tsp. freshly grated lemon zest
- 1/4 cup celery leaves are finely diced and divided.
- 1/4 cup light olive oil
- Twotbsps.Small brined capers drained and unrinsed.

Instructions

1. Custom instruments: pastry ring 3 3/4-inch, food processor (optional)
2. Slice the steak into 1-inch pieces and set aside for 10 mins in the refrigerator.
3. In a small bowl, mix dry mustard, egg yolks, and vinegar. Stir continuously until caramelized while streaming in the oil, then whisk in the salt, shallots, capers, parsley, and around 2/3 of the celery leaves.
4. Cut the meat to your preferred shape through the hand. (Likewise, distribute the meat in 4 quantities and pulse each batch in the food processor bowl fitted with the regular S-blade 3 to 4 times separately.)
5. With neat hands, bend the meat and flavorit easily. Plate and garnish with the lemon zest and reserved herbs using a 3 3/4-inch pastry ring.

5. Low-Carb Beef Bourguignon Stew

It is likely to obtain this dish of Low-Carb Beef Bourguignon Stew in an Instant Pot or slow cooker. It can be enjoyed by those on Atkins, low carb, keto, diabetics, gluten-free, Paleo, grain-free, or Banting Diet.

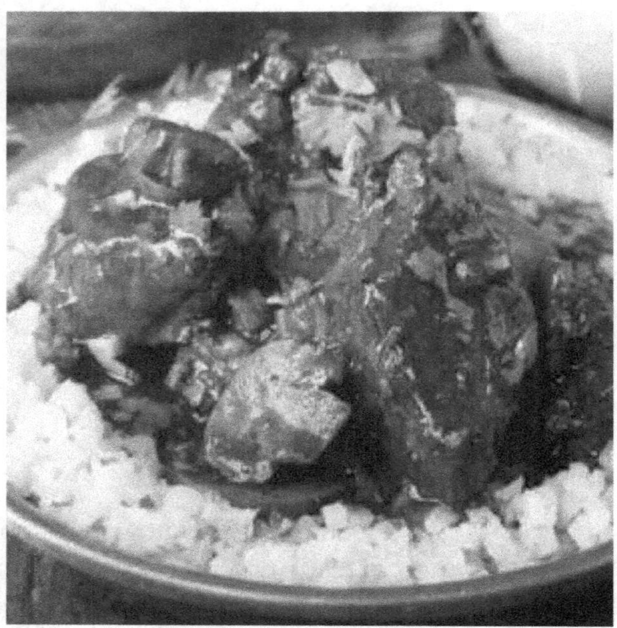

Prep Time: 30 minutes

Cook Time: 30 minutes

Total Time: 1 hour

Servings: 6

Ingredients

- Four ounces white onion (about 1 small)
- Two stalks celery sliced.
- Eight ounces of mushrooms thickly cut into pieces.
- 1 1/2-pound stew meat diced into 1 1/2 -2-inch cubes and drywith a paper towel.
- Four pieces of bacon cut crosswise.
- 1/4 tsp. Black pepper freshly ground.
- 1/2 tsp. sea salt (or to taste)
- 1 cup dry burgundy wine
- 1/2 tsp. dried thyme
- 1 tbsp. Fresh parsley chopped.
- One clove of garlic crushed.
- Half tsp. Xanthan gum.

- One cup beef stock or,you can use low-salt broth.
- Two tbsps. tomato paste
- One bay leaf

Instructions

Instant Pot instructions

1. As the Instant Pot covers off, select the sauté mode. Add the bacon when the "hot" sign appears. Cook the bacon till crispy, mixing frequently. Remove it to a plate lined with paper towels. Do not remove grease comprising bacon.
2. To an Instant Kettle, add half of the beef. Use the pepper and salt to sprinkle. Before flipping, make the first side brown. Brown both ends of it and pull it to a tray. For the other half of the beef, repeat. If during this process, the Instant Pot switches off, set again to Sauté.
3. Discharge of all but one tablespoon of the pot's drippings. (Add around a tablespoon of recommended oil or butter to the Instant Pot if there is less than one tablespoon) Continue with the sauté setting and add the celery and onion to the pot. Please enable it to cook until it starts to soften. Add the mushrooms. Cook the vegetables until they begin to soften the mushrooms. Stir in the garlic and cook for a moment. Transfer to a dish.
4. Add about a teaspoon if there's no oil left in the pot. To the pot, add the xanthan gum. Stir through the xanthan gum to spread the oil. Pour the burgundy in and mix, scraping the brown pieces together. Simmer until the wine begins to thicken. Add broth of beef. Whisk in the tomato paste, thyme, and bay leaf. Just take it to a simmer. Enable to boil until the broth thickens enough for a spoon to stick. Send browned chunks of beef (including the drippings) and bacon to the pot of vegetables. Stir in the salt and pepper.
5. Cover Instant Pot. "Steam release location handle for "Sealing." To change the time to 30 minutes, select the Meat/Stew feature and press the +/- button. Used this Quick Release method (follow Instant Pot instruction book) to vent the Instant Pot when the stew is finished. Press Cancel. When opening the lid, be sure the float valve is down.
6. Taste the seasoning and adjust. Until serving, cut the bay leaf and sprinkle it with parsley.

Slow cooker instructions:

(add 5 hours and 30 minutes to cooking time)

1. On moderate flame, heat the Dutch oven or large soup pot. Add the bacon when the pot is hot. Cook the bacon till crisp, stirring occasionally. Lift to a plate lined with paper towels to clean and transfer to the slow cooker.
2. To the pot, put 1/2 of the beef. Chunks shouldn't harm you. Using pepper and salt to sprinkle. Before flipping, cause the first side to brown. Then brown flip both sides to the slow cooker. For the other part of the meat, return.
3. Discharge of all but 1 tbsp of the pot's drippings. If less than a tablespoon is available, add a little of the oil of your choice. Cl Continue to add the celery and onions to the pot over moderate temperature. Please enable it to cook till it starts to soften. Add the mushrooms. Cook the vegetables until they begin to soften the mushrooms. Stir in the garlic and boil for a minute. Place the vegetables in a crockpot.
4. Add about a teaspoon of your oil choice if there is no oil left in the tank. To the jar, add the xanthan gum. Stir in the oil to spread it. Pour the burgundy in and stir, scraping the brown bits together. Simmer and simmer until the wine begins to thicken. Add broth of beef. Stir in the tomato paste, bay leaf, and thyme. Just bring it to a simmer. Enable to boil until the broth thickens enough for a spoon to coat. Stir in the pepper and salt. Shift the bacon, beef, and vegetables to the slow cooker and mix.
5. Then seal the slow cooker. Process the stew for six-eight hours or until meat is cooked.
6. Taste and change the seasoning when served. Before serving, extract the bay leaf and sprinkle it with parsley.

6. Lunch Meat Roll-Ups

Lunch Meat Roll-Ups seem to be simple to create, adaptable enough to suit everyone's different interests, and make an ideal keto lunch or healthy meal! As specific and over the edge as you prefer, you can also make these roll-ups!

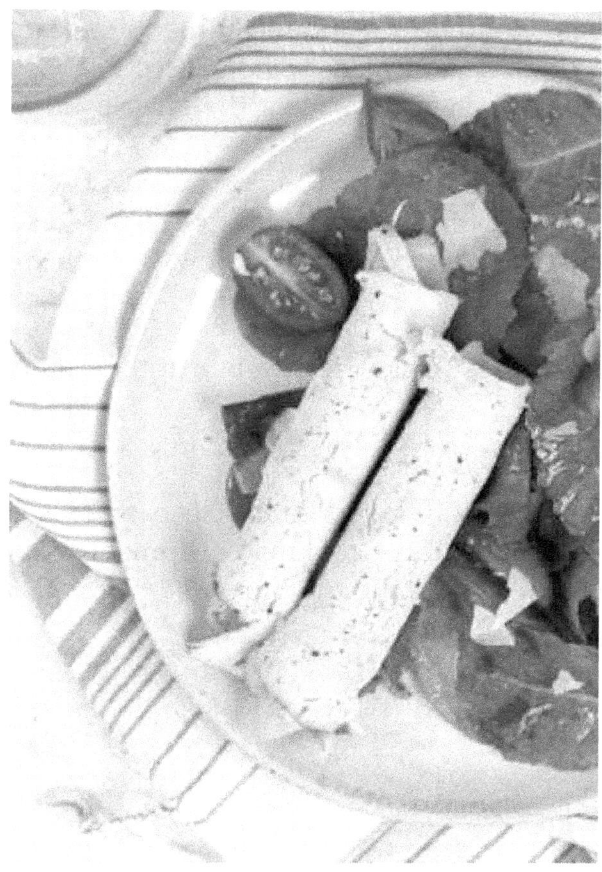

Prep Time: 5 minutes

Total Time: 5 minutes

Servings: 2

Ingredients

- Four pieces of cheese
- Four pieces of lunch meat
- garnishes of your preference if you want shredded lettuce, herb cream cheese, guacamole.
- black pepper and sea salt

Instructions

1. On the workplace surface, put your meat pieces and garnish them with a cheese slice.

2. Note: This would be a wonderful time to guacamole or dressings of your choice on top, herb spread cream cheese,
3. Wrap your lunch meat across the cheese till you have a log, starting from the bottom.
4. Continue to roll up your rolls of meat and cheese until you reach the amount you would like. Use black pepper and sea salt to sprinkle.
5. Serve with a leafy green salad or bowl of bone broth.

Note

Please press on your lunch meat's thicker side to be cut to be smoother to roll and remain together.

7.Carnivore Braised Beef Shank

It's a highly versatile recipe that can be made from a cast-iron skillet or Dutch oven to a crockpot to an instant pot with multiple cooking equipment. You can also slow-cook it in the oven rather than cooking on the stovetop. You get a deliciouslunchtime recipe!

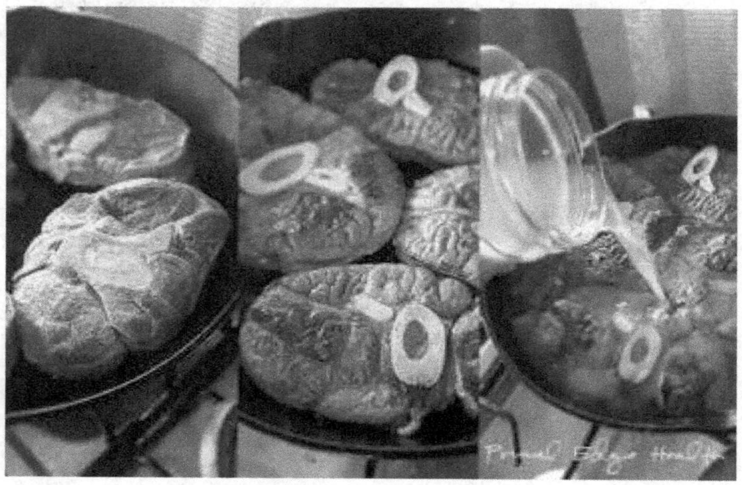

Prep Time: 5 Minutes

Cook Time: 3 hrs.

Total Time: 3 hrs. 5 mins

Servings: 4

EQUIPMENT

Cast iron skillet.

Dutch oven

INGREDIENTS

- Two-three cups of bone broth or water
- One tbsp ghee, beef tallow butter or other cooking fat.
- Four pieces beef shank 1-inch thick, eight ounces each
- One tsp. Salt or as you required.

INSTRUCTIONS

1. In the Dutch oven or cast iron or heavy bottom skillet with cover, burn the cooking fat. Brown from both sides of the beef shanks till a golden-brown crust forms, about 2-3 minutes each side.
2. Over shanks, pour the broth. Use 2 cups of broth, at least. The considerable broth will be acceptable 1/2 to 3/4 of the way up the side to cover the meat, with salt, season. Bring a boil to it.
3. Reduce heat and cover the pot and let the steam escape from a tiny hole.
4. Cook for 3 hours, over a low flame, till the meat begins to fall off the bone. Serve warm in liquid.

NOTES

- Over the last 30 minutes of the cooking process, add any of the vegetables and herbs mentioned above and cook with the meat.
- Oven method Follow steps 1-2, then place the lid on after broth is simmering and switch to the oven for 2 hours for the roast.
- Crockpot Method put meat in a slow cooker's bottom, pour broth over and sprinkle with salt. Cover it with your cover and turn it down. Cooked for 4-6 hours before the bone breaks down easily.
- Seasoning the meat with the instant pot method. Turn the Instant pot on and choose to sauté. When heated, add the cooking fat to the pot and cook the meat until golden brown, around 2-3 minutes on each side. Add some broth. Close the sealing valve and lid. Put the high pressure in order and cook for 35 minutes. For 15 minutes, the normal release pressure releases the remaining pressure gradually.

8. Herb Roasted Bone Marrow

Marrow is an outstanding substitute of the omega-3s essential for safe brain growth and anti-inflammation. It's very, very beneficial for everyone.

It's fairly affordable if you prepare it straight away (versus having it at a fine dining restaurant).It's incredibly tasty.

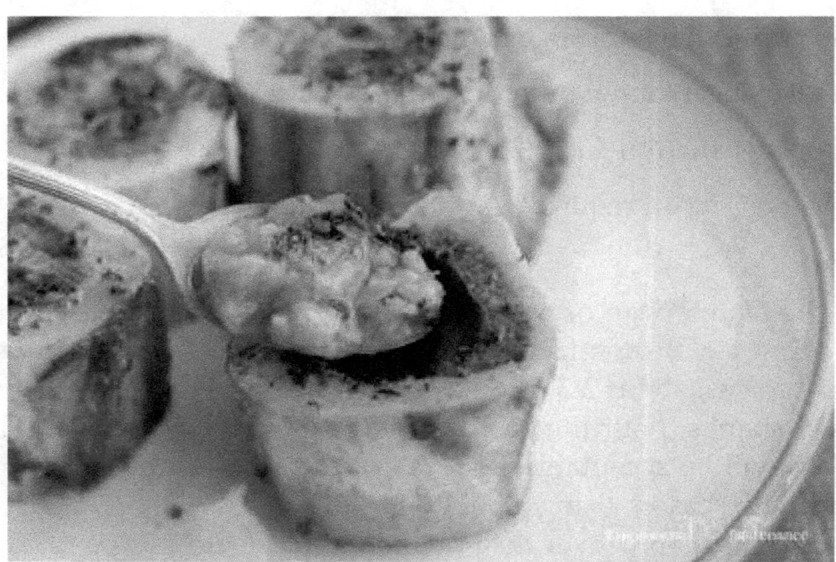

Prep time: 5 mins

Cook time: 15 mins.

Total time: 20 mins

Servings:1-2 marrow bones

INGREDIENTS

- Fresh rosemary
- Marrow bones from grass-fed/pasture-raised beef, 1-2each person
- black pepper and salt
- Fresh thyme

INSTRUCTIONS

1. For one person, the marrow with one or two pieces of bone is quite enough.
2. Defrost it properly if the bones are frozen.
3. To 400 degrees, set the oven. In a baking dish, put the bones. Spacing does not matter - closely or loosely, it is spaced.
4. Finely chop the thyme and fresh rosemary into equal parts. Use 1/2 teaspoon of chopped herbs for four marrow bones. Over the marrow bones, sprinkle the spices.
5. Roast for around fifteen min, until the inside is no longer pink. Until the marrow starts to "cook out" of the bones, you had to catch them.
6. Serve hot and season with salt and pepper. Scoop out the marrow using a spoon.

7. Save any drippings in an airtight jar in the refrigerator for a few days, as well as the remaining marrow. Chop the leftover marrow finely and toss it for a flavor and nutrient boost with hot, cooked vegetables.

Chapter 4: Desserts and Snack Recipes for the Carnivore Diet

After all, it's all about satisfying the soul with food for dessert enthusiasts that allows them to realize like they've reached Paradise on earth at last. Eating dessert does not indicate that you have little or no control over yourself. It just means you've got a clear idea of what you want (it's just a delicious blueberry cheesecake sometimes), and you've got what it takes to satisfy these cravings.

1. Bacony CarnivoreWomelletes

This one is excellent topped with cinnamon butter as well as a pour of pancake syrup without sugar. For sandwiches, it also stands up very well.

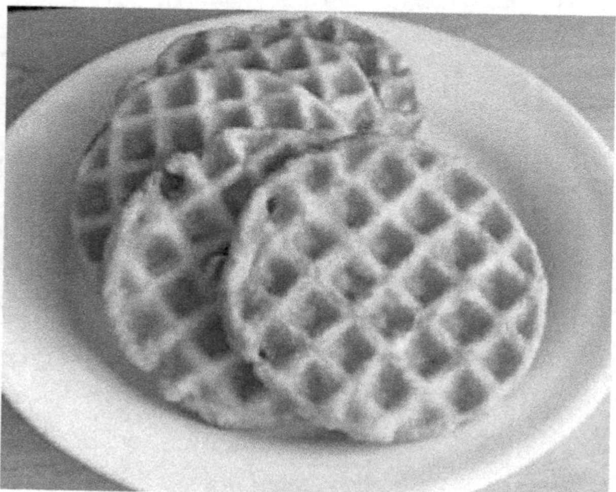

Prep Time: 2 minutes

Cook Time: 8 minutes

Total Time: 10 minutes

Servings: 2 womelletes.

INGREDIENTS

- One large egg.
- One slice of bacon (raw)
- hefty pinch of any spices or flavorings as you want.
- Splash maple extract, if required.

INSTRUCTIONS

1. Put the bacon in a food processor or blender and turn it on.

2. Put any seasonings and egg down the chute until the bacon is ground up and start operating the machine till liquified and well-in incorporated. It is your womelletes slurry.
3. As per its directions, warm your mini-waffle machine.
4. In a waffle maker, add half the slurry and place the cover around.
5. Cook for around 3-5 mins max till golden or to your preferred level of flavor and texture.
6. Take away from the waffle maker, and with the leftover slurry, repeat the procedure 4 and 5.
7. Enjoy the womelletes warm or as you are delighted.

2. Carnivore Cake

While you follow the carnivore diet strictly and sometimes seem to desire a dessert, well, we have nothing sweet for you, but we've got a cake.

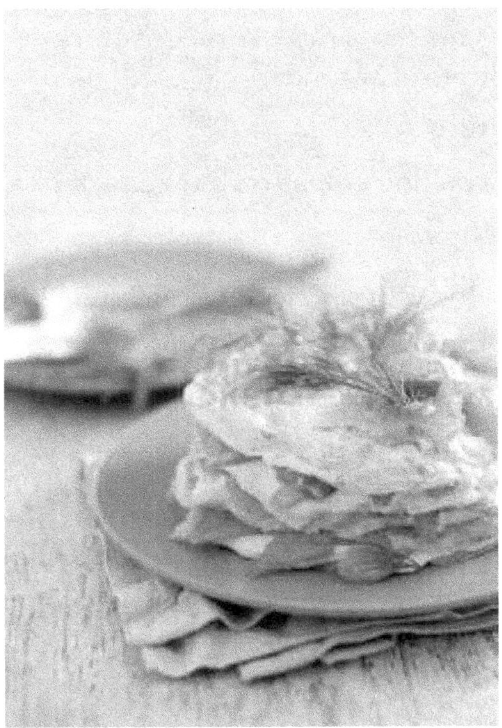

Prep Time: 5 minutes

Cook Time: 10 minutes

Total Time: 25 minutes

Servings: 8

INGREDIENTS

- Seven oz creamy cheese
- One pinch of dill for decoration
- Ten oz smoked salmon
- Eight eggs
- One pinch salt

INSTRUCTIONS

1. Inside a small bowl, beat the salt and eggs until mixed.
2. Heat skillet or 6-in nonstick pan over the moderate flame while heated.
3. To coat the pan's base, pour 1⁄4 cup of the mixture into the pan and whisk. Adjust the pan to the flame and allow the eggs to cook.
4. Cooked the egg crepes till they are just set (about 30 seconds) on the bottom, so there is no browning on the sides. Turn gently over the crepe and cook on the opposite side for a couple of seconds.
5. Repeat till all the mixture is used.
6. To cool off, place the cooking crepes on a wire rack or a plate.

Let usbring everything together.

- Bring one crepe upon this plate and cover it with a thin coating of cream cheese.
- Layer cream cheese with diced smoked salmon and top with next crepe.
- Continue layering till all components are being used.
- Customize and serve with dill.

NOTE:

In the refrigerator, let the cake stay for 1 hour; it'll be smoother to break. For decorative purposes, utilize fresh dill.

3. Egg Custard

With its elegant yet mild taste and its creaminess, this traditional dessert is still a highlight. Preferably sized for a children's treat yet mature enough for a formal dinner, it requires just 15 minutes to prepare and can be kept for up to 3 days in the fridge, sealed. (The evening once you've made this is much better.)

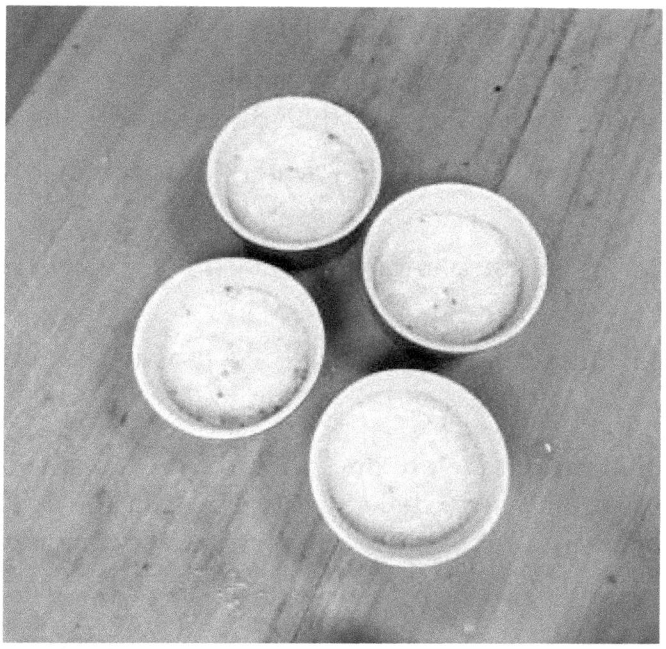

Prep Time: 10 minutes

Cook Time: 2 hours.

Servings:6

INGREDIENTS

- Two eggs
- Two cups whole milk
- Two egg yolks
- 1/3 cup sugar
- Freshly shredded or ground nutmeg
- Onetsp. of vanilla extract

PREPARATION

1. Heat the oven around 300 degrees.
2. Placed in a deep baking pan broad enough to accommodate six 4-ounce ovenproof cups (you can use coffee cups or ramekins marked as oven-safe).
3. Get the milk to a boil with moderate flame in a medium-size saucepan.
4. In the meantime, mix the yolks, sugar, vanilla, and eggs in a distinct dish.

5. Through boiling milk, stir the egg mixture, stirring gently to incorporate.
6. Pour the mixture into the cups via a fine strainer (unless the strainer clogs, choose a spoon to scrape it clean), then drizzled with the nutmeg gently.
7. In the pan, pour hot (not boiling) water till it hits half the way up the cups' ends.
8. Bake for 30 to 35 minutes until the custard is just finished (it can still be a bit loose).
9. Before served, just let the custard cool in cold water for around 2 hours.

4. Carnivore Chaffle Recipe

Because of the sauce, this meal has only one net carb. With a small salad aside, it can be served. It is very satisfying and tastes delicious! 1 serving in the oven renders this recipe.

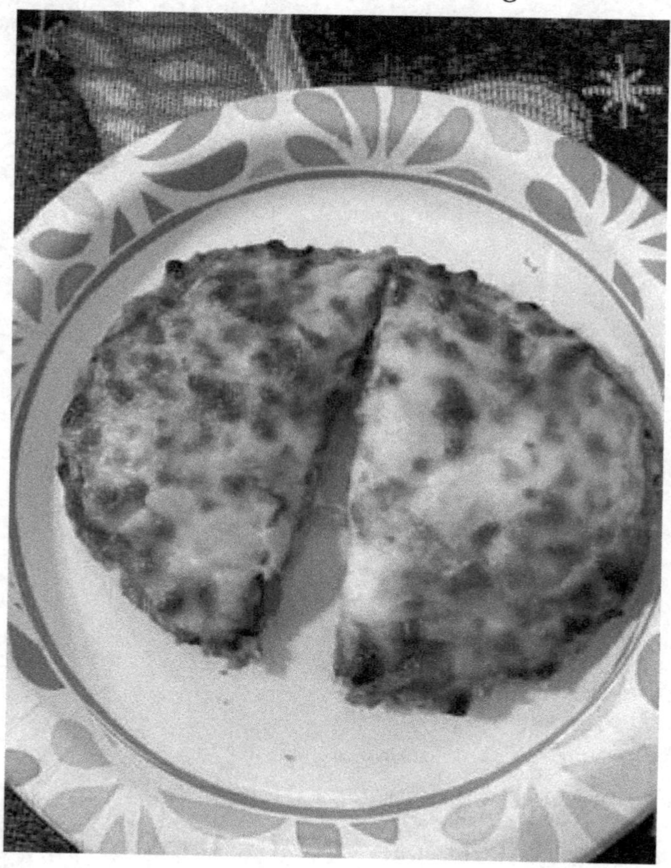

Prep Time: 3 minutes

Cook Time: 8 minutes

Serving: 1

INGREDIENTS

- 1/4 cup parmesan cheese shredded.
- 1/4 cupchopped pork rinds.
- One egg is well beaten.
- One tsp. Grill mate roasted garlic and herb flavoring.

INSTRUCTIONS

1. In a small bowl, mix all the ingredients and incorporate until thoroughly mixed.
2. Cover it with a silicone sheet or parchment paper using a small baking sheet.
3. Through wet hands, tap the mixture into a small circle or use a silicone spatula to create the pizza crust.
4. The oven baking duration is bake around each side for 10 minutes at 350 degrees in the oven.
5. Mini Dash Waffle Maker: Split the mixture into two and cook every other serving for at least 4 minutes before a crust forms (it could take longer if you are using a large waffle iron)
6. Air Fryer Baking Time: Cook on each side at 300 degrees for eight minutes.
7. If you prefer to remove the carnivore pizza crust with any seasonings and place the keto-friendly sauce of choice on. Mostly prefer black olives and Italian sausage.
8. Place 1/3 of mozzarella cheese on top.
9. Place the cheese in the oven, air fryer, or microwave until it becomes crispy, just long enough to melt. It takes just 1 minute for the microwave or 3 to 4 minutes for the oven or air fryer.

5. Meat Bagels

A meat bagel is meat that has been molded into a bagel pattern and served like a bagel. For the keto, Paleo, low carb, and for those on the carnivore diet, it is the ideal bagel!

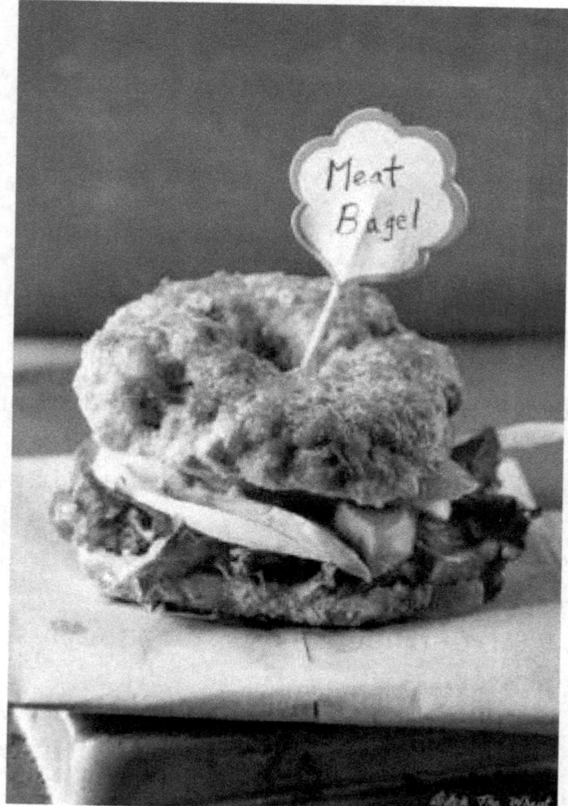

Prep Time:15 minutes

Cook Time:40 minutes

Total Time:55 minutes

Serving: 6

INGREDIENTS

- Two pounds ground pork
- 2/3 cup of tomato sauce
- Two large eggs
- 1 ½ onion, finely diced.
- 1/2 tsp ground pepper
- One tablespoon butter/bacon/ grass-fed ghee fat etc.
- One teaspoon sea salt
- One teaspoon paprika

INSTRUCTIONS

1. Heat the oven to 400°F. Create a parchment paper baking dish.
2. Sauté the onions with some cooking fat over a moderate flame, like grass-fed ghee butter etc. Sauté once they're transparent. Before placing them in the meat, allow the onions to chill.
3. Adjust all the components in a dish, along with the fried onions. Blend enough to disperse the spices uniformly.
4. Distribute the meat into six pieces. Roll a piece into a ball utilizing the hands, shape the center, and straighten gently to create a bagel.
5. Put the meat-looking bagel in the dish and proceed with each of the meat parts.
6. Bake until the meat is completely cooked, or for 40 minutes.
7. Enable the cooling of the meat bagels. Just like a normal bagel, slice the meat bagel. Load the meat bagel with salads such as slices of onions, tomato, spinach, etc.

Chapter 5: Dinner Recipes for the Carnivore Diet

Dinner is also an essential meal, and with a variety of amazing foods, you can try new things. Better sleep, greater stress resilience, reduced inflammation, lower anxiety, improved digestion, and steady sugar levels are connected to a nutritious meal.

1.Pot Roast Recipe with Gravy

Without lots of vegetables such as onions and garlic, you think you can't make Carnivore Diet Pot Roast because you are on the carnivore diet and can't consume vegetables. Here is the recipe, which is full of nutrition and quite easy to make.

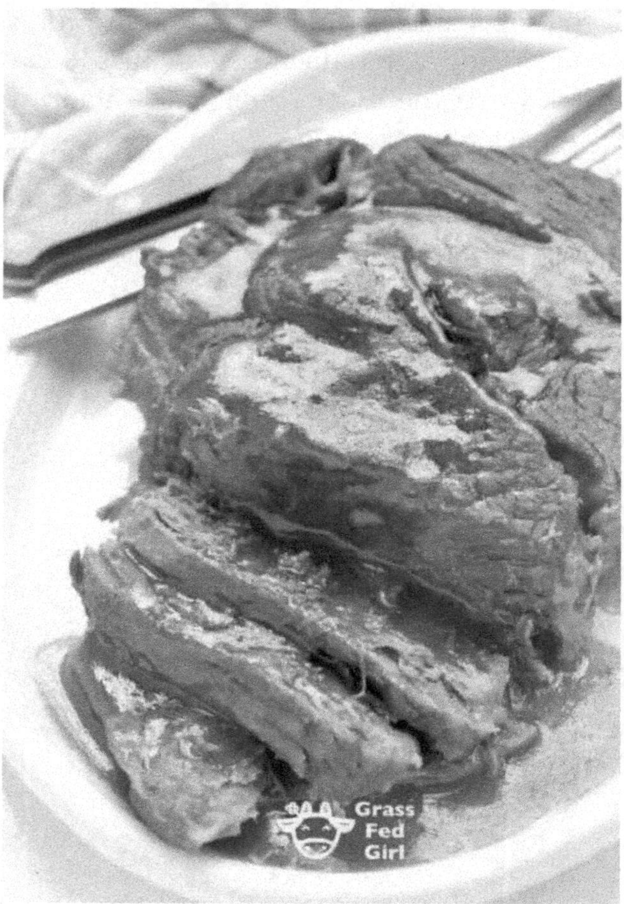

Prep Time: 10 minutes

Cook Time: 3 hours.

Servings: 4

Ingredients

- 1 4-5- lbs. pot roast

- Four tbsps. Butter or ghee.
- Two tsps. Sea salt.
- Three to Six cups of beef broth

Instructions

Recipe Notes

Cooking Time:

90 minutes Instant Pot

7 hours Slow Cooker

Stove Top

1. Heat the oven to 325°C. On both sides, salt the roast. On moderate temperature, heat the heavy bottom pan with a cover and put two tbsp of ghee.
2. Once the pan seems to be very hot, brown both sides of the roast from the surface for around 1-2 minutes.
3. From each side, whenever the pot roast is cooked, add the broth till the pot roast is coated and Put the cover and cook in the oven.
4. Bake in the oven for 2-3 hours, while enclosed, till itis fork-tender. Take it out of the oven and set off.
5. On moderate flame, place a small saucepan, add 1.5 cups of the remaining broth and the leftover 2 tbsp of ghee.
6. For 5-6 minutes, whisk the saucepan constantly till the broth decreases and thickens.
7. On a large dish, put the slice and roast crosswise. On over pot roast, put the thickened sauce.
8. Start serving and have a pleasant time.

Instant Pot

1. Turn on the device to sauté mode and dissolve the ghee.
2. For around two min each, add the pot roast and cook it on every side.
3. When the meat is wrapped, add the broth, and fix the cover, ensuring that the vent is covered.
4. Cooked for 90 minutes over high temperature.
5. Let the pressure automatically escape and ensure that it is a fork-tender.
6. Under moderate flame, put a small saucepan and pour 1.5 cups of the Instant Pot's remaining broth and two leftover tbsp of ghee.
7. For 5-6 mins, whisk the saucepan constantly till the broth decreases and thickens.
8. In the representing tray, move the pot roast and cut it crosswise.

9. Over the pot roast, spill the sauce. Start Serving and enjoy the meal.

Slow Cooker

1. Heat the frying pan on moderately high heat and dissolve the ghee.
2. Put the pot roast and cook it for about 2 minutes on every side till it is browned.
3. To the slow cooker, add the roast and add in the broth till it covers the meat.
4. About 6 hours, cooked on high heat as well as the meat is fork-tender.
5. Add 1.5 cups of broth and the leftover two tablespoons of ghee to a medium saucepan at moderate temperature.
6. For 3-5 minutes, stir the saucepan constantly until the broth decreases and thickens.
7. Move the pot roast to a serving dish and slice it crosswise into pieces.
8. On over pot roast, spill the thickened sauce. Present the meal and enjoy.

2. Carnivore Skillet Pepperoni Pizza

A quick and simple Carnivore Skillet Pepperoni Pizza will fulfill the desire for pizza! Also, when you are on the Carnivore diet, no need to skip family pizza evening. One pan and just a couple of supplies!

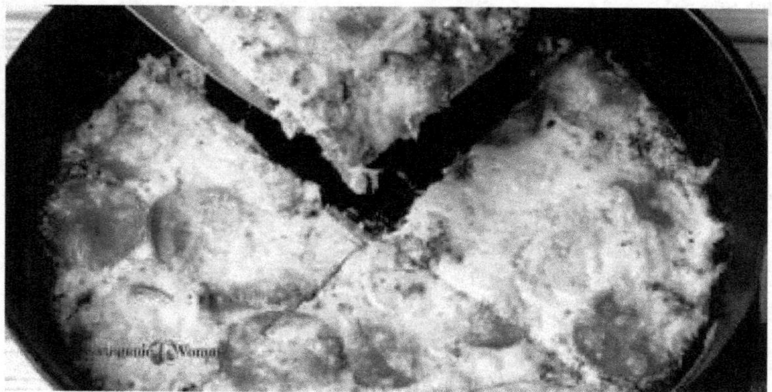

Prep Time: 10 Minutes

Cook Time: 15 Minutes

Total Time: 25 Minutes

Servings: 4

Ingredients

- 2 oz (1/2 cup) mozzarella cheese, grated.

- Four eggs.
- Pizza Base.
- Two tablespoon mayonnaise or melted butter, tallow, or lard.
- Pepperoni slices to cover the pizza.
- One tsp each garlic and onion powder.
- Pinch of salt for thetaste.
- One teaspoon Italian seasoning.
- More Italian seasoning you canuse if you need it.
- More cheese to sprinkle on top as you want it.
- Pizza Topping.
- 2 oz shredded parmesan.

Instructions

1. Heat the oven around 375°C.
2. Oil the cast iron frying pan.
3. Mix the cheese, eggs, seasoning and 2tbsp fat, all ingredients in a dish.
4. Into cast iron pan, add the mixture.
5. Sprinkle with some flavorings, cheese, and pepperoni on top.
6. Cook for 15 minutes in the oven or till the pizza is swollen and the layer starts to brown.
7. Slice it into four parts and try it!

3. Carnivore Ham and Cheese Noodle Soup

A Carnivore diet noodle recipe!? Cheese, bacon, bone broth, ham and fresh carnivore noodles are mixed in this rich cheesy, comforting nutritional soup! A pleasant change of style of the regular entry for the carnivore diet!

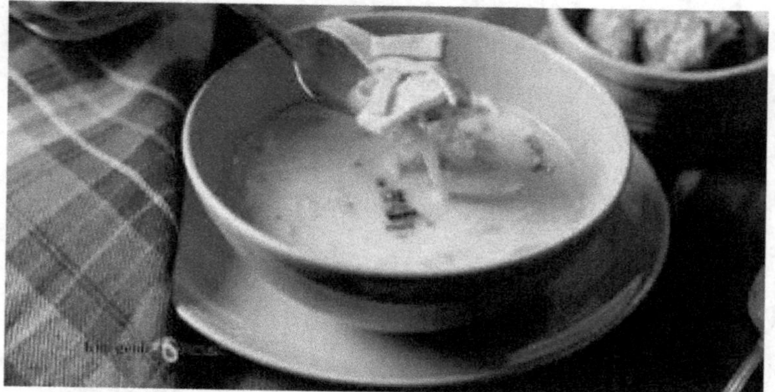

Prep Time: 15 Minutes

Cook Time: 15 Minutes

Total Time: 30 Minutes

Servings: 4

Ingredients

- 2 oz cream cheese cut into small pieces.
- 10-12 oz cubed cooked ham
- 1/4 cup bacon chopped or 3-4 pieces of cooked crisp bacon finely diced
- Two cups of bone broth or regular broth
- One cup Carnivore Noodles if you want it.
- Two cups cheddar cheese, shredded (save 1/2 cup for garnish)
- half cup heavy cream
- Pepper and Saltaccording to your taste.

Instructions

1. Heat the broth in a large medium pot until it almost begins to boil. Hold the broth at a reasonable volume.
2. Mix in the cubes of cream cheese and whisk until the broth is mixed and the chunks are removed.
3. Whisk in the finely chopped cheese till it mixes into the combination, about half a cup at a time.
4. Add the noodles and cubed ham and bring to a boil until fully cooked.
5. Mix in heavy cream and boil for a further min on low flame.

6. Cover each bowl with crumbled or chopped bacon and saved shredded cheddar cheese. Split into four wide bowls.

4. Carnivore Moussaka

It is a high-calorie meal, especially when it comes to high-fat sheep yogurt, aged cheese, and butter. In contrast, please remember that the only thing that contributes carbohydrates to this meal is sheep yogurt. Suppose when it falls to the taste. Just try this recipe because it can satisfy your tastebuds.

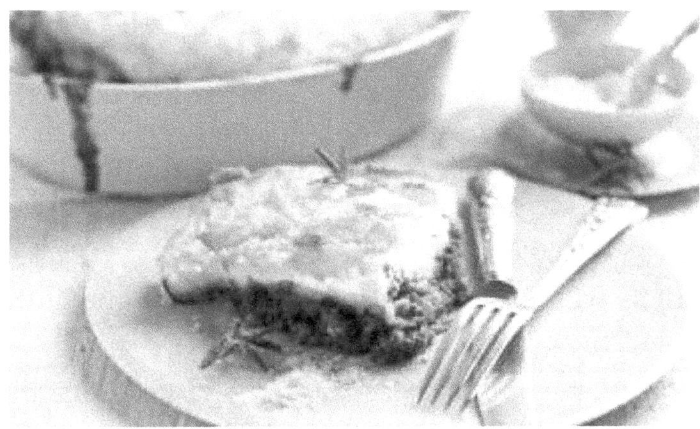

Prep Time: 30 minutes

Cooking Time: 40 minutes

Servings: 4

INGREDIENTS

- 250g (8,8 oz) chopped lamb.
- 250g (8.8 oz) dicedbeef or veal.
- Eight medium eggs
- 400g (14 oz) Sheep yogurt - strained Greek type (As a substitute use sour cream)
- 500g (1 Lb.) thin veal cutlets
- 50g (1,7 oz) butter or ghee (we always use sheep or goat butter)
- 100g shredded kefalograviera cheese

Spice mixture (amounts to your liking)

- powder rosemary
- dry oregano

- red, white, and black pepper freshly ground.
- dry peppermint
- smoked red paprika powder.
- Ceylon cinnamon
- garlic powder
- sea salt
- ground bay leaves

Instructions

1. Get your chopped meat layer prepared first. In a saucepan or deep-frying pan, dissolve the butter and brown your meat paste in it. Put all the seasoning, except for the oregano, from the list to your taste. In the final moment, you can put oregano so that it does not get sour. Take from heat once the meat sauce is prepared and add one egg. Stir rapidly. Set it down.
2. Roll the veal cutlets with either a sliding pin Grease some butter or ghee to ceramic baking dish or clay.
3. Using a pinch of pepper and sea salt to mix one egg. Dip the egg into each veal slice and put that on the base of the baking dish.
4. Bake at 180oC (350oF) for 10 minutes in the oven.
5. Mix the sheep yogurt or sour cream with six eggs use an electric blender. To your taste, add a pinch of salt.
6. Put the meat sauce over the veal's slices and put the Carnivore moussaka back in the oven. Around ten min, bake. Then coat it with the paste of yogurt or cream and eggs and move it to the oven. Proceed to bake for the next 10 minutes.
7. Then coat it with finely chopped Kefalograviera cheese and layer it uniformly. Please put it back in the oven and cook for ten more minutes. By switching on just the upper heater in the oven, you may use the top process roasting.
8. Represent with a little more finely chopped cheese or a little bit more sour cream. Using fresh parsley or some other texture.

NOTES

You can only use chopped meat sauce for a slightly quicker recipe and cover it with cheese and fluffy topping.

Do not slice till it has cool down at least half the way. It will help you to slice sharp sides with neat pieces.

5. AIP Chicken BaconSauté

A delight for the Carnivore's diet: These

AIP chicken bacon sautés indeed a tasty dish that gratifies and best serves you.

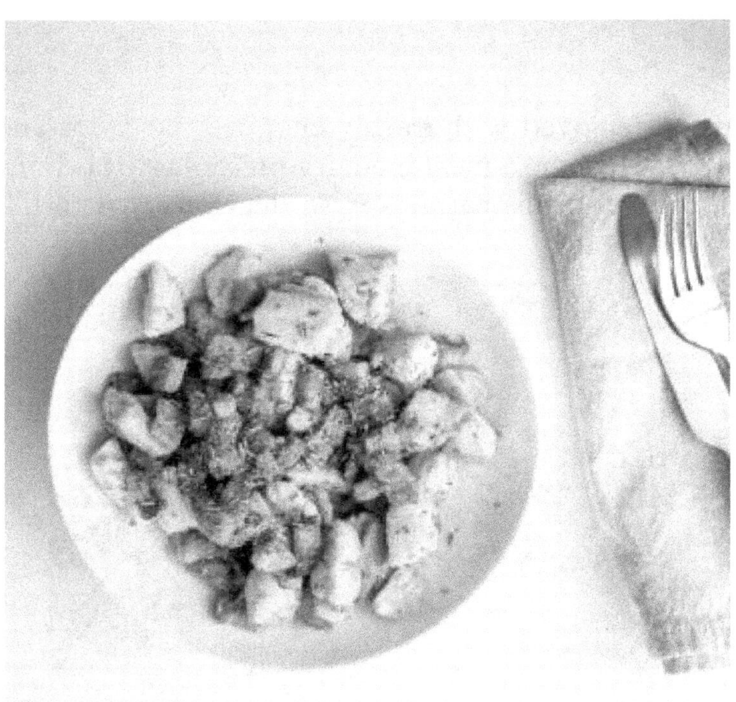

Prep Time: 10 minutes

Cook Time: 20 minutes

Servings: 2

INGREDIENTS

- Fourpieces of bacon, diced.
- Onetbsp. garlic powder
- Onetbsp avocado oil for cooking
- One chicken breast smalldiced.
- Salt according to taste.
- 2 tbsps. Italian seasoning

INSTRUCTIONS

1. In a frying pan, add the avocado oil and cook the bacon and chicken. Cooked for approximately 10 min.
2. For seasoning, use Italian seasoning, garlic powder and salt according to your taste.

Pointtonote All nutrition information is calculated and concentrated on quantities per serving.

6. Low Carb Carnitas

Cooked at home carnitas enjoyed with freshly chopped avocados and crunchy onions a quick low carb meal, but it can be a meal memory pretty fast! It is indeed chosen easily to low-carb lifestyle choices, and this carnitas is so delicious that tortillas ought not to be missed in the end.

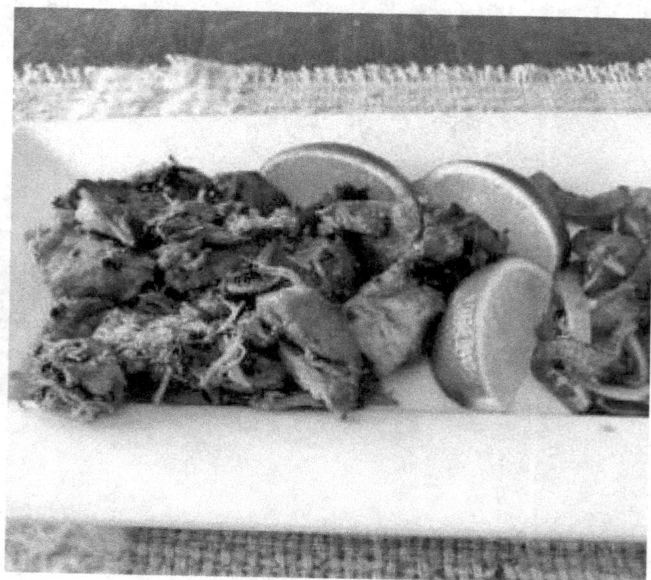

Prep Time: 30 minutes

Cook Time: 2 hrs. 15 minutes.

Servings: 10

Ingredients

- 3 lb. boneless pork shoulder roast cut into 1–2-inch pieces.
- Four sprigs of fresh thyme
- Two cups of water.

- Half cup finely diced onion.
- Oneteaspoon chipotle spice chooses the spice that suits your taste.
- One orange.
- Prefer onetablespoon lard or oil.
- Twotablespoon lard olive oil if you don't want lard.
- Two bay leaves, one teaspoon dry oregano
- Oneteaspoon salt.
- Three cloves garlic finely diced.

Instructions

1. Take the orange and then suck the orange juice out of it. In a bowl, bring it together and put it aside.
2. Heat 2 tablespoons of lard above medium-high heat in a heavy bottom pot or large Dutch oven. To line the pot's base, put some sliced meat in one layer, be careful not to create a mess. Cook the first layer of meat till it is browned, flipping both sides brown using tongs. Transfer to a plate if that meat layer is browned and apply the new layer of meat and cook till browned, then switch to the plate. Rinse until all the meat is browned, then modify.
3. Add the garlic and onion to the Dutch oven pot when the meat is browned, then take away from the pan. Cooked for about 5 minutes or so, frequently mixing, till the onions are crispy and crunchy. Getting back to meat.
4. Utilize the preserved orange zest and juice to the Dutch oven and the next six ingredients (through the Chile pepper). Take it to a boil, lower the heat and cover it. For 2 hours, boil.
5. Take the pot back to a gentle simmer after 2 hours and cook disclosed for 15 to 20 minutes or until most of the liquid has vanished, moving constantly. Take away the bay leaves and thyme sprigs and go to the next stage or store the meat till it is ready. The meat can be stored in the fridge for up to 3 days at this stage.
6. Heat One Tablespoon of lard over the moderate temperature in a big skillet while cooking the carnitas. Remove the meat from the sauce using a slotted spoon and place it over a thin line in the skillet. Cooked for five min or till the meat begins to crust, slightly flipping (you may need to do this in batches).
7. Offer with lime wedges, guacamole (or sliced fresh avocados), refried beans, jalapeno pepper, lime wedges, and caramelized onions.

7. Carnivore's Lasagna

For meat lovers, it is stuffed with Italian sausage, ground beef, meatballs, and pepperoni.

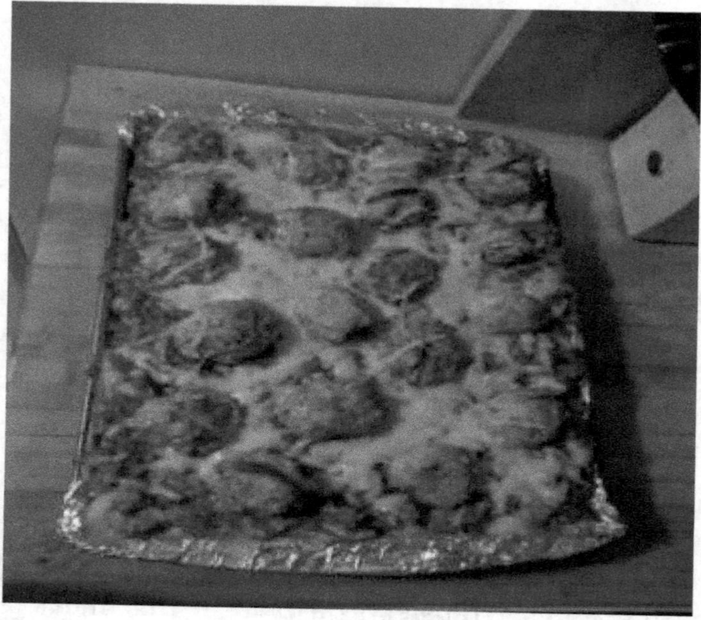

Prep Time: 1 hour 10 minutes.

Cook Time: 1 hour.

Servings: 1 lasagna

INGREDIENTS

- Half onion finely chopped.
- 1lb. hot Italian sausagesliced.
- Four garlic cloves crumbled.
- 1 1/2 cups parmesan cheese, grated.
- One tsp.Dry oregano, divided.
- 1/2 cup oatmeal
- 3 (15 ounce) cans tomato sauce
- 2 tbsps.Brown sugar
- 18 lasagna noodles
- Onetbsp.Fennel seed, divided.
- Onetsp.Dried thyme, divided.

- Two lbs. Lean ground beef, divided.
- Two tsps.Salt, divided.
- One tbsp. Olive oil
- One tsp.Black pepper.
- One tsp.Dry basil, divided.
- 2⁄3 lb. Pepperoni chopped into small pieces.
- Twotbsps.Dry parsley, divided.
- Two eggs.
- 32 ounces ricotta cheese
- Half tsp. ground nutmeg
- 8 -16 ounces mozzarella cheese, grated.

Instructions

1. Heat the oven to 350 degrees.
2. Heat the olive oil in a large pan at moderate temperature. Put garlic, onion, Italian sausage, and half of the ground meat. Cook for approximately 10 minutes.
3. If required, remove the meat mixture. Put 1/2 teaspoon basil, thyme, oregano, fennel seed, salt, black pepper and 1tbsp of brown sugar, one tablespoon parsley, tomato sauce. Mix, carefully wrap and allow to boil for 1 hour on low flame.
4. Start preparing the ricotta cheese mixture, lasagna noodles and meatballs while the sauce is cooking. Then, in a wide bowl, break one egg. Add the 1/2 cup of Parmesan, oatmeal and the remaining ground meat, basil, fennel, black pepper, thyme, oregano, and salt according to your taste. Merge properly.
5. Shape the meat into balls that have a size of around 1 inch. Please put it on a sprayed pan and bake for 20 minutes, rotating half the way through the cooking time over the meatballs. In the bowl, put the ricotta cheese in it. Add the remaining nutmeg, egg, and the remaining parsley. Merge and set it aside.
6. Then, boil the lasagna noodles for at least 15 minutes in a big pan full of very hot water.
7. The lasagna is placed in a deep 9x3-inch pan till the sauce is cooked. On the base of the pan, pour 2 cups of the sauce. Just lay down six noodles. Layer half of the ricotta on the noodles and top with 1/3 of the parmesan and mozzarella. Place half the pepperoni on top of that.

8. Similarly, make another layer, beginning with 2 cups of sauce. Lay down the remaining portion of the lasagna noodles on top afterward.
9. Blend the rest of the sauce into the cooked meatballs and scatter on top of the lasagna. Cover with a cheese layer.
10. Wrap in foil and bake for 25 minutes at 350F. Let us remove the foil and bake for 25 minutes. Take it out and cool it for 15 minutes before served.

Conclusion

If you've made it on the carnivore diet this far, you finally are noticing some beneficial effects.As a result of your metabolism having shifted completely to ketosis and blood sugar levels remaining consistent, you can feel a lot more physically active with excessive concentration levels. When you undergo the carnivore diet, this is what happens to your body.

While being on the carnivore diet, some individuals even undergo blood sugar drops because carbohydrates' consumption is inaccurate. For patients with Type 2 diabetes, this has to be a preventative measure.

You should also find that one's desires for high carbohydrates will have decreased because you are now better prepared to get all the energy from protein and fat you want.

Rebuild and create every cell in the body; meat has all the nine essential amino acids you consume. And it has some other good things that you will need, too.

Josh Axe, DC, DNM, CNS, and author of Eat Dirt, says that meat is filled with vitamin B12, a nutrient vital for generating long-lasting strength. "Meat also provides your body with a variety of other essential vitamins and minerals many of which are more bioavailable and easier to absorb than the nutrients found in plant sources."There are plant-based foods, of course, as most vegans will say, containing all the essential nutrients (quinoa, for example), and you can combine foods to get everything you need.

Reasonably Set Your Goals

Stick to them and make them accessible. Later or Sooner, you will be confronted with all of the delicious carnivore diet recipes in the world. This one needs a serious effort, like any permissive form of diet. Look ahead, choose the meals for the entire week in advance, and make a grocery list and keep to it as much as practicable to avoid cravings.

Don't start with very wide segments. Although the carnivore diet is in the form of "eat until fulfilled," that does not mean you should strive to explore, especially if weight loss is your target. Go gently and, if necessary, raise the quantities. Using your meal plan as an opportunity to listen more closely to your body's needs, avoiding what it doesn't want.

The Carnivore Diet meal plan will help you meet your goals safely and sustainably if you want to boost your health by avoiding refined foods, achieve your gym goals by underpaying your calorie intake or can't get enough meat.

The Ultimate Electric Smoker Cookbook

25+ Recipes and 13 Tricks to Smoke Just Everything

Haile Banister

Table of Contents

Introduction

Barbeque is a huge part of American cuisine and culture. Smoked meats are a favorite among the entire country. Barbeque becomes a must in summers when families get together on long summer weekends, spending quality time together. Nowadays, this has become nearly impossible because of the tough work-life balance and people's desire to grab an easy bite. No one has the time and energy to set up the conventional-style barbeque. Some people might still be up for doing all the hard work, but most of the population would welcome a quick and easy way to enjoy the smoked flavors of barbequed meat.

Technology has made this difficult feat possible. Electric Smokers are a great appliance that makes our job simple. There was a time when you had to spend the whole day in front of the Smoker to prepare a good smoked steak. With the electric Smoker, you can enjoy the authentic flavor of barbeque with little effort. What the electric Smoker does is that it uses the same conventional method for cooking, but you do not have to do all the hard work manually; the electric Smoker does it for you. All you must do is prepare the meat, set up the electric Smoker, pour in some water in the water tray, throw in some wood chips, turn up the heat according to your needs and set the timer.

Meanwhile, you go about your business, run your errands, have a chat with your friends, and your yummy food is being prepared all on its own. You do not need to worry about temperature control or about managing the charcoal. The electric Smoker fits best with the modern way of life. Another huge advantage of electric smokers, apart from them being super easy to operate, is that they are easy to clean. They are just like little closets which have removable racks. You can remove every part, clean it, and place it back. Also, because the temperature and the smoke can be regulated and controlled, the result is perfect most of the time. The chances for mishaps are rare, unlike the traditional style, where things can get tricky quite often.

If you want to enjoy a delicious barbeque with the least effort, you should read on about this amazing appliance, making you a pro at family barbeques in no time. Enjoy reading!

Chapter 1: What is an Electric Smoker?

In this chapter, the basic introduction and working of the electric Smoker will be discussed. Before understanding the Electric Smoker, we must first understand the meaning of the cooking method that the Electric Smoker uses.

This technique is known as 'Smoking,' and it is a type of process related to barbeque.

1.1. What is Smoking?

Smoking is a more specialized and extreme type of barbecuing. You will be using the smoke from different types of aromatic wood chips or wood chunks in smoking. You may use wood chips of cherry, apple, hickory, mesquite, and many others. These impart their unique flavor and smoky aroma to the meat being smoked.

The process of smoking takes longer than barbecuing. The temperature is also lower than barbecue. The temperature is usually set between 125 to 175◦F. The temperature is kept lower because if the temperature is turned up, then the meat's outer layer will be cooked and will not allow the smoke to reach throughout the meat and impart its rich aroma and taste.

Smoking is an advanced technique, and it required a much longer time for food preparation than grilling and normal barbeque. This method also requires a maximum amount of expertise to understand the texture of different types of meat and how they will be perfectly smoked.

The Electric Smoker

An electric smoker is a cooking appliance that is used outside. Smoking is an advanced type of variation of barbecue. The electric Smoker uses an electric source and heating rods to produce heat for cooking and smoking. The conventional way to smoke is to burn charcoal to produce the required heat, but the electric Smoker is easier to use and simple to operate. The whole process is cleaner as compared to the conventional style. The body of the electric Smoker is either made of stainless steel or cast iron.

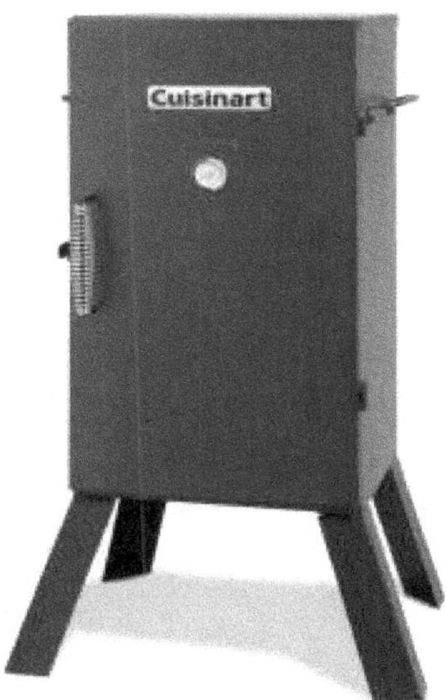

(An electric smoker)

There are numerous different types of electric smokers available in the market. You have an option to choose a smoker that is according to your requirements. Different models vary in their specific features, size, number of cooking racks present, temperature control features, number of cycles, preheat options, keep warm option, manual settings, automatic settings, digital displays, and control panels.

Sometimes variety can also overwhelm a buyer. To buy an electric smoker, it is recommended to first determine your requirements and then research the market too but the proper kind of Smoker for yourself. In the following pages, you will also find guidelines to help you decide whether you even need an electric smoker or not. Before that, we will briefly discuss the common features present in almost all electric smokers.

Working of an Electric Smoker

Normally, when you see an electric smoker, it looks like a cabinet; it is quite efficient in smoking the meat with relatively few components. The basic heating function is that the electric rods heat the entire cooking chamber, and the heated air is spread throughout the chamber. This causes the meat to cook by convection. There are six basic components of the electric Smoker:

- Cooking Chamber
- Woodchip tray
- Electric Heating rods or other heating elements
- Racks or grills to place the meat.
- Water Pan

Cooking Chamber

Like the gas smokers and the charcoal smokers, the electric smokers also have a vertical alignment. The space designated for cooking is at the top. The electric heating rods are placed at the bottom of the cooking chamber. Above the heating, rods are the grills, wood chips drawer and the water pan.

Electric Heating Rods:

The electric rods are placed at the base of the electric Smoker. They are the main source of heat for cooking. Some models of the electric Smoker have one heating rod, and some have more than one rods. This depends on the shape and size of the electric Smoker.

Wood Chip Tray

This is a specific space or tray provided above the electric rods to place the wood chips or wood chunks within the heating chamber. When the woodchips burn slowly, they cause smoke, which spreads within the cooking chamber and surrounds the meat. This smoke gives the meat a smoky and rich flavor. The woodchip tray is sometimes called the firebox as well.

Different types of hardwood are available to put in the electric Smoker. You can use various wood chips and chunks of mesquite, oak, alder, apple, cherry, maple, and hickory.

Water Pan

This is like a slightly deep pan or tray, fixed like a rack in the electric Smoker. Before starting the Smoker, this tray is filled with cold water. The main function is that when the heating rods are turned on, this cold water keeps the temperature from rising quickly inside the heating chamber. The other function is that steam is created when the water is heated up to a boiling point, which helps cook the meat. The steam helps the convection cooking process.

Grills or Racks

Above the water, the tray has placed the racks or grills. These are made of stainless steel. The food is placed on these for cooking. You can put the meat directly on the grill, or you can use heatproof skillets or barbecue utensils.

Vents and Dampers

the vents are usually placed at the top part of the electric Smoker. When the Smoker's temperature gets too high, the vents are opened to release some hot air and bring the temperature down.

The dampers are there for exactly the opposite reason. They are placed at the bottom part of the electric Smoker. When you open the dampers, oxygen enters the cooking chamber. The flames of the woodchips feed on this oxygen and increase the temperature inside the chamber.

Chapter 2. Why buy an Electric Smoker?

If you are someone who loves barbecue and the rich flavor of smoked meat, you might have thought about investing in an electric smoker. Even though you think about it, you are not quite sure whether you should invest in an electric smoker or not. You cannot deny that it is an expensive appliance and if you only occasionally barbecue, this appliance is not for you. Having said that, if you enjoy preparing delicious barbecue now and then, you might want to consider the electric Smoker. Using an electric smoker is easier than the conventional barbeque method, and it is much easier to clean. If you enjoy the smoky aroma and taste in each bite of meat, you might want to ditch the conventional method and adopt electric smoking. This is perfect for that tender, aromatic, and rich smoke flavor. However, you must be warned against the prejudice that surrounds electric smokers. The die-heart conventional barbecue community may argue that the electric Smoker does not give off the meat's authentic smoky flavor. You may agree or not to this argument but investing in an electric smoker would be your best bet if you are new to smoking.

In this chapter, we will discuss the top five reasons to buy an electric smoker. The five arguments in favor of the electric Smoker are:

- Perfect choice for beginners
- The cost
- The easy usage
- You can set it up where conventional barbeque grills might not be allowed.
- The option to cold smoke

2.1. Perfect Choice for Beginners

Investing in an electric smoker is a safe choice for beginners. Smoking is a slightly tricky technique. If you go by the conventional way, it might take you longer to learn and maybe you might give up early on. With the electric Smoker, you can operate it with ease. The temperature and length of cooking can be regulated, and the best part is that the results are almost always perfect. Getting perfect results in cooking is a huge plus because it further motivates you.

Using the electric Smoker, you can learn and become familiar with the basic method and technique involved. Once you have learned the basics, you can either move on to the more conventional style or even decide to stick to the electric Smoker.

2.2. The Cost

If you survey the market, you will find that electric smokers are cheaper than their conventional counterparts. When you look closely, the amount of food they can cook in one session is quite commendable. Another reason the electric Smoker might feel more appealing is that it needs only a one-time setup. After the initial setup, no maintenance is required. Cleaning is easy. To operate is easy. So, in the long run, this seems to be a better investment.

2.3. The Easy Usage

If you see the conventional system of smoking and barbecue, you have a lot to manage. You must control the optimum temperature, need the expertise to light the charcoal, maintain airflow to keep a smooth temperature and manage any temperature spikes or accidents during the entire procedure. In short, you will be on your toes the whole time. Now, flip the situation to the electric Smoker. You prepare your food items, place them on the grills, fill in the water tray, put them in the woodchips, and turn on the heating rods. You can even set the time. It is as easy as this. In case you are hosting a few people over, you will have plenty of time to set up the area and interact with your guests.

2.4. Can Carry the Electric Smoker Anywhere with Power Supply

The appliance comes in handy in two situations. Many states have a fire ban in summers, meaning you cannot set up a charcoal grill or do any cooking outside. There is a fear of forest fires due to the dry summer air. You can take out your electric Smoker and enjoy proper smoked food with friends and family in such a situation.

Another situation where the electric Smoker comes in handy is in small houses and apartments where space is an issue. In apartments, there is a prohibition on barbequing and smoke. You can easily set up your electric Smoker on your balcony and enjoy your favorite food in this situation.

2.5. The Option to Cold Smoke

Sometimes you want to cold smoke some food items like cheese and bacon. It is not easily possible on conventional smokers. It would help if you bought the cold smoke attachments with an electric smoker, generally available easily with all-electric smoker models. This attachment can be used to prepare a variety of preparations like meatloaves, deserts, dried meat, and fish sausages.

Chapter 3. Proper Usage of the Electric Smoker

After you have purchased the Electric Smoker, comes to the process of setting it up. Most electric smokers are easy to install and setup. It is best to read the manual to understand the working of the specific model.

This chapter will discuss step-by-step how we should prepare our food items and the correct method and sequence to smoke our desired food product.

3.1. Preparation of Meat

The meat preparation will be done the same way you would do for conventional barbecue and smoking as usual. Some people follow their family recipes passed down through generations. Some people prefer a marinade kept overnight; some perform a dry rub to season and prepare the meat. It is entirely up to you how you want to season the meat you want to prepare. The electric Smoker can smoke every kind of meat, so do not be shy and prepare your favorite meat for smoking. Be sure that the electric Smoker will prepare the same flavor and texture you expect from the traditional style smoker will give.

3.2. Setting up the Electric Smoker

Few points should be kept in mind when setting up the electric Smoker. The first and most important is that this is an outdoor appliance. Please keep it in a properly ventilated space. It cannot be kept indoors. It must be set up outside. It should be set up on a flat and strong surface that can withstand high temperatures. Sometimes the appliance can heat-up up to high temperatures. Please keep it in an open space with room to move about so that the appliance is in no danger to be tripped over and become a hazard. Keep children away from the electric Smoker while operating and afterward until it cools down after one or two hours.

3.3. Read the Electric Smoker Manual

Different models of Electric Smokers have a different set of instructions. The basic working of thee the Electric Smokers is the same, but there is a slight difference in how each Smoker is operated. It would help if you had a complete understanding of how your appliance is turned on and off, how to regulate temperature, when is it safe to open the appliance, what temperatures are suitable for which meat, how much time it requires for specific meats. It will help if you read up about all such details to use your Electric Smoker to its fullest.

3.4. Seasoning the Electric Smoker

This is an important process. You only need to do this once when your electric Smoker is brand new. To get rid of any harmful chemicals left in the Smoker during manufacturing, this procedure is done. All manuals have detailed descriptions of the seasoning. You must follow the exact instructions of your Electric Smoker because they are model specific.

However, a common procedure followed for seasoning is that you apply any cooking oil on all the electric Smoker's inner surfaces such that the surfaces are completely coated. Now turn on the Electric Smoker and let it operate empty for 2 to 3 hours. Then let it cook, and then your appliance is ready for use.

3.5. Preparing the Cooking Chamber

First, make sure that the cooking chamber is clean. Fill the water tray with water. This must be done before turning on the heat. Fill in the wood chip tray with wood chips or woodchucks that you wish to use. Usually, the wood chip compartment should be filled if the meat will be smoked for 3 to 4 hours. Next, set up the temperature and time for smoking. Always remember that the heating chamber should be preheated. Do not put the meat in the cold chamber and turn on the heat afterward. It is always recommended to put the meat in a well-heated chamber. This is a pro tip for the best results.

3.6. Putting in the meat

First, let the cooking chamber reach a certain temperature, then place the meat on the grills. You will need to open the chamber, place the meat, and then close it. Take care of that you put in the meat swiftly so that less heat is lost from within the chamber during this action. Temperature and the correct amount of heat are essential for the meat to be prepared to perfection. It is also recommended not to open the chamber when the meat is being smoked. This might disrupt the smoking process and bring the temperature down. The same rule applies to smoking as the one that applies in baking. Optimum temperature is essential.

3.7. The Process of Smoking

This is a slow process. It usually takes three or more hours. Only fish takes a shorter while to smoke. Otherwise, all other meats take much longer. Always take care to replenish the woodchips during the smoking process.

The smoking process will be carried out on its own, so there will be no other precaution except for keeping an eye on the wood chips.

Another thing to lookout for will be the water. This water serves as the steam that gives the meats the required moisture that does not let them dry out. If the water isdried up, the meat will also become dry and difficult to chew on. So, it is always important that there is enough moisture circulation in the heating chamber. Always keep an eye out for the water tray. It should not be dry.

3.8. Taking out the meat

Before taking out the meat from the heated chamber, always check if the meat is cooked properly. Every meat has an internal temperature that indicates its doneness. So before bringing the meat out, insert the thermometer to the thickest part of the meat can see that the optimum temperature has been achieved or not. If you think the meat is undercooked, keep it in the chamber for 20 more minutes and check again. If all seems well, take out the Smoker's rack and place it on the counter to let it rest and then slice your meat.

Serve the meat with traditional side dishes like coleslaw, corn on the cob or baked potatoes. With the electric Smoker, you do not need to worry about the meat not being cooked properly. With the temperature regulation, the chance for accidents is reduced significantly.

Chapter 4. Tips and Tricks to Smoke Anything

Knowing some tricks and hacks about appliances always helps in preparing perfect meals. The same is the case with an electric smoker. This chapter discusses a few tricks and tips to help you in preparing smoked meats and foods. Usually, we start learning with experience but learning from other's experiences can give you a head start. Here is a list of tried and tested tricks and tips for the usage of an Electric Smoker. These tips and tricks will help you along your journey with the electric Smoker. Read all the points carefully to get the best results.

4.1. Do not Over Smoke the Food

When you first buy an electric smoker, you might be tempted to use many strong aromatic woodchips. But the reality is that you do not need an overpowering smoke flavor to make the barbecue delicious; only a mild smoky flavor will do the job. It is also true for poultry that over-smoked chicken becomes bitter and inedible. So always be careful about the amount of smoke you want for your food. In the case of smoke, the less is more saying is true.

4.2. Smoke Chicken at High Temperature

Chicken is not one of those meat groups which need a lower temperature for a longer time to be perfectly cooked. The chicken cooks at a higher temperature. The rule of thumb is to take the temperature to 275◦F and smoke the chicken for around one to two hours. To check the chicken for doneness, insert a probe inside the chicken thigh and see that the internal temperature is about 165◦F. The proper cooking of chicken is important because undercooked chicken can cause harmful effects and infections to the body.

4.3. Do not Soak the Wood Chips

It is common practice to soak woodchips in water before use. What happens is that when we soak the wood chips and put them in the Smoker and the smoking starts, white smoke is created. We think that this white smoke gives a smoky, rich flavor to the meat, but it is not true. This white smoke is just steam that dilutes the smoke's flavor and interferes with the temperature inside the chamber.

What you should do is that use the wood chips directly. The smoke that will be created will be thin blue smoke, which is the type of smoke that imparts a rich aromatic flavor to the smoked dishes.

4.4. Season your Electric Smoker before Use

This point is more of a health concern rather than a tip or trick. Seasoning is the process performed before cooking anything in the Smoker. This is usually done to eliminate all factory residue, chemicals, and dust from inside the cavity that has been left over from the manufacturing plant.

This process also has a good effect on subsequent smoking as well. After the seasoning, a black layer of smoke is formed on the electric Smoker's inner surfaces. So, after seasoning, whatever you will smoke, the black coating will impart the smoky flavor.

4.5. Preheat the Cooking Chamber

Always preheat the cooking chamber. Turn on the electric heat rods before putting in the meat and wait till the optimum temperature is reached; only then should you put in the meat. This will ensure that the meat will neither remain undercooked or overcooked.

4.6. Put Poultry in Oven to Finish

Most of the electric smokers have a maximum temperature of 275◦F. This temperature is enough to cook poultry to perfection, but the desired crispy skins cannot be achieved at this temperature. So, if you want crispy skins, take out the chicken from the Smoker and place it in the oven at around 300◦F for 10 minutes. You will have yummy crispy skins.

4.7. Cover the Racks and Grills with Aluminum Foil

This tip is more for cleanliness than the taste of the smoked good. It would help if you covered all your racks and trays with aluminum foil. This will protect the racks and grills, and whenever the aluminum gets dirty, it can be replaced with a fresh layer of aluminum foil.

4.8. Do not use the Wood Chip Tray

In the electric Smoker, you fill the wood tray with woodchips. Often, people have experienced that they must refill the wood chip tray repeatedly, and it can be a bit inconvenient. Rather than wood chips, you can use a pellet smoker. A pellet smoker is a separately available tube that gives off thin blue smoke, which gives the aroma and amazing flavor to the smoked meats.

4.9. Leave the Vent Open

It is a good idea to keep the vent of the Electric Smoker completely open. This is to prevent the accumulation of creosote. Creosote is a substance in smoke that gives a smoky flavor to the foods. This substance is good to impart a smoky flavor to the dish, but a high quantity of this substance can accumulate over the meat and gives off a bitter flavor.

4.10. Control the Temperature Swings

The temperature swings are phenomena that are seen in all heating appliances using heating rods. What happens is that if you set the temperature of the appliance at 220◦F, the rod, when it reaches this temperature, will turn off; however, the temperature still keeps rising and is risen to about 240◦F and then starts coming back, it gets lower and lower about 210◦F, and then the rods turn on again, and it takes a while to get to 220◦F. you need to learn to manage this situation by keeping the temperature selection about 10◦F lower than the desired temperature. This way, the temperature swings will be controlled.

4.11. Invest in a Good Thermometer

In smoking, you can often be confused if the meat is done or not. Sometimes you can be fooled but the appliance's internal thermostat. But the doneness of meat is determined by the internal temperature of the meat. So, to check the internal temperature of the meat, you should have a separate thermometer. Such thermometers are commonly known as probes. You can insert the probe into the thickest part of the meat and determine the internal temperature. We must understand that the thermostat of the electric Smoker and the meat's internal temperature are different, and the doneness of the meat depends on the meat's internal temperature. Different meats have the different internal temperature that determines that they are fully cooked. Some meats are done at lower internal temperatures, such as fish and seafood. Some meats require high temperatures, like beef and lamb. Understanding this is especially important, and the first step towards this understanding is investing in a good thermometer.

4.12. Keep the Meat Overnight Before Smoking

To achieve the meat's full flavors, it is always a good idea to keep the meat overnight. It does not matter if you decide to marinate, dry rub, or brine the meat; leaving it in the refrigerator overnight will cause the flavors to fully absorb in the meat, and the meat will also become tender before smoking. The meat will be cooked even if you decide not to let it stay overnight, but the results might not be as good as the meat that has been kept overnight. In smoking and barbecue, patience plays an important role. The more patient you are, the better your food will cook and taste.

4.13. Do not Hurry.

Smoking is a long process. It takes time for meats to properly smoke. Whenever you decide to smoke meat, always keep in mind that you must have the patience to let the meat cook completely. Sometimes the temptation to check on our dishes can be harmful to the recipe. When you open the electric smoker door, the temperature is disrupted, and the recipe might be affected. Even opening the door for one or two minutes can even have such an effect. So, you must be patient while the Smoker is working. This is an amazing appliance, and you should trust it to work its wonder. All you must do is sit back and relax.

Chapter 5. Ultimate Electric Smoker Recipes

In this chapter, you will find easy-to-follow recipes that you can make in your Electric Smoker. You must follow all recipes exactly according to the instructions for the best results.

5.1. Beef BBQ Brisket

This is an easy recipe for BBQ brisket that you will prepare in your Electric Smoker. Be assured that you will enjoy the original BBQ flavor. The meat will have a beautiful texture on the outside and will be tender inside. Just follow the instructions carefully, and you are in for a treat. They this recipe and you will not be disappointed.

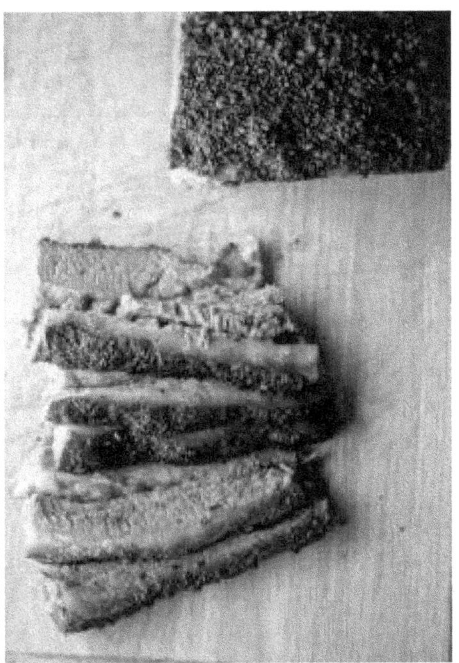

- Course: Dinner
- Cuisine: American BBQ

- Total Time: 8 hours 50 minutes
- Preparation Time: 30 minutes
- Cooking Time: 8 hours
- Rest Time: 20 minutes
- Serving Size: 2 servings
- Nutritional Value Per Serving
    - Calories: 564 calories
    - Carbohydrates: 0 g
    - Protein: 77.3 g
    - Fats: 27.4 g

Equipment Used:

- Electric Smoker

Ingredients:

1. BBQ rub (store-bought) 5 tbsp.
2. Beef Brisket ½ kg.

Instructions:

- Preheat the electric Smoker at 225◦F.
- Then prepare the beef brisket. Wash the meat and pat it dry.
- Trim all the excess fat from the brisket, leaving only one-fourth of an inch of fat on the meat.
- Next, remove the excess skin from the underside of the meat cut.
- Now, apply the BBQ rub on the beef on both sides generously.

- Put the brisket in the Electric Smoker and insert the probe in the thickest part of the beef.
- Smoke the beef until the temperature has reached 160◦F. This usually takes six hours. It might take longer, so you must see when the temperature reaches a certain point.
- At this stage,please take out the brisket very carefully and wrap it tightly in aluminum foil.
- Place it back into the Smoker and wait until the brisket's temperature reaches 190◦F. This usually takes additional 2 hours. The time might be a bit more depending on the brisket.
- When the beef is at 190◦F, take it out of the Smoker.
- Let it rest for 20 to 30 minutes.
- Then unwrap the brisket and slice it.
- Enjoy the delicious BBQ brisket.

5.2. Smoked Salmon

The best thing about this recipe is that it is easy to make and quick to prepare. Minimum ingredients are used to achieve perfection with this smoked salmon. Try this recipe, and you will be in for a mouthwatering treat.

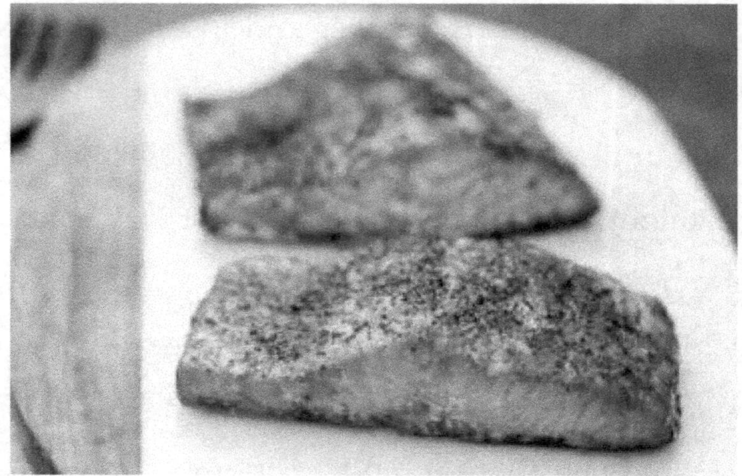

- Course: Lunch
- Cuisine: American
- Total Time: 2 hours 10 minutes
- Preparation Time: 10 minutes
- Cooking Time: 1 hour
- Rest: 20 minutes
- Serving Size: 3 servings
- Nutritional Value Per Serving
    - Calories: 454 calories
    - Carbohydrates: 0 g
    - Protein: 57.5 g
    - Fats: 24.2 g

Equipment Used:

- Electric Smoker

Ingredients:

1. Fresh Salmon 1 kg.

2. Brown Sugar 2 tbsp
3. Dried Dill 1 tsp
4. Pepper 1 tsp
5. Salt 1tsp

Instructions:

- Wash and pat dry the fish carefully. You must be careful with raw fish meat because it is delicate and can break.
- Mix the salt, pepper, sugar, and dill in a bowl.
- Rub this sugar mixture on the top side of the fish.
- Put it in the refrigerator for one hour. This will allow the fish to dry brine.
- Preheat the Electric Smoker at 250◦F.
- Place a probe into the thickest part of the meat.
- Let it smoke until the meat reaches 145◦F. It takes about 45 minutes to one hour.
- The dish can be served at room temperature or even cold.
- For this specific dish, you can use pecan, cherry, or oak wood for a subtle flavor.

5.3. Smoked Chicken

Chicken is one of the most widely popular food throughout the world. This recipe gives smoked chicken a spicy and flavorful twist. The brown sugar used in the rub gives it a caramelized look and texture and adds richness to the taste. Try this recipe out and you will not be disappointed.

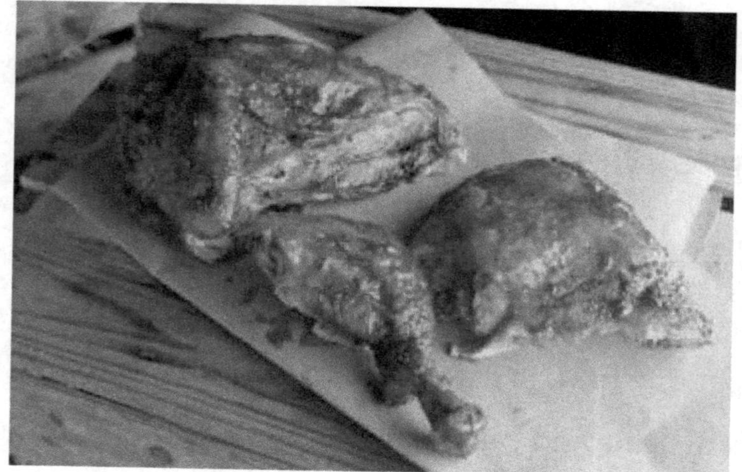

- Course: Dinner
- Cuisine: American BBQ
- Total Time: 5 hours
- Preparation Time: 30 minutes
- Cooking Time: 4 hours
- Rest Time: 30 minutes
- Serving Size: 4 servings
- Nutritional Value Per Serving
    - Calories: 240 calories
    - Carbohydrates: 0 g
    - Protein: 21 g
    - Fats: 17 g

Equipment Used:

- Electric Smoker

Ingredients:

1. Medium sized whole chicken with skin

2. Thyme 1 tbsp
3. Cayenne Pepper 2 tbsp
4. Garlic Powder 1 tbsp
5. Chili Powder 2 tbsp
6. Salt 1 tbsp
7. Sugar 2 tbsp
8. Onion Powder 1 tbsp
9. Black Pepper 2 tbsp
10. Olive Oil 3 tbsp

Instructions:

- Arrange the woodchips in the electric smoker tray. You can use peach, apple, or cherry woodchips. Then turn on the electric Smoker to preheat at 225°F.
- In a medium-sized mixing bowl, mix the thyme, cayenne pepper, garlic powder, chili powder, salt, sugar, onion powder, and black pepper. This will make the perfect rub for the chicken.
- First, rub the whole chicken with olive oil. All sides and inside the hollow cavity of chicken as well.
- After that, apply the prepared rub on the chicken generously. Rub it on the entire surface of the chicken.
- Put the skin over the breast of the chicken and apply the rub under the skin as well.
- Put the prepared chicken in the electric Smoker and insert a probe in the thigh.

- Check the chicken after every hour and take it out when the meat's internal temperature reaches 164◦F. The whole process takes about 4 hours.
- Served the smoked chicken warm.

5.4. Smoked Corn on the Cob

Corn on the cob is a crowd'sfavorite side dish. It is popular among kids and adults alike. These complement all sorts of meats in a barbecue and give us that much-needed light and sweet flavorsin the middle of a high protein barbecue. Try this easy recipe, and you will not regret preparing some smoked corn on the cob.

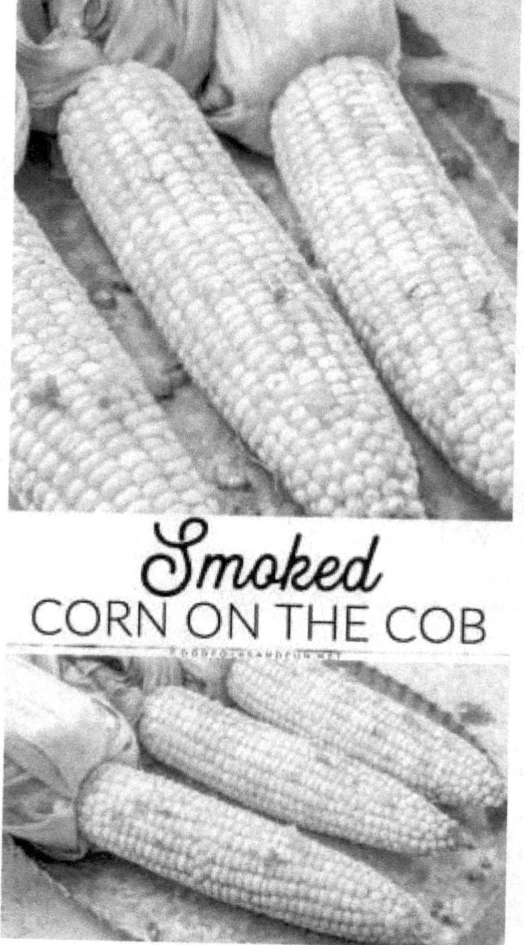

- Course: Side Dish
- Cuisine: American
- Total Time: 5 hours 10 minutes
- Preparation Time: 4 hours
- Cooking Time: 1 hour
- Rest Time: 10 minutes
- Serving Size: 6 servings
- Nutritional Value Per Serving
    - Calories: 142 calories
    - Carbohydrates: 16.6 g
    - Protein: 2.7 g
    - Fats: 8.6 g

Equipment Used:

- Electric Smoker

Ingredients:

1. Ear corn with husks 6 pieces
2. Brown sugar 2 tbsp
3. Salt ½ tsp
4. Garlic powder ½ tsp
5. Melted butter ¼ cup.
6. Onion powder 1 tsp
7. Sliced green onion 3 pieces.

Instructions:

- Take a large roasting pot and fill it half with room temperature water.
- Pull the husks of all the corn cobs and remove the silks. Let the husks remain attached to the cob but just pulled back.
- Soak the corn cobs in the water and if needed, fill the pot with more water to completely immerse the cobs into water.
- Soak for 4 hours.
- After that remove, the cobs from the pot and place them on paper towels and let them dry.
- Preheat the electric Smoker at 225°F. Place the woodchips inside the electric Smoker.
- In a mixing bowl, mix the butter, sugar, salt, onion powder, and garlic powder to make a rub for the corn on the cob.
- With the help of a brush, apply the rub generously to the corn cobs.
- Pull the husks back on the corn cobs. Place them in the electric Smoker.
- Leave for 60 minutes and then take them out.
- Let them rest for 10 minutes, and then serve them as a delicious side dish.

5.5. Grilled Chicken Thighs with Asparagus

This delicious chicken recipe is perfect for enjoying on the weekend. It is easy to make and takes only 2 hours to prepare. The juicy chicken with the light smokiness is a success with kids and adults alike. This dish will be a crowd favorite. Try out this recipe and enjoy it with friends and family.

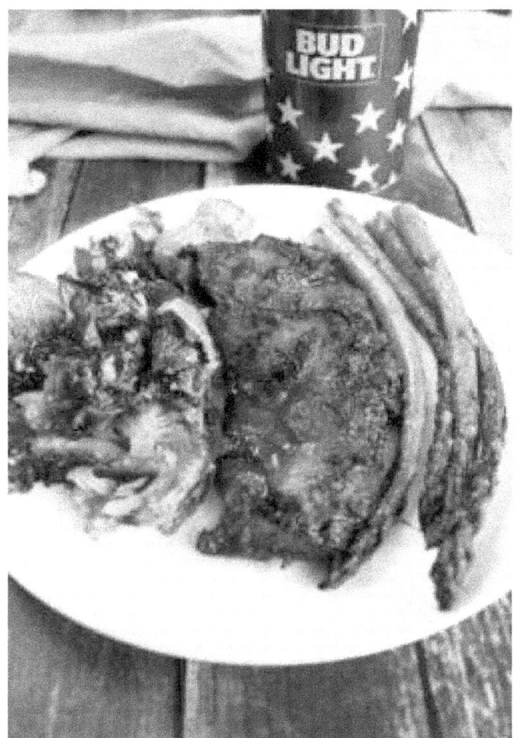

- Course: Lunch
- Cuisine: American
- Total Time: 5 hours
- Preparation Time: 3 hours
- Cooking Time: 2 hours
- Rest Time: 10 minutes
- Serving Size: 3 servings
- Nutritional Value Per Serving
    - Calories: 482 calories
    - Carbohydrates: 58.8 g
    - Protein: 58.5 g
    - Fats: 19.3 g

Equipment Used:

- Electric Smoker

Ingredients:

For Chicken:

1. Chicken thighs 3 to 4 pieces
2. Store-bought BBQ rub 5 tbsp.
3. Water as required.
4. Sugar 1 tsp
5. Salt 1 tsp
6. ¼ cup apple cider vinegar

For Asparagus

1. Asparagus 1 bunch
2. Red pepper flakes 1 tsp
3. Balsamic Vinegar ¼ cup
4. Pepper 1 tsp
5. Salt 1 tsp

Equipment Used:

- Electric Smoker

Instructions:

- Prepare to brine the chicken thighs. Put the chicken in a large zip lock bag, then add Vinegar, salt, and sugar.
- Then, fill the bag with water such that the chicken pieces are completely soaked. Put it in the refrigerator for 2 to 3 hours.

- The brining process will ensure that the chicken does not dry out while in the electric Smoker.
- Similarly, prepare a marinade for the asparagus bunch as well. Please put it in a large zip lock bag. Add the balsamic vinegar, salt pepper, pepper flakes and water to soak the asparagus. Please leave it in the refrigerator for 3 hours.
- Prepare a small BBQ spray bottle having one part vinegar, two parts water and 1 tsp sugar. Mix it properly. This will be used to spray on the chicken while it is being smoked.
- Take the chicken out of the refrigerator after 2 hours and wash and dry the pieces.
- Apply the BBQ rub generously on the chicken pieces.
- Preheat the electric Smoker at 225◦F for 15 minutes. Put the apple woodchips in the wood tray.
- Place the chicken thighs in the electric Smoker.
- Spray with the BBQ spray bottle after every 20 to 30 minutes. This will prevent the chicken from drying.
- Smoke the chicken for about two hours.
- Take the chicken out of the Smoker and let it rest for 10 minutes.
- Meanwhile, please take out the asparagus and spread it on a paper towel and pat dry.
- Put the asparagus in the electric Smoker and leave for 10 minutes, and then take it out.
- Serve the chicken with a side of asparagus.

- This is a good pairing to serve, and the asparagus complements the smoked chicken beautifully.

5.6. Smoked Turkey Breast

Turkey has often been bland and boring meat. This recipe gives the turkey a tasty and spicy twist. The BBQ sauce mixed with hot sauce and honey gives the smoked turkey a rich flavor and an amazing texture. Try out this mouthwatering and delicious recipe and enjoy the aromatic and tender turkey meat. This recipe never disappoints.

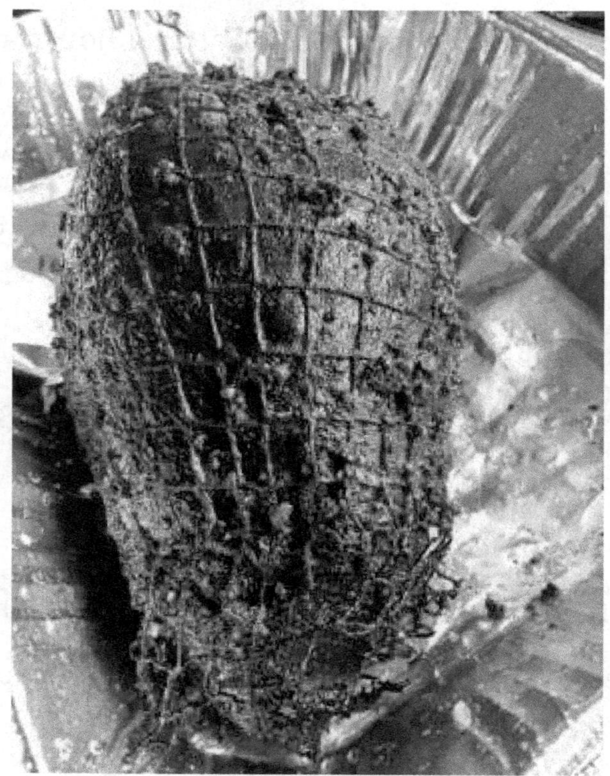

- Course: Lunch
- Cuisine: American
- Total Time: 3 hours 20 minutes

- Preparation Time: 5 minutes
- Cooking Time: 3 hours
- Resting Time: 10 minutes
- Serving Size: 3 to 4 servings
- Nutritional Value Per Serving
    - Calories: 380 calories
    - Carbohydrates: 16.5 g
    - Protein: 28.2 g
    - Fats: 20.8 g

Equipment Used:

- Electric Smoker

Ingredients:

1. Turkey breast 1 piece
2. Store-bought BBQ rub 4 tbsp.
3. Olive oil 3 tbsp.
4. Butter 100 g
5. Hot Tabasco sauce 2 tsp
6. Honey 1tsp

Instructions:

- First, preheat the electric Smoker at 250°F for at least 15 minutes.
- Put in the mesquite woodchips in the Smoker.
- Next, prepare the turkey meat. Cover the whole meat with a layer of olive oil. Rub the oil generously.

- Then apply the BBQ rub on the whole meat piece. Rub the mixture generously so that the whole turkey breast is covered with the BBQ rub.
- In a heatproof cup, prepare the basting mixture for the turkey. Add the butter, cut into small cubes to the cup. Put in the honey, hot sauce and ¼ teaspoon BBQ rub.
- Put the turkey and the cup in the electric Smoker and let it remain closed for approximately 45 minutes. Put a probe in the turkey meat at the thickest part of the meat.
- When you open the electric Smoker after 45 minutes, you will see that the basting mixture is prepared and is steaming.
- Pour the basting mixture about 2 tbsp on the meat and let it smoke.
- Repeat the procedure with the basting mixture after every 20 minutes.
- When the internal temperature of meat is near 170◦F, raise the electric Smoker's heat to 270◦F for the last 10 minutes.
- Take out the meat when the internal temperature reaches 170◦F.
- Let the meat rest for 15 minutes and then slice it.
- Serve this mouthwatering and delicious meal to your friends and family.

5.7. Smoked Potatoes

Baked potatoes are an all-time favorite side dish. They go well with all meats, especially chicken. They can be served as it is or with a rich sour cream. This is an easy and useful recipe to smoke potatoes perfectly. This recipe is simple and easy to prepare and goes well with almost anything. You can even make this and have it on its own. It is great comfort food. Try it out and you will not be disappointed.

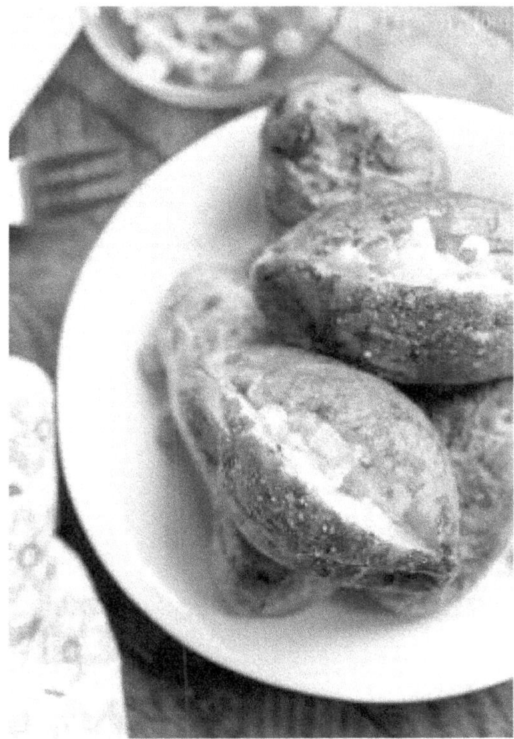

- Course: Side Dish
- Cuisine: American
- Total Time: 2 hours 20 minutes
- Preparation Time: 10 minutes
- Cooking Time: 2 hours
- Rest Time: 10 minutes
- Serving Size: 4 servings
- Nutritional Value Per Serving
    - Calories: 119 calories
    - Carbohydrates: 10 g
    - Protein: 1.8 g
    - Fats: 8.5 g

Equipment Used:

- Electric Smoker

Ingredients:

1. Medium sized potatoes 4 pieces
2. Olive oil ¼ cup
3. Granular Salt ¾ cup

Instructions:

- Preheat the electric Smoker at 275°F. Put in the wood chips of your choice. Preheat for at least 15 minutes.
- Wash the potatoes and dry them on a paper towel.
- Poke each potato with a fork 5 or six times at different places on the potato surface. This will prevent the potato from exploding when it is exposed to a high temperature in the electric Smoker.
- Pour the oil in an open cup and coat each potato with a thin layer of oil.
- Next, pour the salt into a shallow dish. Coat the potatoes with this salt.
- Place the potatoes in the electric Smoker and wait for approximately 2 hours.
- After 2 hours, check the potatoes for doneness. The potatoes should be cooked and soft.
- Take the potatoes out and let them rest for 10 minutes.
- Slit the potatoes from the entrance and fill them with American-style chili if you want to serve as a main dish.
- Another serving idea is to slit the center and fill it with sour cream and top it with sliced green onions. This makes a perfect side dish.

5.8. Smoked Burgers

Burgers are a staple food in American cuisine. These smoked beef burgers have a smoky flavor and are perfect for a quiet weekend lunch with the family. The burgers do not have a sauce but are still delicious and mouthwatering. The best part about this recipe is that it is easy to make, and it takes less time for preparation and cooking. Try this recipe and enjoy it with friends and family.

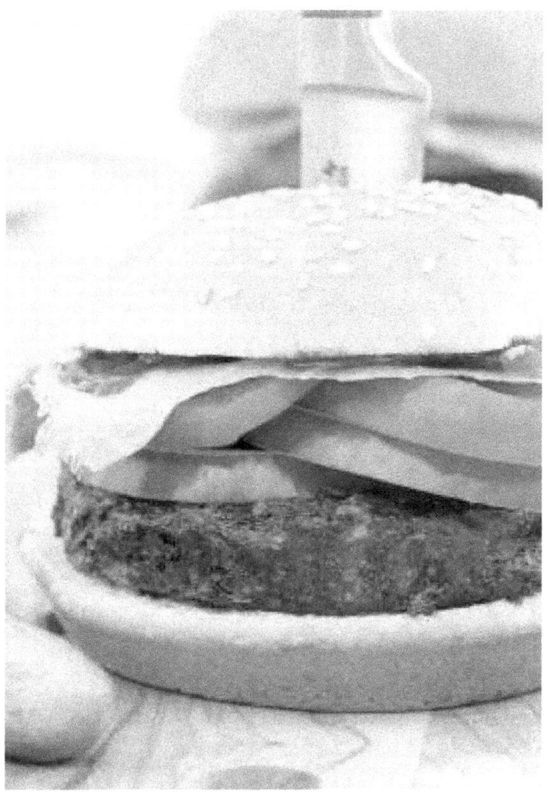

- Course: Lunch
- Cuisine: American
- Total Time: 1 hour 20 minutes
- Preparation Time: 10 minutes
- Cooking Time: 1 hour

- Rest Time: 10 minutes
- Serving Size: 6 servings
- Nutritional Value Per Serving
    - Calories: 160 calories
    - Carbohydrates: 1 g
    - Protein: 11 g
    - Fats: 11 g

Equipment Used:

- Electric Smoker

Ingredients:

1. Pre-prepared beef burger patties 6 pieces
2. Salt 2 tbsp
3. Garlic Powder ½ tbsp
4. Pepper 1 tbsp
5. Dehydrated onion ½ tbsp

Instructions:

- Make sure that the burger patties are at room temperature.
- In a mixing bowl, add the salt, pepper, garlic powder, and dehydrated onion. Mix these ingredients well such that a rub is formed.
- Apply this rub on the burger patties. Cover both sides of the burger patty with the rub.
- Preheat the electric Smoker at 275◦F for 15 minutes. Add the woodchips to the electric Smoker.

- Next, place the burger patties in the Electric Smoker.
- If you want your burger to be medium-well done, smoke for 45 minutes and if you want it to be well done, smoke for 60 minutes. This depends entirely on your preference.
- Once the patties are cooked, take them out of the Smoker and let them rest for 10 minutes.
- Next, prepare the buns and put them in the burger patties. These can be served as it is or some raw vegetables and sauce can be added.

5.9. Smoked Chicken Drumsticks

This is a recipe for mouthwatering and flavorful drumsticks. The flavors are sweet and spicy. This recipe is prepared in 2 ½ hours, and you can enjoy these tasty drumsticks with BBQ sauce. Do try this recipe; this is a hit among kids and adults alike.

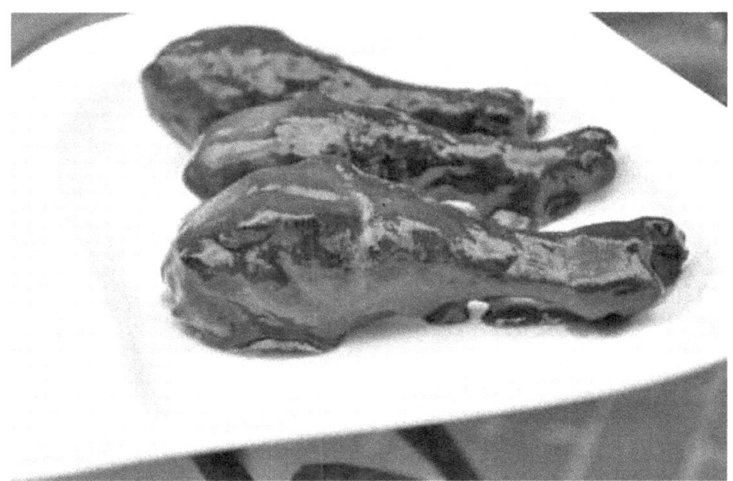

- Course: Dinner
- Cuisine: American
- Total Time: 3 hours

- Preparation Time: 15 minutes
- Cooking Time: 2 hours 30 minutes
- Serving Size: 6 persons
- Nutritional Value Per Serving
    - Calories: 180 calories
    - Carbohydrates: 8 g
    - Protein: 17 g
    - Fats: 8 g

Equipment Used:

- Electric Smoker

Ingredients:

1. Chicken Drumsticks 1.5 kg.
2. Store-bought Steak Rub ½ cup.
3. Cayenne Pepper 1 tsp
4. BBQ sauce ½ cup
5. Tabasco sauce 5 tbsp

Instructions:

- Wash and pat dry the drumsticks.
- Do not remove the skins from the chicken drumsticks.
- Rub the drumsticks with the store-bought steak rub and the cayenne pepper. Keep the drumsticks in the refrigerator for 2 hours.
- After a while, prepare the Electric Smoker.
- Put in the apple woodchips for a mild smoky flavor.

- Fill in the water tray with cold water.
- Turn on the electric Smoker at 250◦F to preheat.
- In the meanwhile, arrange the drumsticks in a stainless-steel wings rack.
- Put in the drumsticks in the Smoker and leave for 2 hours.
- At the end of 2 hours, check the internal temperature of drumsticks. The drumsticks are ready when the thermometer shows 160◦F as the internal temperature of the meat.
- Take out the drumsticks and let them rest for 5 minutes.
- Meanwhile, mix the BBQ sauce and tabasco sauce in a bowl.
- Dip all the drumsticks in the sauce one by one and arrange them on a platter.
- Serve hot.

5.10. Smoked Mac and Cheese

Mac and cheese as comfortable as comfort foods get. It serves as a great side dish with your barbeque. It is conventionally made in an oven, but you can also use a smoker to prepare this dish to give an extra smoky richness.

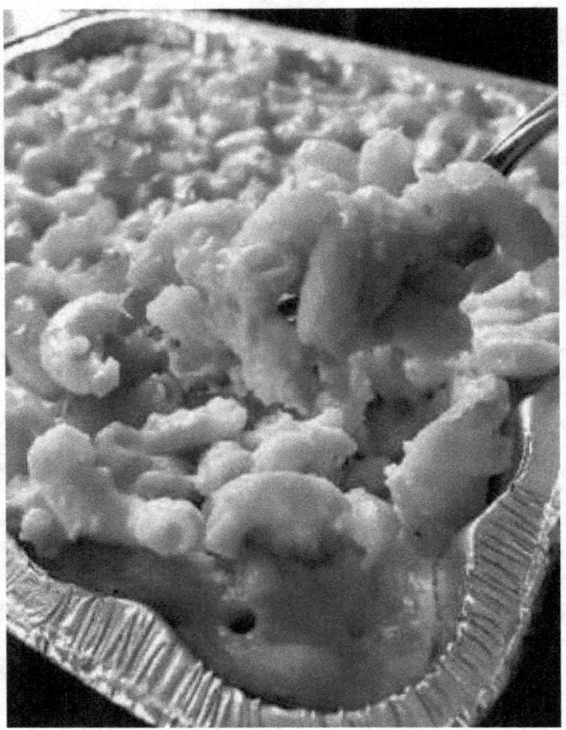

- Course: Side Dish
- Cuisine: American
- Total Time:2 hours 30 minutes
- Preparation Time: 30 minutes
- Cooking Time: 2 hours
- Serving Size: 4 servings
- Nutritional Value Per Serving
    - Calories: 380 calories
    - Carbohydrates: 50 g
    - Protein: 8 g
    - Fats: 4 g

Equipment Used:

Electric Smoker

Ingredients:

1. Elbow Macaroni 1 packet, about ½ kg
2. Milk 3 cups
3. Flour ¼ cup
4. Cheese of your choice (grated) 500 g.
5. Cream cheese 250 g
6. Butter ¼ cup
7. Salt to taste
8. Pepper to taste

Instructions:

- First, boil 12 cups of water in a medium cooking pot. When the water comes to a boil, add the elbow macaroni, and let it boil for 8 to 10 minutes. When the macaroni is boiled, remove all the water, and put the macaroni aside.
- Next, you will prepare the cheese sauce.
- In a medium-sized pan, put in the butter in melt it over the flame. After the butter is melted, add the flour, and mix it. Cook for about two minutes till the flour starts to brown.
- Next, add the milk and cook for five minutes with constant stirring or whisking to not form lumps. Let the milk thicken. When the milk starts to thicken, take the saucepan off the flame, and add cream cheese.
- Mix the cream cheese and make a smooth mixture.
- In a heat-resistant bowl, add the cheese. Pour this mixture over the cheese and mix well.

- At this point, prepare the electric Smoker and put it to preheat at 225◦F.
- Now take an aluminum tray and spread the cooked macaroni in its base.
- Pour the cream and cheese mixture over the macaroni such that it is fully immersed in the mixture.
- Put the aluminum tray in the Smoker for two hours.
- Take out the dish after two hours. The upper layer will come out crusty with cheesy and gooey richness beneath.
- Enjoy your mac and cheese separately or with barbequed chicken or meat.

5.11. BBQ Smoked Ribs

If you are someone who enjoys the ribs on the bone, this recipe is just for you. You will enjoy the rich smokiness of the ribs flavored with mild herbs served with BBQ sauce. Preparing BBQ ribs might be a bit tricky if you go the conventional way, but the ribs prepared in the electric Smoker save you all the hassle, giving you the same flavor.

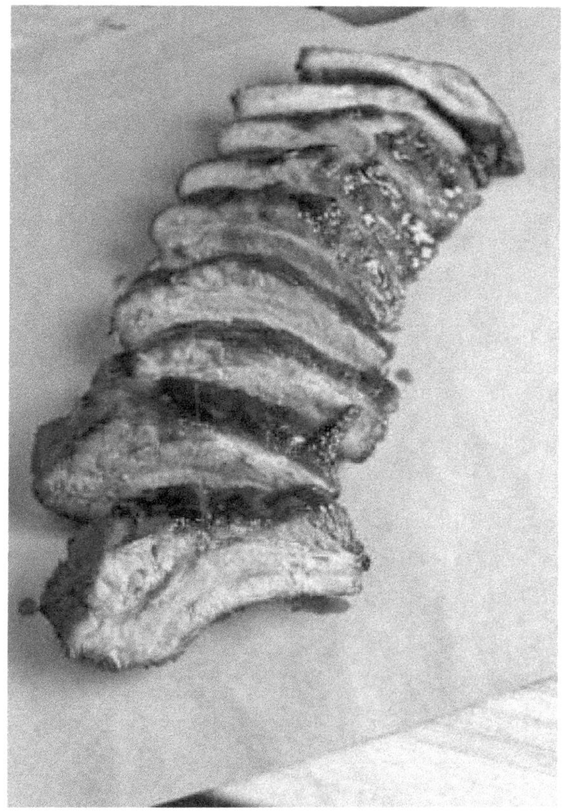

- Course: Dinner
- Cuisine: American
- Total Time: 4 hours 30 minutes
- Preparation Time: 30 minutes
- Cooking Time: 4 hours
- Rest Time: 15 minutes
- Serving Size: 4 servings
- Nutritional Value Per Serving
    - Calories: 302 calories
    - Carbohydrates:0 g
    - Protein: 22 g

- Fats: 23 g

Equipment Used:

- Electric Smoker

Ingredients:

1. One cut of ribs 1.5 kg
2. Black pepper 1 tsp
3. Paprika 1 tsp
4. Garlic Powder 2 tsp
5. Brown Sugar ¼ cup
6. Salt 1 tsp
7. BBQ sauce ¼ cup

Instructions:

- Prepare the ribs. Trim the extra fat and cut the ribs to easily fit on the Electric Smoker grills.
- Next, prepare the rub for the ribs. In a bowl, mix the pepper, paprika, salt, garlic powder, brown sugar, and salt.
- Rub this mixture on the ribs generously such that all parts of the ribs are rubbed with the herbs.
- Put the ribs in a large zip lock bag and put them in the refrigerator overnight.
- The next day, prepare the electric Smoker with applewood chips. Fill the water tray and turn on the Smoker at 225◦F.
- Let the Smoker preheat for 20 minutes.

- Bring out the ribs and arrange them in the smoker racks.
- Place them in the Smoker and let them smoke for 2 hours.
- After 2 hours, take them out,wrap them in aluminum foil, and put them back in the Electric Smoker.
- Let them smoke for a further two hours.
- Take the ribs out and let them rest for 15 minutes.
- After that, unwrap the ribs and serve.

5.12. Smoked Beef Jerky

Commercially prepared beef jerky is commonly available in the market. But there is nothing as flavorful and delicious as homemade beef jerky. In this recipe, we will learn how to prepare beef jerky from scratch.

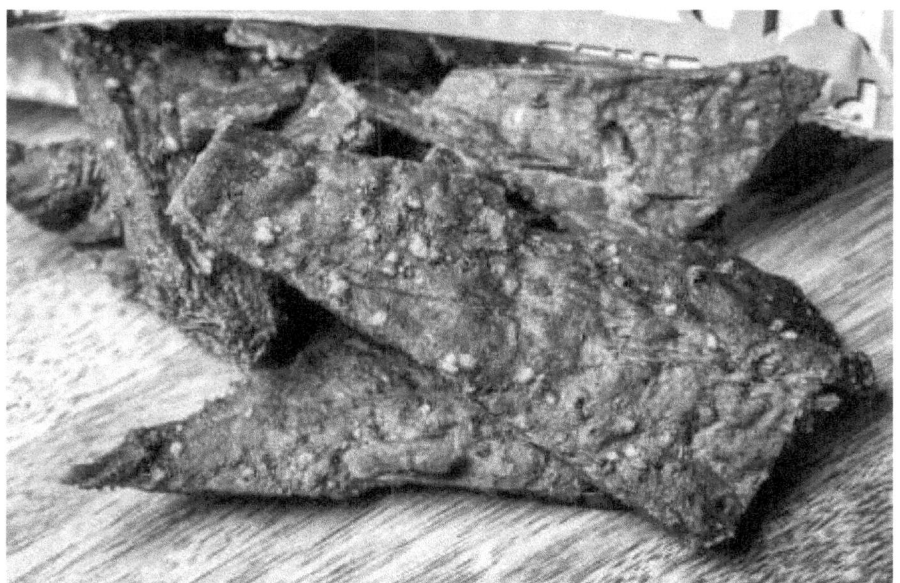

- Course: Snack
- Cuisine: American
- Total Time:5 hours

- Preparation Time: 30 minutes
- Cooking Time: 3 hours
- Resting Time: 1 hour
- Serving Size: 5 servings
- Nutritional Value Per Serving
    - Calories: 240 calories
    - Carbohydrates:1 g
    - Protein: 50 g
    - Fats: 4 g

Equipment Used:

- Electric Smoker

Ingredients:

1. Round beef steak 1.5 kg
2. Honey ¼ cup
3. Soy sauce ¼ cup
4. Worcestershire sauce ¼ cup
5. Brown sugar ¼ cup
6. Garlic Powder 2 tsp
7. Red pepper flakes 1 tbsp
8. Salt 1 tsp
9. Onion Powder 2 tsp

Instructions:

- First, prepare the beef by trimming the extra fat and skin from the meat.

- Next, cut the meat into ¼ inch slices. Make sure that the slices are evenly cut.
- Set the meat aside.
- In a medium-size saucepan, add the honey, soy sauce, Worcestershire sauce, pepper, salt, garlic powder, onion powder, and sugar. Simmer it over the flame until a uniform mixture is formed.
- Let the mixture reach room temperature. Apply the mixture generously on the beef slices and put them in a zip lock bag.
- Pour the remaining sauce into the zip lock bag. Let it in the refrigerator overnight.
- The next day, prepare the electric Smoker with wood chips and water. Turn on the heat at 175◦ F and preheat for 10 minutes.
- Meanwhile, take out the beef slices and set them on a tray and let them reach room temperature.
- After that, arrange them in an aluminum tray and put them in the Smoker.
- Let the beef smoke for 3 hours.
- Take it out after three hours and rest for about 2 to 3 hours until it becomes dry.
- You can consume it as a snack and store it in an airtight container for up to 2 weeks.

5.13. Striped Bass Recipe

This is a delicious recipe having a mouthwatering flavor. Smoking the fish gives a much better flavor than just grilling. The smokiness makes this dish worth enjoying on a warm summer day. You can have it with a rich tartar sauce, or a little lime juice drizzled on it. If you try this recipe, you are in for a treat.

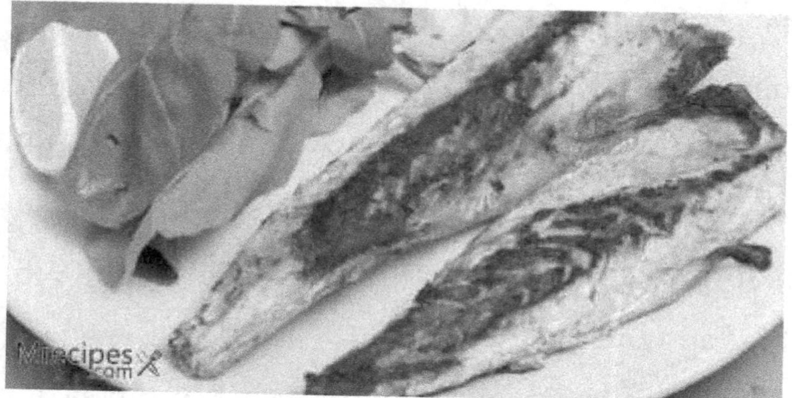

- Course: Lunch
- Cuisine: American
- Total Time: 3 hours
- Preparation Time: 45 minutes
- Cooking Time: 2 hours
- Serving Size: 6 servings
- Nutritional Value Per Serving
    - Calories:154 calories
    - Carbohydrates: o g
    - Protein: 4 g
    - Fats: 28 g

Equipment Used:

- Electric Smoker

Ingredients:

1. Striped Bass Fillets 1 kg

2. Brown Sugar ¼ cup
3. Water 4 cups
4. Salt ¼ cup
5. Bay leaves 2 leaves.
6. Black pepper 2 tsp
7. Lemon 5 to 6 slices
8. Dry wine ½ cup for brine ½ cup for Smoker
9. Olive oil 3 tsp

Instructions:

- Clean and wash the fish fillets.
- Heat the four cups of water and dissolve salt and sugar in them. Let it come to room temperature.
- When it is at room temperature add, bay leaves, pepper, wine, and lemon slices.
- Put in the fish fillets inside this brine such that they are completely soaked.
- Cover them and leave them overnight.
- The next day prepares the Electric Smoker. Put the alder woodchips in the tray. Fill the water tray half with water and half with white wine.
- Turn on the burner at 180◦F.
- Bring out the fish fillets and take them out of the brine and wash them with cold water. Ste them on the counter on a tray lined with paper towels. Let them dry and come to room temperature.
- Meanwhile, coat the smoker grills with olive oil.

- When the fish fillets have reached room temperature, set them on the grills and smoke for two hours.
- The doneness is checked by inserting a thermometer; the internal temperature should be 145∘F.
- Please take out the fish and let it rest for 10 minutes before serving.

5.14. Smoked Cajun Shrimp

Shrimps are a crowd favorite seafood. They are easy to make, and preparation also takes a few minutes. Either you are using fresh shrimps or frozen ones, this recipe works best for both. The only thing is that for frozen shrimps, you will have to defrost them first. This recipe is easy and simple to follow and seldom goes wrong. You will thank us when you have tried this one.

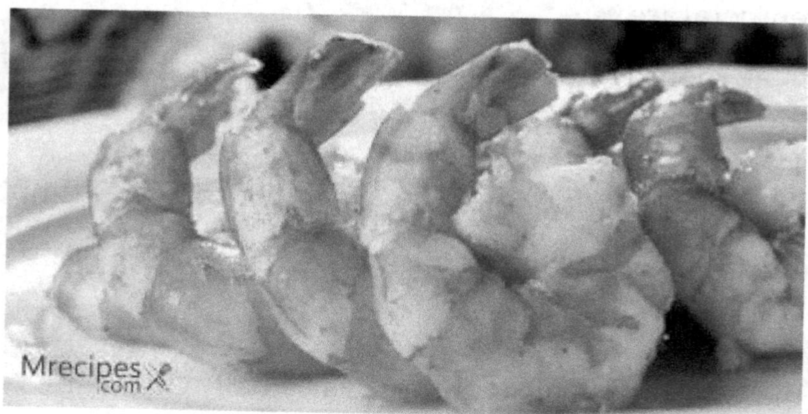

- Course: Appetizer
- Cuisine: American
- Total Time: 1 hour
- Preparation Time: 20 minutes
- Cooking Time: 30 minutes
- Serving Size: 6 servings

- Nutritional Value Per Serving
    - Calories: 92 calories
    - Carbohydrates: 2.2.g
    - Protein: 4.6 g
    - Fats:7.6 g

Equipment Used:

- Electric Smoker

Ingredients:

1. Jumbo Shrimps 1 kg
2. Salt ¼ cup
3. Dried thyme 2 tbsp
4. Paprika 3 tbsp
5. Cayenne Pepper 2 tsp
6. Onion Powder 2 tbsp
7. Black Pepper 3 tbsp
8. Garlic Powder 2 tbsp
9. Olive Oil 3 tbsp
10. Lemon Juice ¼ cup
11. Fresh Parsley 1 bunch chopped.

Instructions:

- Prepare the shrimps. Take out the shells and devein them. Wash and pat them dry.
- In a bowl prepare the dry rum. Add salt, sugar, cayenne pepper, paprika, garlic powder, thyme, and onion powder. Mix this carefully.

- Next, prepare an aluminum tray by greasing it with olive oil.
- Place the shrimps on the tray in a single layer.
- Apply the dry rum to the shrimps generously.
- Start the electric Smoker at 225◦F. Put in the wood chips and water.
- Let it preheat for 20 minutes.
- Meanwhile, pour lemon juice over the shrimps.
- Put the shrimps in the oven for thirty minutes, moving them after every ten minutes.
- Please take out the shrimps after 30 minutes or as soon as they start turning pink.
- This dish can be served warmed or even at room temperature.

5.15. Smoked Scallops

Scallops are juicy and delicious, either grilled or cooked. In this recipe, we have smoked the scallops to give them a rich smokiness. The scallops can be enjoyed with a side of a fresh green salad. This is the ultimate healthy dish to eat for lunch. Do try it out for a different and mouthwatering experience. You will not be disappointed.

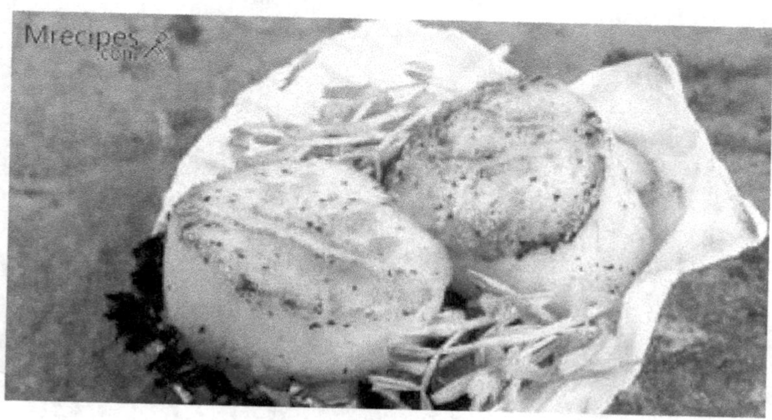

- Course: Appetizer
- Cuisine: American
- Total Time: 50 minutes
- Preparation Time: 5 minutes
- Cooking Time: 30 to 40 minutes
- Serving Size:5 servings
- Nutritional Value Per Serving
    - Calories: 105 calories
    - Carbohydrates: 5 g
    - Protein: 8.7 g
    - Fats: 5.3. g

Equipment used:

- Electric Smoker

Ingredients:

1. Sea Scallops 1 kg
2. Olive oil 3 tbsp
3. Salt 1 tsp
4. Garlic 2 cloves minced.
5. Pepper 1 tsp

Instructions:

- Wash the scallops under cold running water and dry them on a paper towel.
- In a bowl, mix the oil, salt, pepper, and lemon juice.

- Apply the mixture to the scallops.
- Turn on the electric Smoker and prepare it with water and add the wood chips.
- Let it preheat for 10 minutes at 225◦F.
- Meanwhile, lightly grease an aluminum pan and place the scallops on it such that the scallops do not touch each other.
- Put the scallops in the Smoker and smoke for 20 to 30 minutes.
- Check the internal temperature of the scallops.
- Take them out when the temperature reaches 145◦F.
- Let the scallops rest for 10 minutes and then serve with a fresh green salad and a vinaigrette.

Smoked Curried Almonds

Almonds are an extremely healthy source of good fats. One enjoys munching them around. This recipe tries a twist on the good old roasted almonds. Let us make snack time fun with these delicious smoked curried almonds. You can keep them for as long as a month and keep enjoying a fistful every day. Heath and taste go hand in hand with this yummy snack.

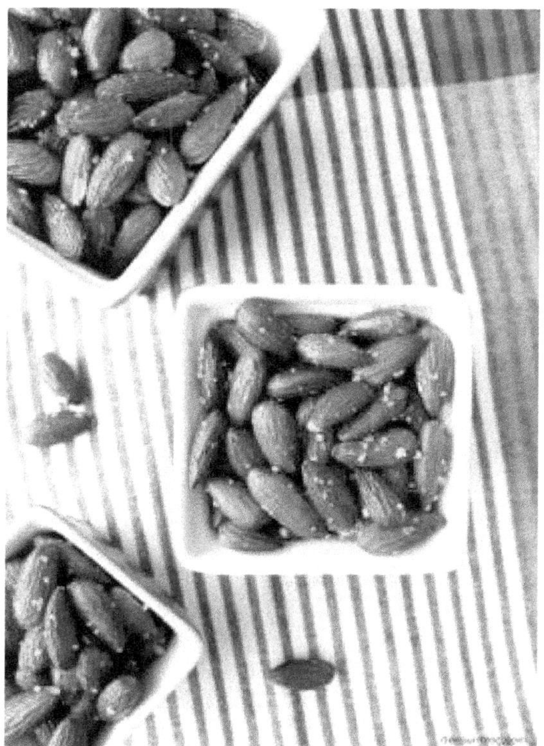

- Course: Snack
- Cuisine: American
- Total Time: 1 hour 5 minutes
- Preparation Time:5 minutes
- Cooking Time: 1 to 2 hours
- Serving Size: 6 servings
- Nutritional Value Per Serving
    - Calories: 170 calories
    - Carbohydrates: 5 g
    - Protein: 6 g
    - Fats: 15 g

Equipment Used:

- Electric Smoker

Ingredients:

1. Raw Almonds with skins ½ kg
2. Butter 2 tbsp
3. Curry powder2 tbsp
4. Raw Sugar 2 tbsp
5. 2 tbsp
6. Salt 1 tsp
7. Cayenne Pepper 1 tsp

Instructions:

- Preheat the electric Smoker at 225°F. Fill the water tray half with water and put in the pecan wood chips.
- In a large bowl, mix the butter, salt, sugar, cayenne pepper and curry powder.
- Toss all the almonds in this mixture.
- Prepare an aluminum tray, spread the almonds in the tray as a layer and put it in the Smoker.
- Leave the almonds for one hour and take them out.
- Delicious, curried almonds are ready.
- Let them rest to reach room temperature and enjoy this rich flavorful snack.
- These can be stored in an airtight container for up to 3 months.

Smoked Apples with Maple Syrup

If you have a sweet tooth and enjoy fruity desserts, this one is just for you. The naturally citrus flavor of apples is balanced perfectly with the sweetness of maple syrup and raisins. Do try out this recipe; you will not regret it.

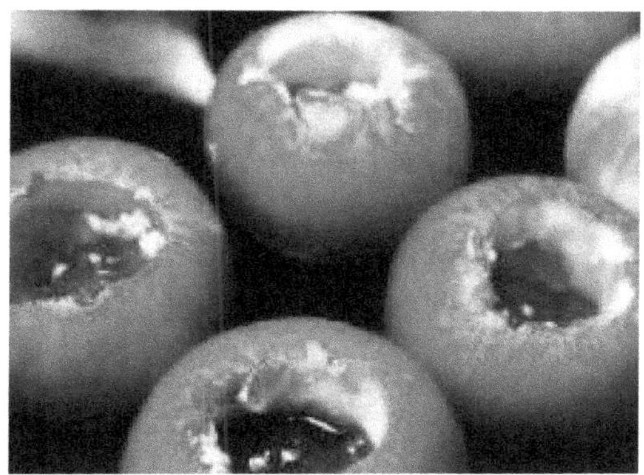

- Course: Dessert
- Cuisine: American
- Total Time: 2 hours
- Preparation Time: 30 minutes
- Cooking Time: 1 hour 30 minutes
- Serving Size: 6 servings
- Nutritional Value Per Serving
    - Calories: 224 calories
    - Carbohydrates: 47 g
    - Protein: 1 g
    - Fats: 5 g

Equipment Used:

- Electric Smoker

Ingredients:

1. Apples 6 pieces
2. Maple Syrup ½ cup
3. Raisins ½ cup
4. Cold Butter ¼ cup cut in small cubes.

Instructions:

- Prepare the electric Smoker with water and pecan woodchips. Turn it on at 250◦F.
- Take the apples, wash them, and pat dry. Core the apples such that their outer shape is maintained, and a small cavity is formed inside. The apple should still be able to stand without support.
- Fill the lower part of each apple with a small number of raisins, followed by some butter and then the maple syrup.
- Grease an aluminum tray and arrange the apples in the tray.
- Put the apples in the electric Smoker and let them smoke for 1 hour 30 minutes.
- Take them out and let them rest for 10 minutes.
- Serve warm with vanilla ice cream.

Smoked Bean Sprouts

Bean sprouts are a great option for a side dish. They can be served with barbecued chicken and are a great source of vitamins and fiber. These are an excellent option for a side dish because they are easy to make and are prepared quickly.

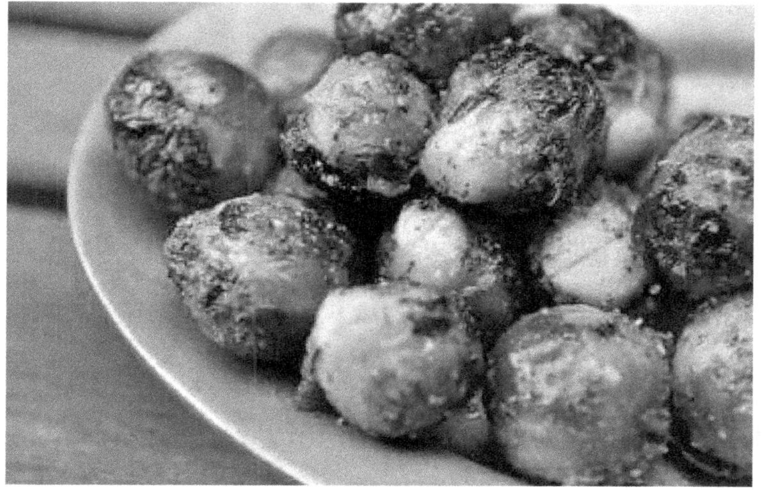

- Course: Side Dish
- Cuisine: American
- Total Time: 1 hour 30 minutes
- Preparation Time: 15 minutes
- Cooking Time: 1 hour
- Serving Size: 6 servings
- Nutritional Value Per Serving
    - Calories: 45 calories
    - Carbohydrates:8 g
    - Protein: 3 g
    - Fats: 0 g

Equipment Used:

- Electric Smoker

Ingredients:

1. Brussel Sprouts ½ kg
2. Olive Oil 3 tsp

3. Salt 1tsp
4. Pepper ½ tsp

Instructions:

- Wash the Brussel sprouts with cold water and dry them out in a colander.
- Remove the base of the Brussel sprouts and the dried-out parts.
- In a bowl, mix the olive oil, salt, and pepper.
- Apply the mixture to the sprouts and put them in a single layer in an aluminum tray.
- Turn on the electric Smoker at 225◦F. Prepare with water and wood chips.
- Let the Smoker preheat for 10 to 15 minutes and then put in the sprouts.
- Let them smoke for 60 minutes.
- Take them out and serve as a side dish with barbeque chicken.

Smoked Cauliflower

Cauliflower is super healthy food. It is a rich source of vitamin C and dietary fiber. It contains eighty percent of the recommended amount of Vitamin C required for a day. It fills up your stomach and is slowly digested, thus keeping the stomach filled for a long while.

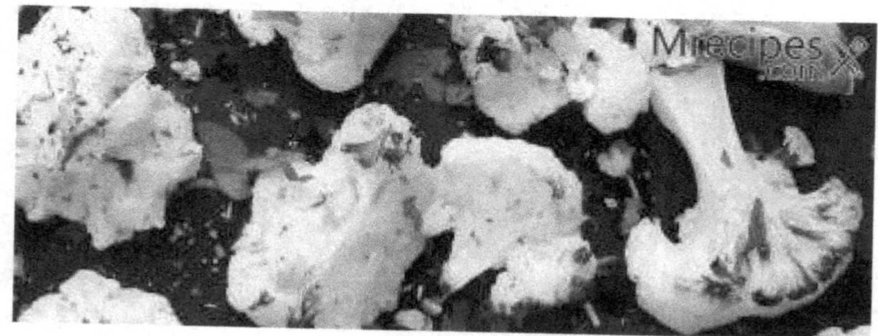

- Course: Side Dish

- Cuisine: American
- Total Time: 2 hours
- Preparation Time: 5 minutes
- Cooking Time: 2 hours
- Serving Size: 6 servings
- Nutritional Value Per Serving
    - Calories: 129 calories
    - Carbohydrates: 8 g
    - Protein: 3 g
    - Fats: 11 g

Equipment Used:

- Electric Smoker

Ingredients:

1. Cauliflower head 1 big
2. Salt 1 tsp
3. Olive Oil 3 tsp
4. Pepper 1 tsp
5. Balsamic Vinegar 3 tbsp

Instructions:

- Preheat the electric Smoker at 225°F. Fill the water tray and the woodchip tray accordingly.
- Cut the cauliflower head into small florets and wash them with cold water.

- In a bowl, mix the olive oil, balsamic vinegar, salt, and pepper.
- Toss the cauliflower florets in the bowl.
- In an aluminum tray, layer the cauliflower florets and put them in the Smoker.
- Smoke for 2 hours, turning the florets once midway.
- Take out after two hours and serve as a side dish.

5.20. Smoked Cherry Tomatoes

Smoked cherry tomatoes are not a dish in themselves but can form a base for other dishes like salads and pasta. This recipe is included here because smoked cherry tomatoes add flavor and richness to the foods they are mixed with. To add a rich smoky flavor to pasta, you can add cherry tomatoes. Adding smoked cherry tomatoes to a salad hive is the required kick to the otherwise boring salad. Smoked cherry tomatoes are uses as a side dish in Middle Eastern food commonly.

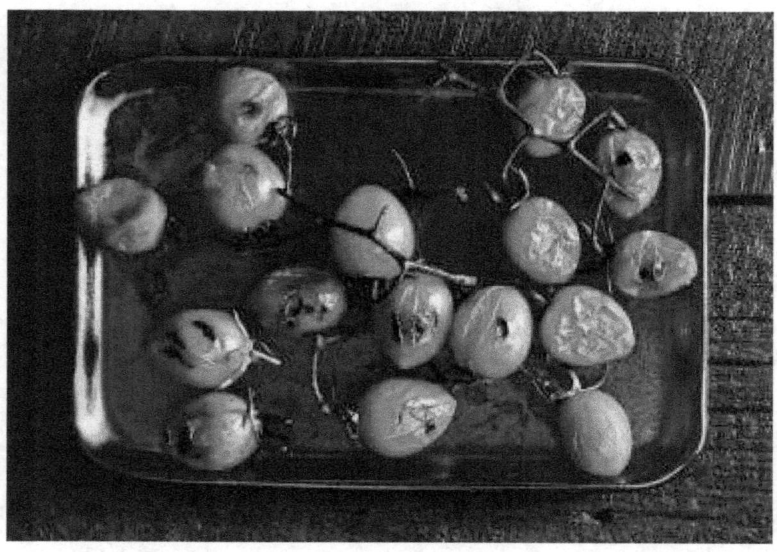

- Course: Side Dish
- Cuisine: American

- Total Time:1 hour 5 minutes
- Preparation Time: 5 minutes
- Cooking Time: 1 hour
- Serving Size: 4 servings
- Nutritional Value Per Serving
    - Calories:25 calories
    - Carbohydrates: 3.6 g
    - Protein: 1.1 g
    - Fats: 0.5 g

Equipment Used:

- Electric Smoker

Ingredients:

1. Cherry Tomatoes 300g

Instructions:

- Preheat the electric Smoker to 225◦F. Fill half of the water tray of the Smoker and fill in the wood chips.
- Wash the cherry tomatoes with cold water and spread them on a paper towel.
- Arrange the cherry tomatoes in the aluminum tray and put them in the Smoker.
- Leave the tomatoes for 60 minutes and then take them out.
- You will observe that the cherry tomatoes have burst open, and the juices are oozing out.

- Do not waste the juices; these juices also give off a smokey and delicious taste to salads and pasta.

5.21. Sweet and Spicy Chicken Wings

Chicken wings are another crowd favorite. This recipe used a lot of spices and cut the overpowering spicy flavor; sugar is used. The sugar gives a sweet taste and a crispy finish with its caramelization. This is a perfect dish if you are planning to host a barbecue party.

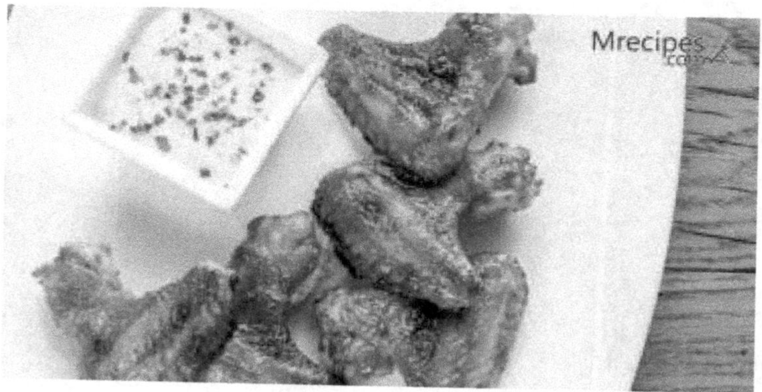

- Course: Lunch
- Cuisine: American
- Total Time: 1 hour 50 minutes
- Preparation Time:20 minutes
- Cooking Time: 1 hour 30 minutes
- Serving Size: 4 servings
- Nutritional Value Per Serving
    - Calories: 356 calories
    - Carbohydrates: 23.9 g
    - Protein: 15.6 g

- Fats:22.7 g

Equipment Used:

- Electric Smoker

Ingredients:

1. Chicken wings 2.5 kg
2. Salt 2 tsp
3. Pepper 1 tsp
4. Onion Powder 1 tsp
5. Garlic Powder 1tsp
6. Paprika¼ cup
7. Cayenne Pepper 1 tsp
8. Brown Sugar ½ cup

Instructions:

- Wash the chicken wings with cold water and trim them.
- If you wish, you can break the wings in half or keep them full. Depends on your preference.
- Next, mix the paprika, salt, pepper, onion powder, garlic powder, sugar, and cayenne pepper in a big mixing bowl.
- Toss the chicken wings into this spice rub. Use your hands to coat the chicken wings with the spice rub.
- Turn on the electric Smoker at 250°F. Put water in the water tray and fill the wood chip tray with wood chips.
- Let the Smoker preheat for 15 minutes.

- Meanwhile, take out the grill from the Smoker and arrange the wings on the grill.
- Put in the wings in the Smoker and smoke for 2 hours. Check the internal temperature of the chicken should be 165◦F.
- Take out the chicken wings and serve them hot.

5.22. Herbal Chicken Wings

This is a delicious recipe of chicken wings that has a strong flavor of herbs and spices. This recipe is inspired by French cuisine. Make this recipe to enjoy the Parisian feel in the comfort of your own house.

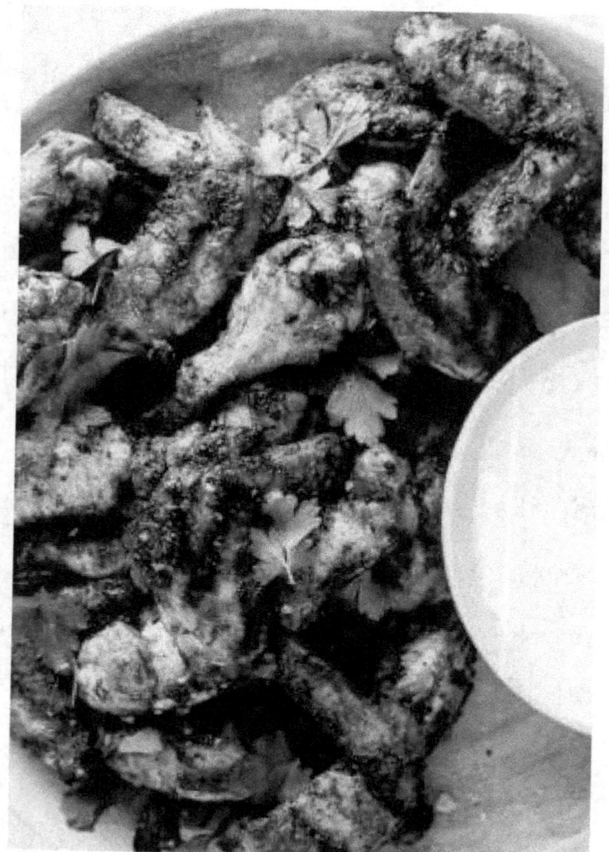

- Course: Lunch

- Cuisine: American
- Total Time:3 hours 20 minutes
- Preparation Time: 10 minutes
- Cooking Time:
- Serving Size: 4 servings
- Nutritional Value Per Serving
    - Calories: 220 calories
    - Carbohydrates:0 g
    - Protein: 18 g
    - Fats: 16 g

Equipment Used:

- Electric Smoker

Ingredients:

1. Chicken Wings 2.5 kg
2. Olive oil ½ cup
3. Garlic 2 cloves minced.
4. Rosemary Leaves 2 tbsp
5. Fresh basil leaves 2 tbsp.
6. Lemon Juice 2 tbsp
7. Salt 1 ½ tsp
8. Pepper 1tsp
9. Oregano 2 tbsp

Instructions:

- Prepare the chicken wings by trimming them. Wash the wings under cold running water.
- It is your choice to break the wings into half or use them as it is.
- In a large mixing bowl,add all ingredients and herbs and make a smooth mixture.
- Save half and toss the chicken wings in the other half.
- Use your hands to toss the wings in the mixture so that it is evenly applied.
- Preheat the electric Smoker at 250◦F and prepare it with water and wood chips.
- Arrange the wings on the smoker racks and smoke them for two hours.
- The doneness is determined by achieving a 165◦F temperature internally.
- Take out the wings and serve them hot.

5.23. Smoked Redfish

In this fish, we are using a dry brine technique. This is an easy and quick recipe;however, it requires the fish to marinate overnight. If you are planning to call guests over, you can prepare the fish fillets in advance.

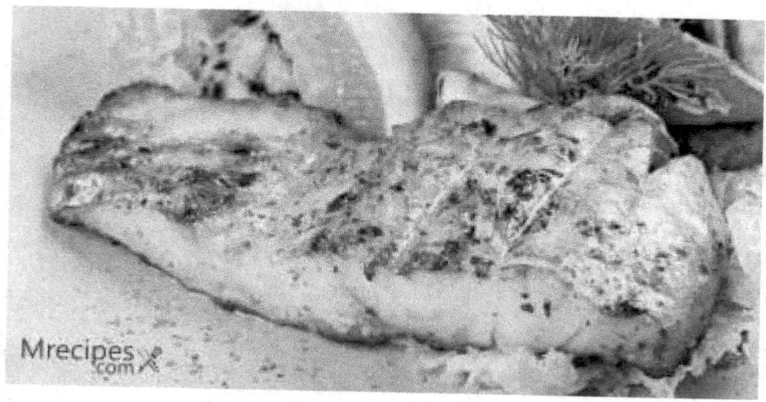

- Course: Lunch

- Cuisine: American
- Total Time: 2 hours 10 minutes
- Preparation Time: 10 minutes
- Cooking Time: 2 hours
- Serving Size: 6 servings
- Nutritional Value Per Serving
    - Calories: 160 calories
    - Carbohydrates: 2 g
    - Protein: 18 g
    - Fats: 4 g

Equipment Used:

- Electric Smoker

Ingredients:

1. 2 redfish fillets with skin 600g
2. Salt half cup
3. Black pepper 1tsp
4. Lemon Zest 1 tsp
5. Garlic powder 1tsp
6. Lemon 2or 4 slices

Instructions:

- Wash the fish fillets with cold running water.
- Next, prepare a rub by mixing all the ingredients and spices.

- Apply the rub on the fish fillets generously. Wrap the fish fillets in cling film and refrigerate them overnight.
- The next day take out the fish fillets and bring them to room temperature.
- Prepare the electric Smoker with wood chips and water. Turn it on at 170◦F.
- When the fillets are at room temperature, wash them and pat them dry.
- Put them in the Smoker for two hours.
- After two hours, check the internal temperature. It should be 140◦F.
- Let the fillets rest for 30 minutes before serving.

5.24. Smoked Dory

This fish is easy to cook and quickly prepared. We will use the dry rub method to prepare the dory fish fillets. This turns out to be a delicious recipe and is a crowd favorite.

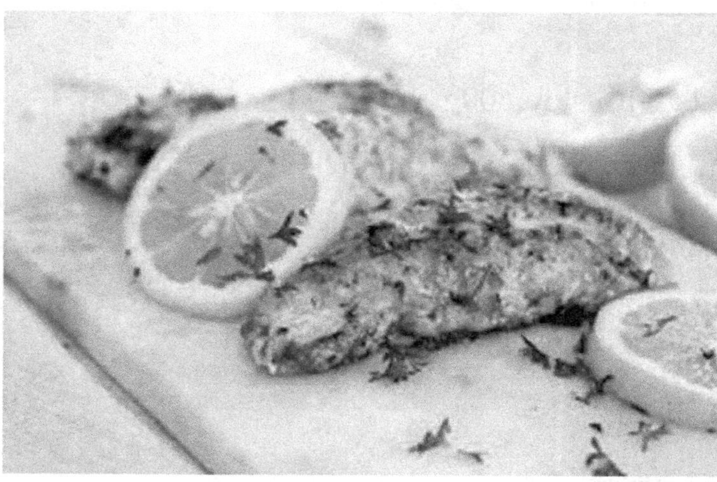

- Course: Dinner
- Cuisine: American
- Total Time: 1 hour 15 minutes
- Preparation Time: 15 minutes

- Cooking Time: 1 hour
- Serving Size: 4 servings
- Nutritional Value Per Serving
    - Calories: 175 calories
    - Carbohydrates: 2 g
    - Protein: 22 g
    - Fats: 8 g

Equipment Used:

- Electric Smoker

Ingredients:

1. 4 fillets of dory fish800g
2. Onion Powder
3. Salt half cup
4. Black pepper 2tsp
5. Ginger powder 1 tsp
6. Garlic powder 1tsp
7. Coriander for garnish
8. Lemon slices for garnish

Instructions:

- Wash the fish fillets with cold running water.
- Next, prepare a rub by mixing all the ingredients and spices.
- Apply the rub on the fish fillets generously. Wrap the fish fillets in cling film and refrigerate them overnight.

- The next day take out the fish fillets and bring them to room temperature.
- Prepare the electric Smoker with wood chips and water. Turn it on at 220◦F.
- When the fillets are at room temperature, wash them and pat them dry.
- Could you put them in the Smoker for two hours?
- After one hour, check the internal temperature. It should be 160◦F.
- Let the fillets rest for 30 minutes before serving.
- Garnish the fish fillets with coriander and lemon slices for serving.

5.25. Herbal Smoked Salmon

Salmon is one fish variety that is consumed very often among people. The reason for this is that it is an excellent source of protein, and it cooks easily. Smoked salmon is something that you can enjoy at family dinners and other gatherings. You can never go wrong with smoked salmon.

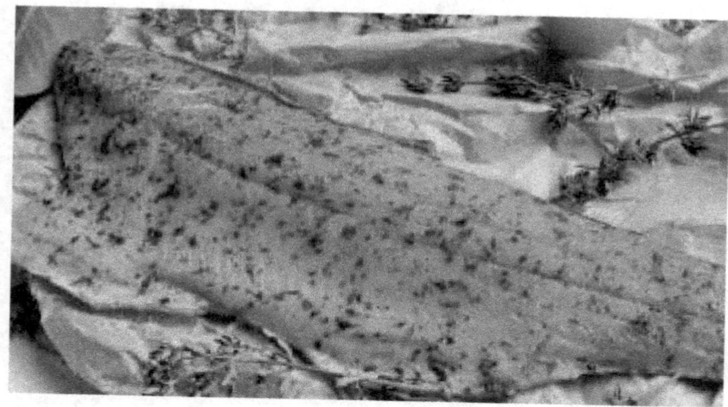

- Course: Dinner
- Cuisine: American
- Total Time: 4 hours 30 minutes
- Preparation Time: 30 minutes
- Cooking Time: 4 hours

- Serving Size: 4 servings
- Nutritional Value Per Serving
    - Calories: 210 calories
    - Carbohydrates: o g
    - Protein: 22.3. g
    - Fats: 12.3 g

Equipment Used:

- Electric Smoker

Ingredients:

1. Salmon fillets 750 g
2. Salt ¼ cup
3. Sugar ¼ cup
4. Water ½ cup
5. Black Pepper 2 tbsp
6. Lemon 2 slices
7. Fresh dill chopped 1 bunch.

Instructions:

- Prepare the marinade for the fish. In a flat dish, pour water, salt, sugar, and pepper. Mix them well.
- Soak the fish fillets in the marinade and cover them with dill and lemon slices.
- Wrap the fillets in cling wrap and refrigerate overnight.

- The next day, prepare the Electric Smoker. Put the wood chips and water in the water tray.
- Turn on the electric Smoker at 180◦F. Put the fish fillets on the grill and smoke for four hours.
- In this recipe, we are smoking the fish at a lower temperature for a longer time. If you have a time constraint, you can use a higher temperature for a shorter period.
- Check the doneness of the fish by inserting the thermometer. The internal temperature must be 130◦F.
- Take out the fish and let it rest for 30 minutes before serving.

5.26. Smoked Stuffed Mushroom

These stuffed mushrooms can be served by themselves and can be served as a side dish as well. Try this recipe, and you will not be disappointed.

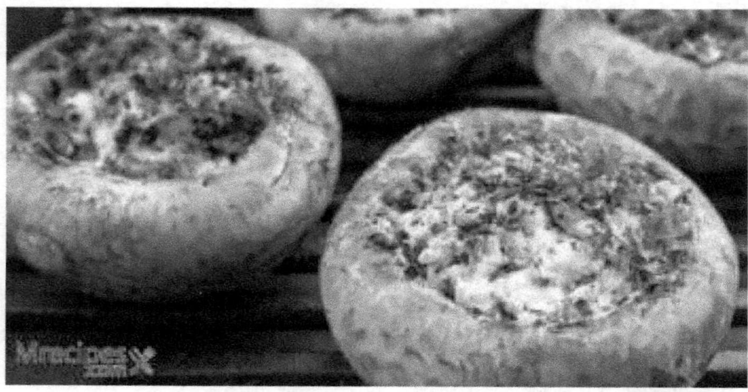

- Course: Side Dish
- Cuisine: American
- Total Time: 1 hour 15 minutes
- Preparation Time:20 minutes
- Cooking Time: 55 minutes

- Serving Size: 6 servings
- Nutritional Value Per Serving
    - Calories:320 calories
    - Carbohydrates: 22 g
    - Protein: 8 g
    - Fats: 7 g

Equipment Used:

- Electric Smoker

Ingredients:

1. Button Mushrooms with stem 24 mushroom
2. Onion 1 minced
3. Garlic 2 cloves minced.
4. Salt ½ tsp
5. Black Pepper 1 tsp
6. Breadcrumbs ¾ cup
7. Parmesan cheese ¾ cup
8. Olive Oil 1/3 cup
9. Parsley ¼ cup

Instructions:

- Preheat the electric Smoker at 250°F. Put the wood chips in the tray and water in the water tray.
- In a saucepan, put in some olive oil and sauté the onion and garlic in it.

- In another mixing bowl, mix the breadcrumbs, cheese and salt and black pepper.
- Cut the stems of the mushrooms and chop them. Add the chopped stems to the saucepan with the onion and garlic and cook for one minute.
- Set an aluminum tray and set the mushroom heads up-side-down in a layer.
- Mix the onion, garlic, and mushrooms into the cheese mixture.
- Put a spoonful of mixture on the mushroom heads.
- Put the mushrooms in the Smoker and smoke for 45 minutes.
- Take out the mushrooms and let them rest for 20 minutes before serving.

5.27. Smoked Chicken Breast

This is asimple recipe and can never go wrong. Easy to make and delicious to taste. You can prepare this overnight and smoke it the next day. Family and friends will enjoy it alike.

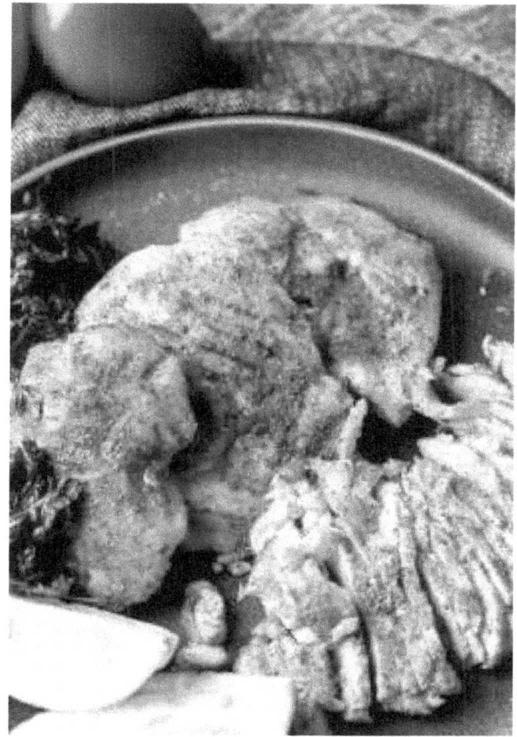

- Course: Dinner
- Cuisine: American
- Total Time: 5 hours
- Preparation Time: 20 minutes
- Cooking Time: 4 hours 30 minutes
- Serving Size: 4 servings
- Nutritional Value Per Serving
    - Calories: 280 calories
    - Carbohydrates: 2 g
    - Protein: 23 g
    - Fats: 4 g

Equipment Used:

- Electric Smoker

Ingredients:

1. 4 chicken breast pieces 1 kg
2. Black pepper 2 tsp
3. Salt 2 tsp
4. Lemon Juice 4 tbsp
5. Paprika 2 tbsp

Instructions:

- Wash the chicken breast pieces. It is your choice to remove the skin or keep it.
- Pat the chicken dry.
- In a flat dish, mix the salt, pepper, paprika and lemon juice.
- Apply the mixture generously on the chicken and wrap the pieces with cling wrap and leave it in the refrigerator overnight.
- The next day, prepare the electric Smoker with the wood chips and water. Preheat the Smoker at 180◦F.
- Bring the chicken fillets at room temperature and wash them under cold running water.
- Pat the chicken dries with paper towels and arrange them on the racks of the Smoker.
- Smoke the chicken for about 4 hours and 30 minutes.
- Check the temperature of the chicken. It will be done when the internal temperature reaches 165◦F.
- Take out the chicken and let it rest for 30 minutes before serving.

- Serve with your choice of side dishes.

Conclusion

This book gives you a detailed overview of the usage and benefits of an Electric Smoker. An electric smoker is a brilliant appliance that has been created following present-day needs. In the busy lifestyle we lead today; no one has the time or energy to sit around a barbeque all day to prepare food. This appliance is a cookery solution keeping up with times. Reading the book will give you clear instructions and illustrations to guide you through understanding the appliance. The recipes shared are precise and straightforward. Tried and tested tips and tricks are shared for your convenience. The beginners and the regular Electric Smoker users will benefit from this book alike.

The recipes mentioned in this book are all tried and tested, and all have amazing results. The quantities mentioned will not disappoint you. Even the first-timeuser of the electric Smoker can create these recipes like a pro. But patience is the key. Most of the recipes take longer than five hours, and the temptation to check on your dishes may ruin the dish. Checking on your dish repeatedly means that you will open the smoker time and again, which will cause the temperature to fluctuate and might cause the recipe to produce unsuccessful results.

Using an electric smoker is a wonderful experience, but sometimes it feels a bit overwhelming. Without guidance, you might feel lost. This book will help you in this situation. Read this book and become a pro at using the electric Smoker.

Air Fryer Cookbook for Summer

Plenty of Succulent Oil Free Recipes to Eat with Style, Save Your Money and Enjoy the Summertime

Mike Byron

Table of Contents

Introduction

Most of the people these days like fried food but are afraid of the excessive use of oil. They do not want to disturb their health but they love dishes like fried chips, chicken wings, fried potatoes, grilled seafood and sandwiches, baked muffins, cakes, etc.

Before Air Fryer

They spent money on a separate oven and a grill and a fryer. But guess what you do not need to spend money in all those. Your three in one fryer is here. Many fryers are uncovered and the popping and exploding of oil results in many burns on your skin and is a mess to clean up after you finish. These things may make you not to cook again but not anymore.

Imagine getting your favorite fried food with fewer fats and more healthy nutrients. Your life will be so much better after getting an Air Fryer.

What is an air fryer?

I'm sure you have come across television ads and infomercials showcasing people using an air fryer, and wondered what it is all about. Well, as the name suggests, an air fryer is a device that makes use of air to cook foods.

It basically works by circulating hot air around the food thereby cooking it effectively. It makes use of a fan that produces and circulates the air around the food.

How Does The Air Fryer Work?

The air fryer is a convenient little device that can be used to cook food at a faster pace. Here is looking at the basic functioning of the air fryer

Must Have Air Fryer Accessories

The air fryer looks like a rice cooker, and comes with 3 distinct parts. The first part is the machine itself, which will work by generating hot air that cooks the food within the fryer. The second is the attachment that will carry the food item. The frying basket is the most commonly used attachment. You will also avail a basic pan and a baking tin. The third component is the container. The container holds on to all unwanted food residue such as oil and spices.

The front of the machine carries the temperature and timer that can be adjusted according to the food to be cooked. The insides of the main machine are made up of 5 distinct parts. The back of the machine comes with the water tank. The top of the machine has 4 parts starting with a heating element at the bottom followed by the heating fan, followed by the cooling fan and then the engine.

The main body of the machine might look a little different depending on the brand but most of them pretty much look the same from the inside.

Chapter 1: Benefits Of Air Frying

There are many reasons to use a fryer.

1. Cook healthier
So, how can frying be healthy? Easy! These units can be used without oil or with a small oil jet.

You can cook fries, onion rings, wings and more while getting really crisp results without extra oil. Compared to using my oven, the fries in the fryer were crisper but not dried out, and their use to cook breaded zucchini was even more impressive!

2. Versatility
Depending on the size of your fryer you can buy many accessories. Cake and pizza pans, kebab skewers and steamer are just some of the accessories I've seen.

3. Space saver
If you have a small kitchen or live in a dorm or shared apartment, you can appreciate this benefit. Most of these units are about the size of a coffee machine. They do not take up too much space on the counter and are generally easy to store or move.

Top Reasons Everyone Should Own An Air Fryer

1. Ease of use
Most fryers are very easy to use. Just choose the temperature and cooking time, add food and shake several times during cooking.

With the baskets you can shake your food easily and quickly and the device does not lose much heat when opened. So do not hesitate to check out if you want! Unlike an oven, you will not slow things down when you do it.

2. Easy cleaning
Part of the cooking that most of us do not appreciate is the cleaning. With an air fryer, you only have one basket and one pan to clean, and you can also use dishwasher. With non-stick coated parts, food does not normally stick to the pan.

It only takes a few minutes to wash after use. It inspires me to cook more often at home, because I'm not afraid to clean!

3. Energy efficiency
These fryers are more efficient than using an oven. I used mine during a heat wave and I love that my kitchen is not hot when I use it. If you're trying to keep your home cool in the summer or worry about your electricity bills, you'll be impressed with the efficiency of these devices.

How To Use An Air Fryer

• Firstly, you are able to set the temperature based on the thing you need and allow it to preheat for just a few minutes before you decide to place the food in.

• Then open it up and put the meals within the air fryer. Close it and allow the food prepare based on the timing you've set. It will not take enough time regardless of what you're cooking.

• You may use a little bit of cooking spray or splash some oil around the food before putting it in. This can help to prevent the meals from getting stuck towards the pan. The oil likewise helps to create food a bit crispier and provides the taste of standard fried food.

• Halfway with the set time or perhaps in between times, provide the air fryer just a little shake so the air inside circulates easily and your meals are completely cooked.

• Other than frying, you can test other cooking methods while using additional parts the air flyers usually include. You should use the grill or baking tray in compliance using the instructions that include the environment fryer.

• Another factor to bear in mind is you shouldn't overcrowd the fryer by putting an excessive amount of food inside it. Put small batches of food within the air fryer to ensure that there's enough room for this all to maneuver and prepare evenly. Overcrowding won't let it move and a few parts is going to be left uncooked. The cooking can also be elevated if you devote an excessive amount of at the same time.

• In the situation of marinated food, allow it to be as dry as you possibly can before placing it within the air fryer. Wet food may cause splattering in addition to an excessive amount of smoke being released in the fryer.

• The separator that will get the environment fryer can be put among layers of food in order to prepare various things concurrently. Just make certain the temperature needed is identical for those products or they will not be cooked evenly.

• Pre-packaged meals may also be made while using air fryer. Lower the suggested oven temperature and hang the environment fryer after your meals are placed within it. Additionally, it cuts down on the normal cooking considerably.

• For baking food, you should use the baking pan provided or purchase one individually. You do not need a stove to bake some muffins any longer and also you have them cooked even faster than in the past.

• Roasting meals are also simpler than using conventional methods. It doesn't take considerable time but you just get individuals healthy and attractive roasted veggies or meats that you simply love. For grilling food, put the grill layer inside as well as your food on the top from it. You don't need to help keep flipping the meals over as with a conventional grill.

This will make things much easier. Give it a shake following a couple of moments for much better air flow. As possible clearly see in the information above, significantly less efforts are needed while the food is cooking. Make use of the simple mechanism and prepare a number of different meals every single day. They get cooked in almost no time and taste great.

Chapter 2: Air Fryer Tips And Tricks

The air fryer makes use of the same technology and causes the amino acids and sugar in the foods to react and develop a brown color.

The mechanism makes the food crispy on the outside, thereby giving it the feeling of a baked or fried food item.

The air fryer is capable of raising the air temperature to up to 200 degree Celsius, which means it permeates through the food to cook it thoroughly.

Here are the different things you can do with an air fryer.

Frying
Now you don't have to worry about deep-frying foods, as it is quite easy to use an air fryer to get the desired results. In fact, you don't need any oil at all to fry the foods, as the fryer makes use of hot air to crisp up foods. All you have to do is add in a little oil to the ingredient mix, which the air fryer will use to both cook and crisp the food. You can, however, brush a little oil on top to make it a little crunchier if you like.

Grilling
It is extremely easy to grill in an air fryer and you only have to expend a little effort towards it. You don't have to worry about constantly flipping the food, as all you have to do is add the food and wait. Once you reach the half way mark, you can give the fryer a gentle shake in order to readjust the food within it. You will have to use the grill attachment, as that will make it easy for you to move the food by using the handle attached to it. The shaking also helps with absorbing or draining the excess oil, thereby making the food healthier.

Baking
Baking is made extremely easy with the air fryer. You don't have to worry about not having a conventional oven, as the air fryer will work well for all your baking needs. It works on pretty much the same rules as an oven and you have to preheat it before baking.

Roasting
This is the most used function of the air fryer. It will be extremely easy for you to roast your foods as the air fryer works very fast. All you have to do is prepare the

vegetables or meats by cutting them into small pieces and then add them to the roasting attachment. You don't have to worry about turning or moving them around, as the air fryer will do all the work for you. The air fryer takes 20% lesser time to roast your vegetables and meats, which makes it great for bachelors, and those in a hurry to cook their food.

Air Fryer Cleaning & Maintenance

It is important for you to clean the air fryer from time to time to ensure that it serves you for as long as possible. Here are the simple steps that you can adopt to clean and maintain the air fryer.

- To clean the cooking basket start by filling a large enough tub with hot water and detergent to generate thick foam.
- Place the attachment within it and allow it to soak for a while before using a brush to clean it thoroughly.
- But be careful so as to not scrub it using harsh brushes as they can leave behind scratches.
- The outside of an air fryer will not get as greasy as a conventional fryer. All you have to do is wipe it with a damp cloth and your fryer will be as good as new.
- You can dip the cloth in hot water if you wish to loosen a stain.
- If there is a tough stain then you can use a toothbrush dipped in salt to scrub over the stain.
- But make sure you don't use a steel mesh or a hard bristled toothbrush as they can leave behind scratches on the body of the machine.
- You must also clean the basket at the bottom that catches the residue. You must empty it as soon as you finish the cooking and pop it into the dishwasher to clean it or follow the same procedure as you would to clean the attachment.

Money saving tips

As Air fryer requires less oil, you wouldn't need to buy huge packets of oils in your monthly groceries. This would lessen your grocery bills. You do not need to buy griller, fryer, and an oven separately. This is your all in one rounder. Remember the dress you wanted to take? But unfortunately, you could not buy it. Not anymore. Not only your grocery bills will decrease, you will witness an immense change in your gas bills. As air fryer makes the oil hot in one-third time of other fryers and your stove will require less gas. The lesser you will utilize gas the lesser your bill will be. This will save the money that you were going to spend on a griller and oven.

A cosmic amount will be saved and you do not need to see your favorite dress cashed by someone else. Not only dresses, you can get whatever you want. Air fryer is an efficient and smart choice for everyone. Air fryer would give you an ease and this would save your time and money even health too. Who would not want to get such an opportunity?

Chapter 3: Air Fryer Breakfast Recipes

No-Bun Breakfast Bacon Burger

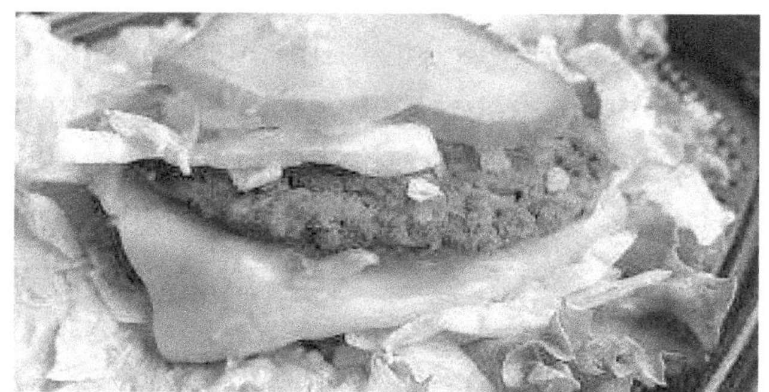

Cook Time: 8 minutes

Servings: 2

Ingredients:

8-ounces ground beef

2-ounces lettuce leaves

½ teaspoon minced garlic

1 teaspoon olive oil

½ teaspoon sea salt

1 teaspoon ground black pepper

1 teaspoon butter

4-ounces bacon, cooked

1 egg

½ yellow onion, diced

½ cucumber, slice finely

½ tomato, slice finely

Directions:

Begin by whisking the egg in a bowl, then add the ground beef and combine well. Add cooked, chopped bacon to the ground beef mixture. Add butter, ground black pepper, minced garlic, and salt. Mix and make burgers. Preheat your air fryer to 370°Fahrenheit. Spray the air fryer basket with olive oil and place the burgers inside of it. Cook the burgers for 8-minutes on each side. Meanwhile, slice the cucumber, onion, and tomato finely. Place the tomato, onion, and cucumber onto the lettuce leaves. When the burgers are cooked, allow them to chill at room temperature, and place them over the vegetables and serve.

Nutritional Values per serving: Calories: 618, Total Fat: 37.8g, Carbs: 8.6g, Protein: 59.4g

Scrambled Pancake Hash

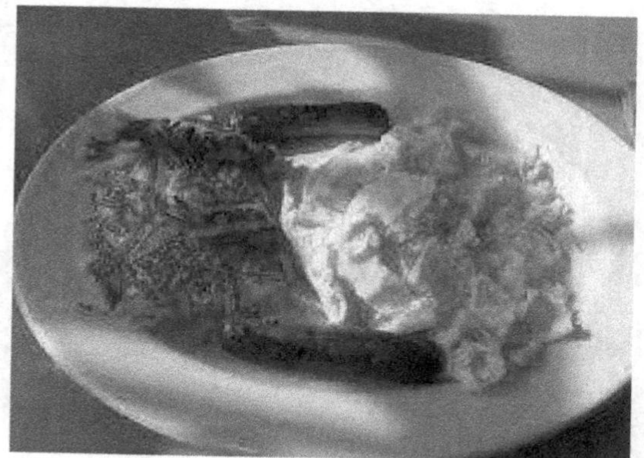

Cook Time: 9 minutes

Servings: 7

Ingredients:

1 egg

¼ cup heavy cream

5 tablespoons butter

1 cup coconut flour

1 teaspoon ground ginger

1 teaspoon salt

1 tablespoon apple cider vinegar

1 teaspoon baking soda

Directions:

Combine the salt, baking soda, ground ginger and flour in a mixing bowl. In a separate bowl crack, the egg into it. Add butter and heavy cream. Mix well using a hand mixer. Combine the liquid and dry mixtures and stir until smooth. Preheat your air fryer to 400°Fahrenheit. Pour the pancake mixture into the air fryer basket tray. Cook the pancake hash for 4-minutes. After this, scramble the pancake hash well and continue to cook for another 5-minutes more. When dish is cooked, transfer it to serving plates, and serve hot!

Nutritional Values per serving: Calories: 178, Total Fat: 13.3g, Carbs: 10.7g, Protein: 4.4g

Morning Time Sausages

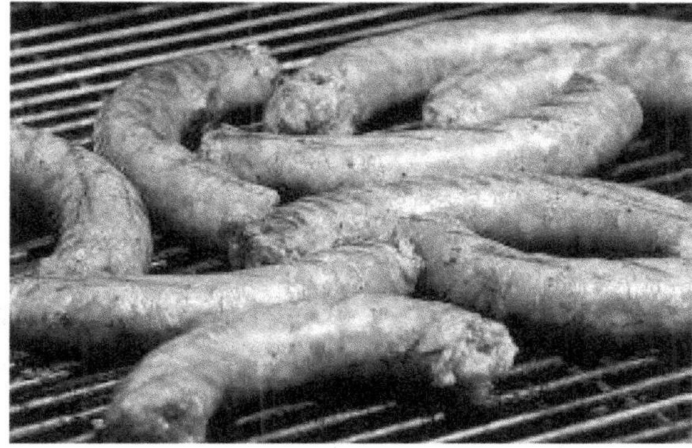

Cook Time: 12 minutes

Servings: 6

Ingredients:

7-ounces ground chicken

7-ounces ground pork

1 teaspoon ground coriander

1 teaspoon basil, dried

½ teaspoon nutmeg

1 teaspoon olive oil

1 teaspoon minced garlic

1 tablespoon coconut flour

1 egg

1 teaspoon soy sauce

1 teaspoon sea salt

½ teaspoon ground black pepper

Directions:

Combine the ground pork, chicken, soy sauce, ground black pepper, garlic, basil, coriander, nutmeg, sea salt, and egg. Add the coconut flour and mix the mixture well to combine. Preheat your air fryer to 360°Fahrenheit. Make medium-sized sausages with the ground meat mixture. Spray the inside of the air fryer basket tray with the olive oil. Place prepared sausages into the air fryer basket and place inside of air fryer. Cook the sausages for 6-minutes. Turn the sausages over and cook for 6-minutes more. When the cook time is completed, let the sausages chill for a little bit. Serve warm.

Nutritional Values per serving: Calories: 156, Total Fat: 7.5g, Carbs: 1.3g, Protein: 20.2g

Breakfast Meatloaf Slices

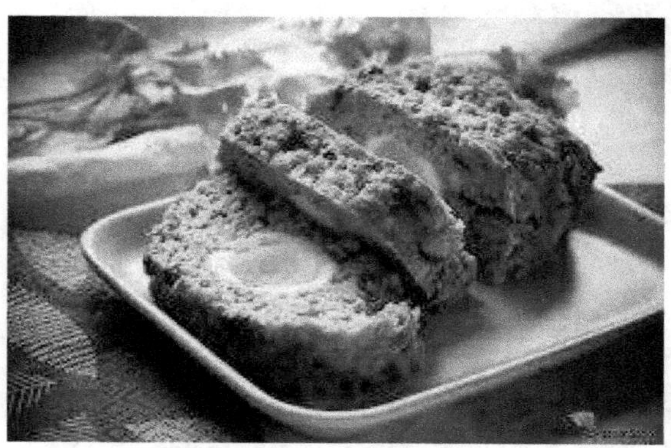

Cook Time: 20 minutes

Servings: 6

Ingredients:

8-ounces ground pork

7-ounces ground beef

1 teaspoon olive oil

1 teaspoon butter

1 tablespoon oregano, dried

1 teaspoon cayenne pepper

1 teaspoon salt

1 tablespoon chives

1 tablespoon almond flour

1 egg

1 onion, diced

Directions:

Beat egg in a bowl. Add the ground beef and ground pork. Add the chives, almond flour, cayenne pepper, salt, dried oregano, and butter. Add diced onion to ground beef mixture. Use hands to shape a meatloaf mixture. Preheat the air fryer to 350°Fahrenheit. Spray the inside of the air fryer basket with olive oil and place the meatloaf inside it. Cook the meatloaf for 20-minutes. When the meatloaf has cooked, allow it to chill for a bit. Slice and serve it.

Nutritional Values per serving: Calories: 176, Total Fat: 6.2g, Carbs: 3.4g, Protein: 22.2g

Egg Butter

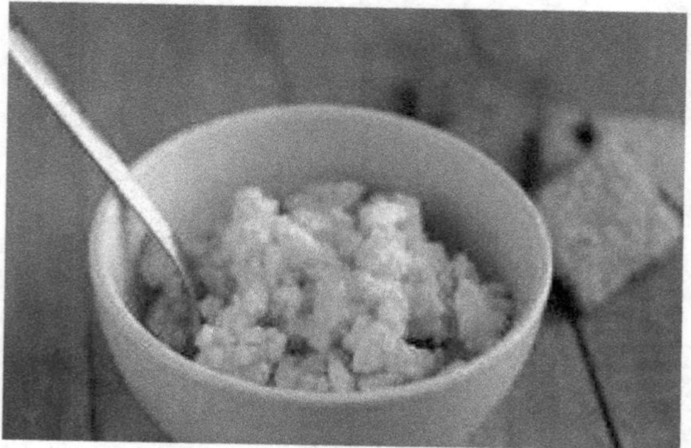

Cook Time: 17 minutes

Servings: 4

Ingredients:

4 eggs

4 tablespoons butter

1 teaspoon salt

Directions:

Cover the air fryer basket with foil and place the eggs there. Transfer the air fryer basket into the air fryer and cook the eggs for 17 minutes at 320°Fahrenheit. When the time is over, remove the eggs from the air fryer basket and put them in cold water to chill them. After this, peel the eggs and chop them up finely. Combine the chopped eggs with butter and add salt. Mix it until you get the spread texture. Serve the egg butter with the keto almond bread.

Nutritional Values per serving: Calories: 164, Total Fat: 8.5g, Carbs: 2.67g, Protein: 3g

Kale Breakfast Fritters

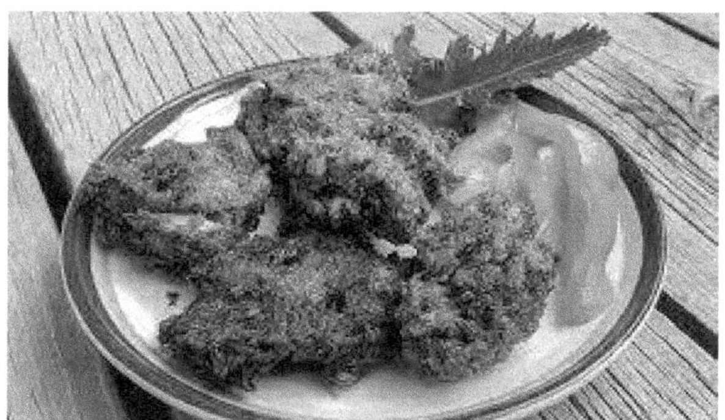

Cook Time: 8 minutes

Servings: 8

Ingredients:

12-ounces kale, chopped

1 teaspoon oil

1 tablespoon cream

1 teaspoon paprika

½ teaspoon sea salt

2 tablespoons almond flour

1 egg

1 tablespoon butter

½ yellow onion, diced

Directions:

Wash and chop the kale. Add the chopped kale to blender and blend it until smooth. Dice up the yellow onion. Beat the egg and whisk it in a mixing bowl. Add the almond flour, paprika, cream and salt into bowl with whisked egg and stir. Add the diced onion and blended kale to mixing bowl and mix until you get fritter dough. Preheat your air fryer to 360°Fahrenheit. Spray the inside of the air fryer basket with olive oil. Make medium-sized fritters with prepared mixture and place them into air fryer basket. Cook the kale fritters 4-minutes on each side. Once they are cooked, allow them to chill then serve.

Nutritional Values per serving:, Calories: 86, Total Fat: 5.6g, Carbs: 6.8g, Protein: 3.6g

Seed Porridge

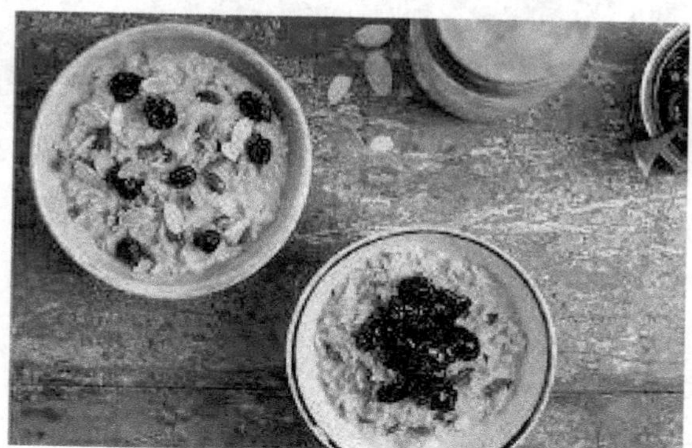

Cook Time: 12 minutes

Servings: 3

Ingredients:

1 tablespoon butter

¼ teaspoon nutmeg

1/3 cup heavy cream

1 egg

¼ teaspoon salt

3 tablespoons sesame seeds

3 tablespoons chia seeds

Directions:

Place the butter in your air fryer basket tray. Add the chia seeds, sesame seeds, heavy cream, nutmeg, and salt. Stir gently. Beat the egg in a cup and whisk it with a fork. Add the whisked egg to air fryer basket tray. Stir the mixture with a wooden spatula. Preheat your air fryer to 375°Fahrenheit. Place the air fryer basket tray into air fryer and cook the porridge for 12-minutes. Stir it about 3 times during the cooking process. Remove the porridge from air fryer basket tray immediately and serve hot!

Nutritional Values per serving: Calories: 275, Total Fat: 22.5g, Carbs: 13.2g, Protein: 7.9g

Keto Bread-Free Breakfast Sandwich

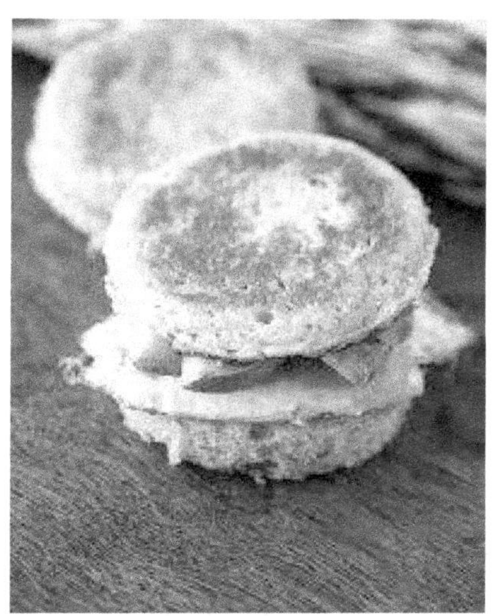

Cook Time: 10 minutes

Servings: 2

Ingredients:

6-ounces ground chicken

2 slices of cheddar cheese

2 lettuce leaves

1 tablespoon dill, dried

½ teaspoon sea salt

1 egg

1 teaspoon cayenne pepper

1 teaspoon tomato puree

Directions:

Combine the ground chicken with the pepper and sea salt. Add the dried dill and stir. Beat the egg into the ground chicken mixture. Make 2 medium-sized burgers from the ground chicken mixture. Preheat your air fryer to 380°Fahrenheit. Spray the air fryer basket tray with olive oil and place the ground chicken burgers inside of it. Cook the chicken burgers for 10-minutes. Flip over burgers and cook for an additional 6-minutes. When the burgers are cooked, transfer them to the lettuce leaves. Sprinkle the top of them with tomato puree and with a slice of cheddar cheese. Serve immediately!

Nutritional Values per serving: Calories: 324, Total Fat: 19.2g, Carbs: 2.3g, Protein: 34.8g

Breakfast Liver Pate

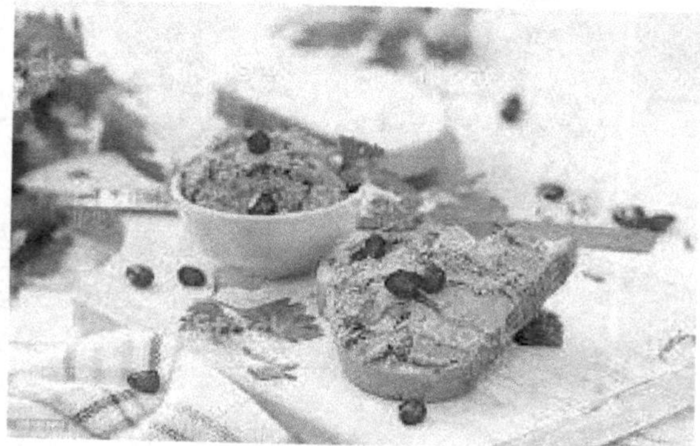

Cook Time: 10 minutes

Servings: 7

Ingredients:

1 lb. chicken liver

1 teaspoon salt

½ teaspoon cilantro, dried

1 yellow onion, diced

1 teaspoon ground black pepper

1 cup water

4 tablespoons butter

Directions:

Chop the chicken liver roughly and place it in the air fryer basket tray. Add water to air fryer basket tray and add diced onion. Preheat your air fryer to 360°Fahrenheit and cook chicken liver for 10-minutes. When it is finished cooking, drain the chicken liver. Transfer the chicken liver to blender, add butter, ground black pepper and dried cilantro and blend. Once you get a pate texture, transfer to liver pate bowl and serve immediately or keep in the fridge for later.

Nutritional Values per serving: Calories: 173, Total Fat: 10.8g, Carbs: 2.2g, Protein: 16.1g

Eggs in Zucchini Nests

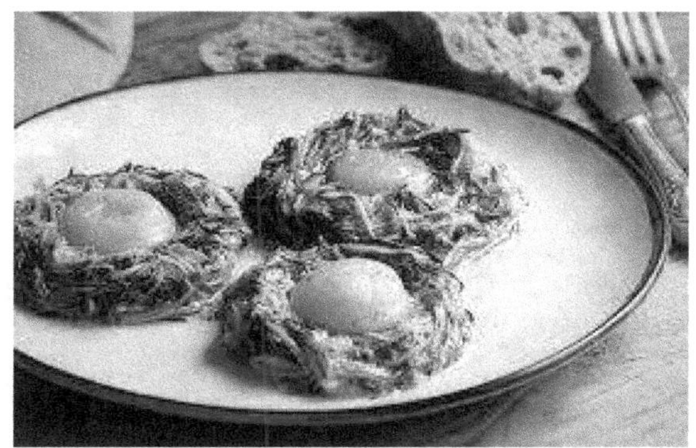

Cook Time: 7 minutes

Servings: 4

Ingredients:

4 teaspoons butter

½ teaspoon paprika

½ teaspoon black pepper

¼ teaspoon sea salt

4-ounces cheddar cheese, shredded

4 eggs

8-ounces zucchini, grated

Directions:

Grate the zucchini and place the butter in ramekins. Add the grated zucchini in ramekins in the shape of nests. Sprinkle the zucchini nests with salt, pepper, and paprika. Beat the eggs and pour over zucchini nests. Top egg mixture with shredded cheddar cheese. Preheat the air fryer basket and cook the dish for 7-minutes. When the zucchini nests are cooked, chill them for 3-minutes and serve them in the ramekins.

Nutritional Values per serving: Calories: 221, Total Fat: 17.7g, Carbs: 2.9g, Protein: 13.4g

Breakfast Chicken Hash

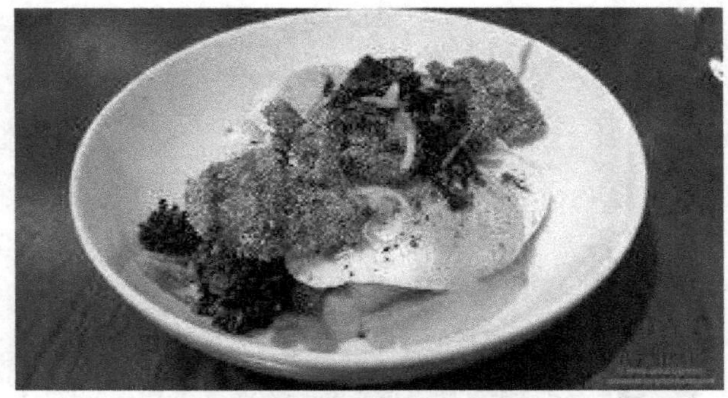

Cook Time: 14 minutes

Servings: 3

Ingredients:

6-ounces of cauliflower, chopped

7-ounce chicken fillet

1 tablespoon water

1 green pepper, chopped

½ yellow onion, diced

1 teaspoon ground black pepper

3 tablespoons butter

1 tablespoon cream

Directions:

Chop the cauliflower and place into the blender and blend it carefully until you get cauliflower rice. Chop the chicken fillet into small pieces. Sprinkle the chicken fillet with ground black pepper and stir. Preheat your air fryer to 380°Fahrenheit. Dice the yellow onion and chop the green pepper. In a large mixing bowl, combine ingredients, then add mixture to fryer basket. Then cook and serve chicken hash warm!

Nutritional Values per serving: Calories: 261, Total Fat: 16.8g, Carbs: 7.1g, Protein: 21g

Flax Meal Porridge

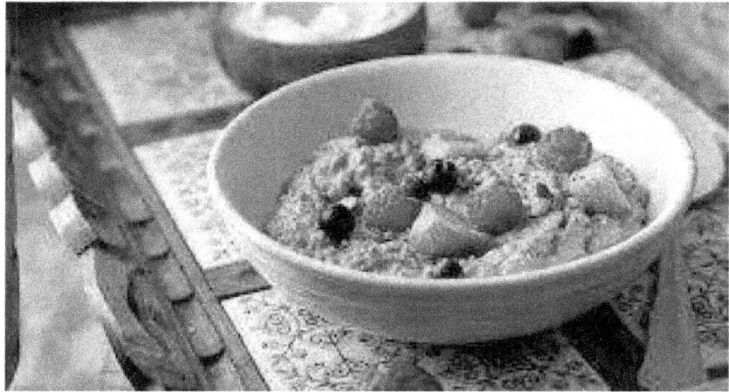

Cook Time: 8 minutes

Servings: 4

Ingredients:

2 tablespoons sesame seeds

½ teaspoon vanilla extract

1 tablespoon butter

1 tablespoon liquid Stevia

3 tablespoons flax meal

1 cup almond milk

4 tablespoons chia seeds

Directions:

Preheat your air fryer to 375°Fahrenheit. Put the sesame seeds, chia seeds, almond milk, flax meal, liquid Stevia and butter into the air fryer basket tray. Add the vanilla extract and cook porridge for 8-minutes. When porridge is cooked stir it carefully then allow it to rest for 5-minutes before serving.

Nutritional Values per serving: Calories: 298, Total Fat: 26.7g, Carbs: 13.3 g, Protein: 6.2g

Breakfast Chicken Strips

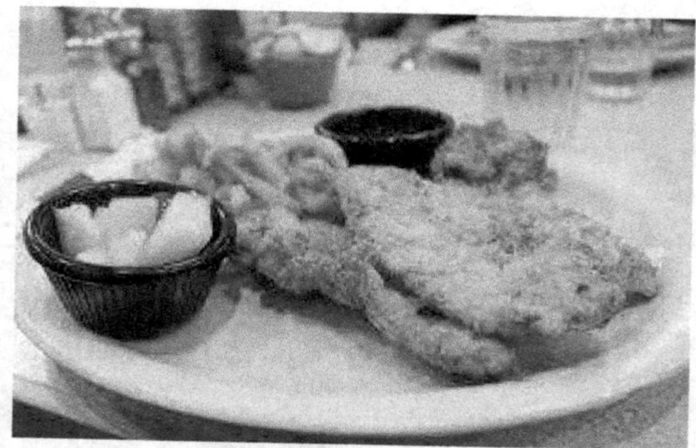

Cook Time: 12 minutes

Servings: 4

Ingredients:

1 teaspoon paprika

1 tablespoon cream

1 lb. chicken fillet

½ teaspoon salt

½ teaspoon black pepper

Directions:

Cut the chicken fillet into strips. Sprinkle the chicken fillets with salt and pepper. Preheat the air fryer to 365°Fahrenheit. Place the butter in the air basket tray and add the chicken strips. Cook the chicken strips for 6-minutes. Turn the chicken strips to the other side and cook them for an additional 5-minutes. After strips are cooked, sprinkle them with cream and paprika, then transfer them to serving plates. Serve warm.

Nutritional Values per serving: Calories: 245, Total Fat: 11.5g, Carbs: 0.6g, Protein: 33g

Breakfast Hash

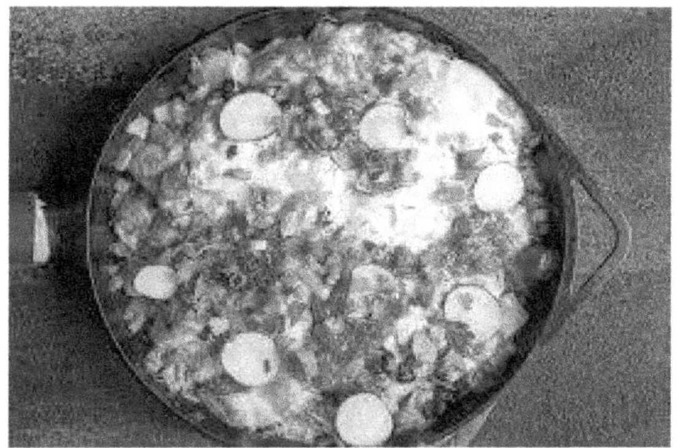

Cook Time: 8 minutes

Servings: 4

Ingredients:

7-ounces bacon, cooked

1 zucchini, cubed into small pieces

4-ounces cheddar cheese, shredded

2 tablespoons butter

1 teaspoon ground thyme

1 teaspoon cilantro

1 teaspoon paprika

1 teaspoon ground black pepper

1 teaspoon salt

Directions:

Chop the zucchini into small cubes and sprinkle with ground black pepper, salt, paprika, cilantro and ground thyme. Preheat your air fryer to 400°Fahrenheit. Add butter to the air fryer basket tray. Melt the butter and add the zucchini cubes. Cook the zucchini cubes for 5-minutes. Meanwhile, shred the cheddar cheese. Add the bacon to the zucchini cubes. Sprinkle the zucchini mixture with shredded cheese and cook for 3-minutes more. When cooking is completed, transfer the breakfast hash into serving bowls.

Nutritional Values per serving: Calories: 445, Total Fat: 36.1g, Carbs: 3.5g, Protein: 26.3g

Keto Air Bread

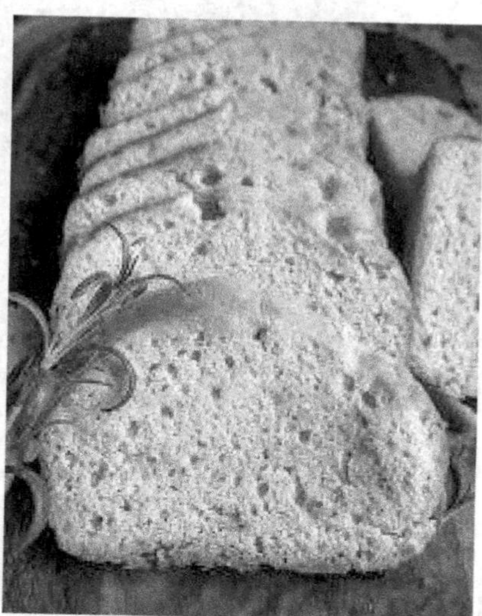

Cook Time: 25 minutes

Servings: 19

Ingredients:

1 cup almond flour

¼ sea salt

1 teaspoon baking powder

¼ cup butter

3 eggs

Directions:

Crack the eggs into a bowl then using a hand blender mix them up. Melt the butter at room temperature. Take the melted butter and add it to the egg mixture. Add the salt, baking powder and almond flour to egg mixture and knead the dough. Cover the prepared dough with a towel for 10-minutes to rest. Meanwhile, preheat your air fryer to 360˚Fahrenheit. Place the prepared dough in the air fryer tin and cook the bread for 10-minutes. Then reduce the heat to 350˚Fahrenheit and cook the bread for an additional 15-minutes. You can use a toothpick to check to make sure the bread is cooked. Transfer the bread to a wooden board to allow it to chill. Once the bread has chilled, then slice and serve it.

Nutritional Values per serving: Calories: 40, Total Fat: 3.9g, Carbs: 0.5g, Protein: 1.2g

Herbed Breakfast Eggs

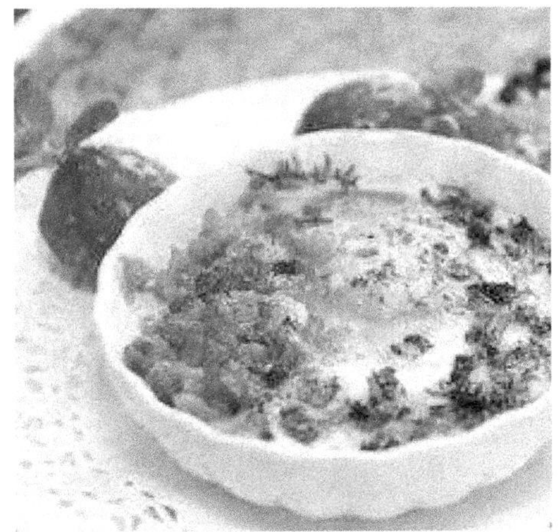

Cook Time: 17 minutes

Servings: 2

Ingredients:

4 eggs

1 teaspoon oregano

1 teaspoon parsley, dried

½ teaspoon sea salt

1 tablespoon chives, chopped

1 tablespoon cream

1 teaspoon paprika

Directions:

Place the eggs in the air fryer basket and cook them for 17-minutes at 320°Fahrenheit. Meanwhile, combine the parsley, oregano, cream, and salt in shallow bowl. Chop the chives and add them to cream mixture. When the eggs are cooked, place them in cold water and allow them to chill. After this, peel the eggs and cut them into halves. Remove the egg yolks and add yolks to cream mixture and mash to blend well with a fork. Then fill the egg whites with the cream-egg yolk mixture. Serve immediately.

Nutritional Values per serving: Calories: 136, Total Fat: 9.3g, Carbs: 2.1g, Protein: 11.4g

Baked Bacon Egg Cups

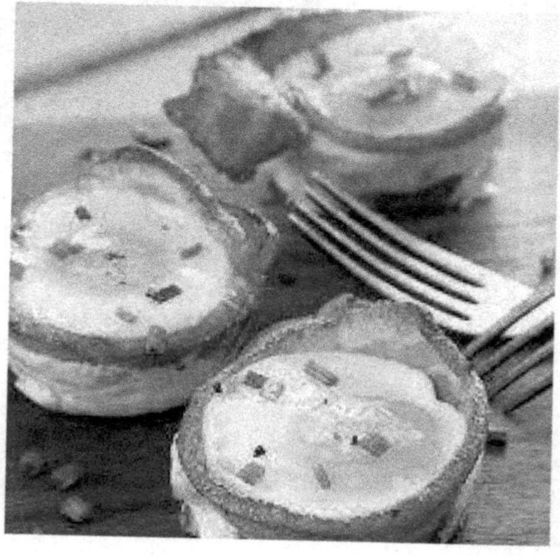

Cooking Time: 12 minutes

Servings: 2

Ingredients:

2 eggs

1 tablespoon chives, fresh, chopped

½ teaspoon paprika

½ teaspoon cayenne pepper

3-ounces cheddar cheese, shredded

½ teaspoon butter

¼ teaspoon salt

4-ounces bacon, cut into tiny pieces

Directions:

Slice bacon into tiny pieces and sprinkle it with cayenne pepper, salt, and paprika. Mix the chopped bacon. Spread butter in bottom of ramekin dishes and beat the eggs there. Add the chives and shredded cheese. Add the chopped bacon over egg mixture in ramekin dishes. Place the ramekins in your air fryer basket. Preheat your air fryer to 360°Fahrenheit. Place the air fryer basket in your air fryer and cook for 12-minutes. When the cook time is completed, remove the ramekins from air fryer and serve warm.

Nutritional Values per serving: Calories: 553, Total Fat: 43.3g, Carbs: 2.3g, Protein: 37.3g

Breakfast Coconut Porridge

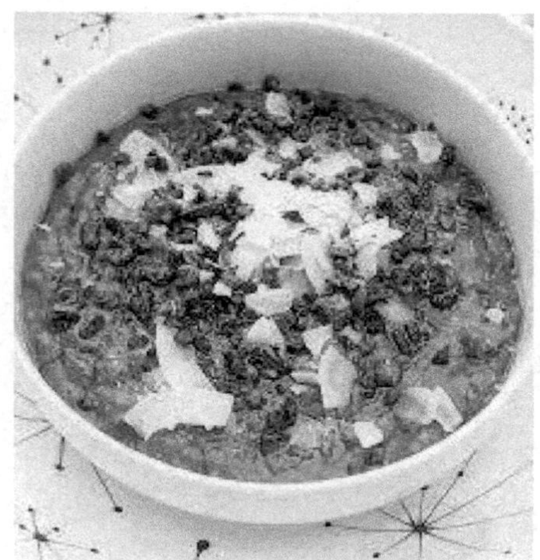

Cook Time: 7 minutes

Servings: 4

Ingredients:
1 cup coconut milk

3 tablespoons blackberries

2 tablespoons walnuts

1 teaspoon butter

1 teaspoon ground cinnamon

5 tablespoons chia seeds

3 tablespoons coconut flakes

¼ teaspoon salt

Directions:

Pour the coconut milk into the air fryer basket tray. Add the coconut, salt, chia seeds, ground cinnamon, and butter. Ground up the walnuts and add them to the air fryer basket tray. Sprinkle the mixture with salt. Mash the blackberries with a fork and add them also to the air fryer basket tray. Cook the porridge at 375˚Fahrenheit for 7-minutes. When the cook time is over, remove the air fryer basket from air fryer and allow to sit and rest for 5-minutes. Stir porridge with a wooden spoon and serve warm.

Nutritional Values per serving: Calories: 169, Total Fat: 18.2g, Carbs: 9.3g, Protein: 4.2g

Keto Spinach Quiche

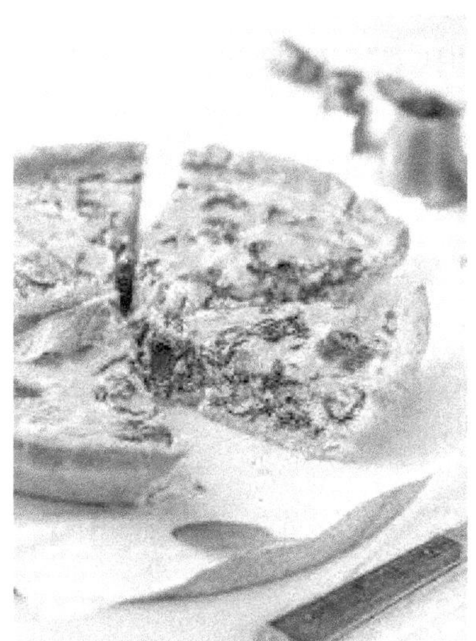

Cook Time: 21 minutes

Servings: 6

Ingredients:

6-ounces cheddar cheese, shredded

1 teaspoon olive oil

3 eggs

1 teaspoon ground black pepper

½ yellow onion, diced

¼ cup cream cheese

1 cup spinach

1 teaspoon sea salt

4 tablespoons water, boiled

½ cup almond flour

Directions:

Combine the almond flour, water, and salt. Mix and knead the dough. Spray the inside of the fryer basket with olive oil. Set your air fryer to 375°Fahrenheit. Roll the dough and place it in your air fryer basket tray in the shape of the crust. Place air fryer basket tray inside of air fryer and cook for 5-minutes. Chop the spinach and combine it with the cream cheese and ground black pepper. Dice the yellow onion and add it to the spinach mixture and stir. Whisk eggs in a bowl. When the quiche crust is cooked—transfer the spinach filling. Sprinkle the filling top with shredded cheese and pour the whisked eggs over the top. Set the air fryer to 350°Fahrenheit. Cook the quiche for 7-minutes. Reduce the heat to 300°Fahrenheit and cook the quiche for an additional 9-minutes. Allow the quiche to chill thoroughly and then cut it into pieces for serving.

Nutritional Values per serving: Calories: 248, Total Fat: 20.2g, Carbs: 4.1g, Protein: 12.8g

Western Omelette

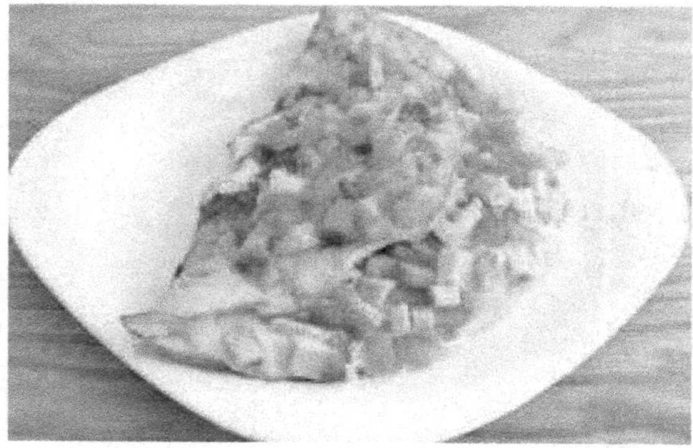

Cook Time: 10 minutes

Servings: 4

Ingredients:

1 green pepper

5 eggs

½ yellow onion, diced

3-ounces Parmesan cheese, shredded

1 teaspoon butter

1 teaspoon oregano, dried

1 teaspoon cilantro, dried

1 teaspoon olive oil

3 tablespoons cream cheese

Directions:

In a bowl, add the eggs and whisk them. Sprinkle the cilantro, oregano, and cream cheese into the eggs. Add the shredded parmesan and mix the egg mixture well. Preheat your air fryer to 360°Fahrenheit. Pour the egg mixture into the air fryer basket tray and place it into the air fryer. Cook the omelet for 10-minutes. Meanwhile, chop the green pepper and dice the onion. Pour olive oil into a skillet and preheat well over medium heat. Add the chopped green pepper and onion to skillet and roast for 8-minutes. Stir veggies often. Remove the omelet from air fryer basket tray and place it on a serving plate. Add the roasted vegetables and serve warm.

Nutritional Values per serving: Calories: 204, Total Fat: 14.9g, Carbs: 4.3g, Protein: 14.8g

Chapter 4: Lunch

Bacon, Lettuce, Tempeh & Tomato Sandwiches

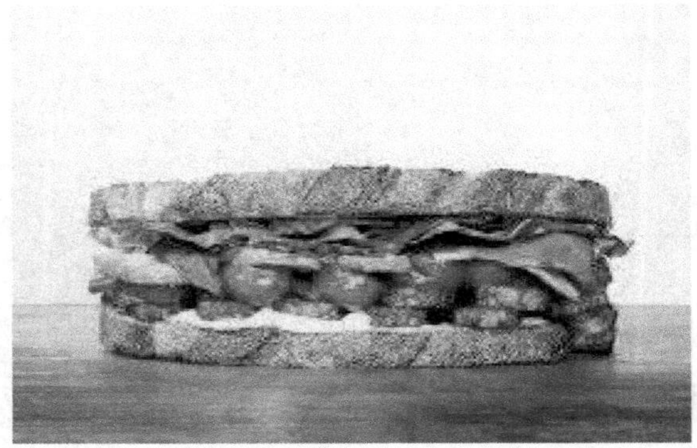

Cook Time: 5 minutes

Servings: 4

Ingredients:

8-ounce package tempeh

1 cup warm vegetable broth

Tomato slices and lettuce, to serve

¼ teaspoon chipotle chili powder

½ teaspoon garlic powder

½ teaspoon onion powder

1 teaspoon Liquid smoke

3 tablespoons soy sauce

Directions:

Begin by opening the packet of tempeh and slice into pieces about ¼ inch thick. Grab a medium bowl and add the remaining ingredients except for lettuce and tomato and stir well. Place the pieces of tempeh onto a baking tray that will fit into your air fryer and pour over the flavor mix. Put the tray in air fryer and cook for 5-minutes at 360°Fahrenheit. Remove from air fryer and place on sliced bread with the tomato and lettuce and any other extra toppings you desire.

Nutritional Values per serving: Carbs: 265, Total Fat: 11.3g, Carbs: 9.2g, Protein: 12.4g

Coconut Chips

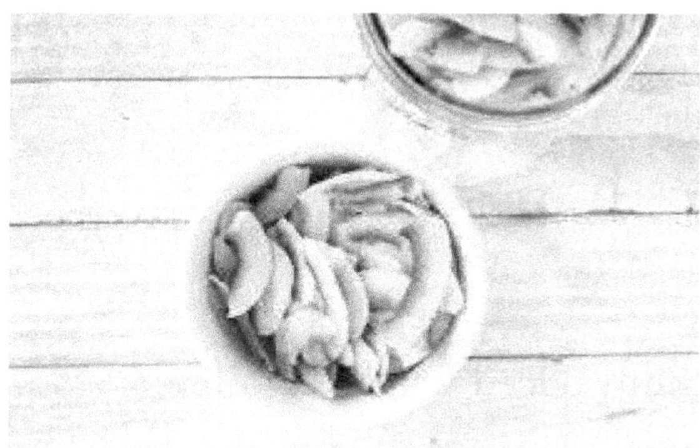

Cook Time: 5 minutes

Servings: 2

Ingredients:

2 cups large pieces of shredded coconut

1/3 teaspoon liquid Stevia

1 tablespoon chili powder

Directions:

Preheat your air fryer to 390°Fahrenheit. Combine the shredded coconut pieces with spices. Cook for 5-minutes in air fryer and enjoy!

Nutritional Values per serving: Calories: 261, Total Fat: 9.2g, Carbs: 7.3g, Protein: 6.2g

Sweet Potato Chips

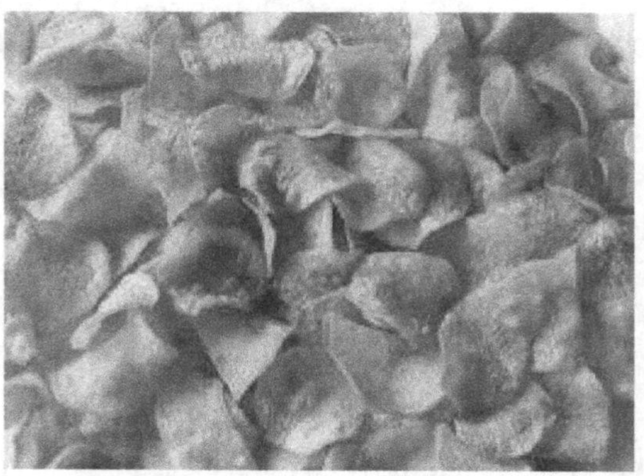

Cook Time: 15 minutes

Servings: 2

Ingredients:

2 large sweet potatoes, thinly sliced with Mandoline

2 tablespoons olive oil

Salt to taste

Directions:

Preheat your air fryer to 350°Fahrenheit. Stir the sweet potato slices, in a large bowl with the oil. Arrange slices in your air fryer and cook them until crispy, for about 15-minutes.

Nutritional Values per serving: Calories: 253, Total Fat: 11.2g, Carbs: 8.4g, Protein: 6.5g

Air Fryer Apple Pork Balls

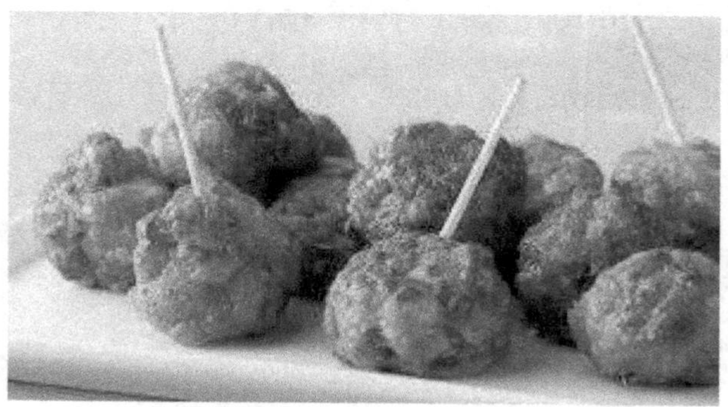

Cook Time: 15 minutes

Servings: 8

Ingredients:

2 teaspoons Dijon mustard

5 basil leaves, chopped

Salt and pepper to taste

2 tablespoons cheddar cheese, grated

4 garlic cloves, minced

1 small apple, chopped

1 large onion, chopped

1 1b. pork, minced

Directions:

Add the minced pork, onion, and apple into mixing bowl and stir. Add mustard, honey, garlic, cheese, basil, pepper, salt and mix well. Make small balls from mixture and place them inside of air fryer basket. Cook at 400°Fahrenheit for 15-minutes.

Nutritional Values per serving: Calories: 267, Total Fat: 12.3g, Carbs: 11.6g, Protein: 16.4g

Air Fryer Pork Loin with Sweet Potatoes

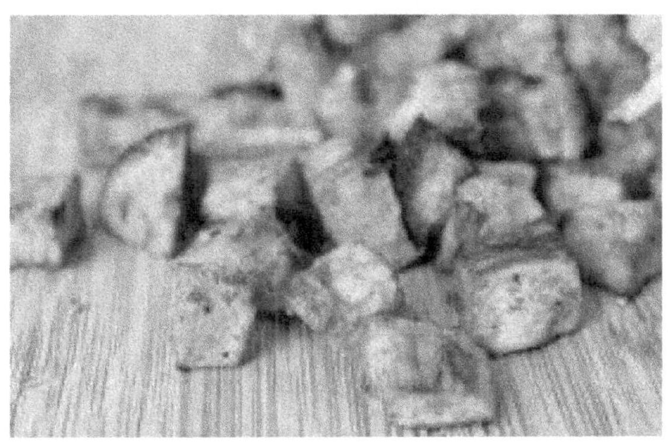

Cook Time: 25 minutes

Servings: 8

Ingredients:

2 lbs. pork loin

2 large Sweet potatoes, diced

1 teaspoon salt

1 teaspoon pepper

½ teaspoon garlic powder

½ teaspoon parsley flakes

Directions:

Add all the ingredients into mixing bowl and mix well. Add bowl with pork and sweet potato mixture into air fryer basket. Cook in air fryer at 350°Fahrenheit for 25-minutes. Carve up the pork into slices and serve with sweet potatoes.

Nutritional Values per serving: Calories: 286, Total Fat: 12.6g, Carbs: 11.4g, Protein: 16.6g

Onion Pakora

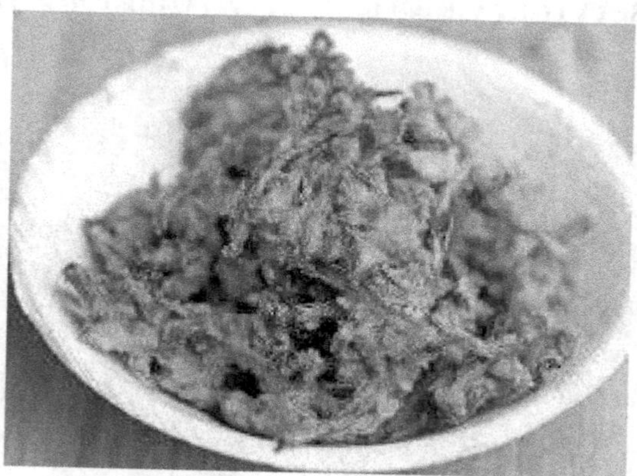

Cook Time: 6 minutes

Servings: 6

Ingredients:

1 cup graham flour

¼ teaspoon turmeric powder

Salt to taste

1/8 teaspoon chili powder

¼ teaspoon carom

1 tablespoon fresh coriander, chopped

2 green chili peppers, finely chopped

4 onions, finely chopped

2 teaspoons vegetable oil

¼ cup rice flour

Directions:

Combine the flours and oil in a mixing bowl. Add water as needed to create a dough-like consistency. Add peppers, onions, coriander, carom, chili powder, and turmeric. Preheat air fryer to 350°Fahrenheit. Roll vegetable mixture into small balls, add to the fryer and cook for about 6-minutes. Serve with hot sauce!

Nutritional Values per serving: Calories: 253, Total Fat: 12.2g, Carbs: 11.4g, Protein: 7.6g

Mushroom, Onion and Feta Frittata

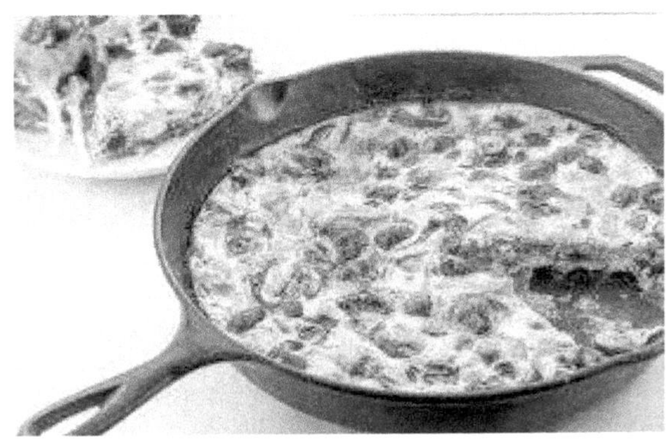

Cook Time: 30 minutes

Servings: 4

Ingredients:

4 cups button mushrooms

1 red onion

2 tablespoons olive oil

6 tablespoons feta cheese, crumbled

Pinch of salt

6 eggs

Cooking spray

Directions:

Peel and slice the red onion into ¼ inch thin slices. Clean the button mushrooms, then cut them into ¼ inch thin slices. Add olive oil to pan and sautė mushrooms over medium heat until tender. Remove from heat and pan so that they can cool. Preheat your air fryer to 330°Fahrenheit. Add cracked eggs into a bowl, and whisk them, adding a pinch of salt. Coat an 8-inch heat resistant baking dish with cooking spray. Add the eggs into the baking dish, then onion and mushroom mixture, and then add feta cheese. Place the baking dish into air fryer for 30-minutes and serve warm.

Nutritional Values per serving: Calories: 246, Total Fat: 12.3g, Carbs: 9.2g, Protein: 10.3g

Curried Cauliflower Florets

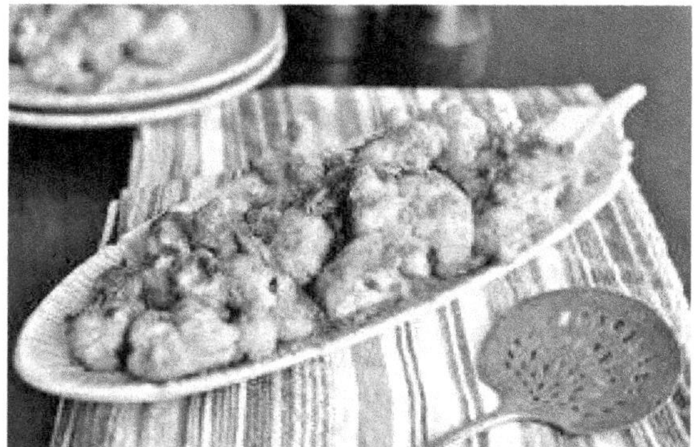

Cook Time: 10 minutes

Servings: 4

Ingredients:

1/4 cup sultanas or golden raisins

¼ teaspoon salt

1 tablespoon curry powder

1 head cauliflower, broken into small florets

¼ cup pine nuts

½ cup olive oil

Directions:

In a cup of boiling water, soak your sultanas to plump. Preheat your air fryer to 350°Fahrenheit. Add oil and pine nuts to air fryer and toast for a minute or so. In a bowl toss the cauliflower and curry powder as well as salt, then add the mix to air fryer mixing well. Cook for 10-minutes. Drain the sultanas, toss with cauliflower, and serve.

Nutritional Values per serving: Calories: 275, Total Fat: 11.3g, Carbs: 8.6g, Protein: 9.5g

Pork Chunks with Sweet & Sour Sauce

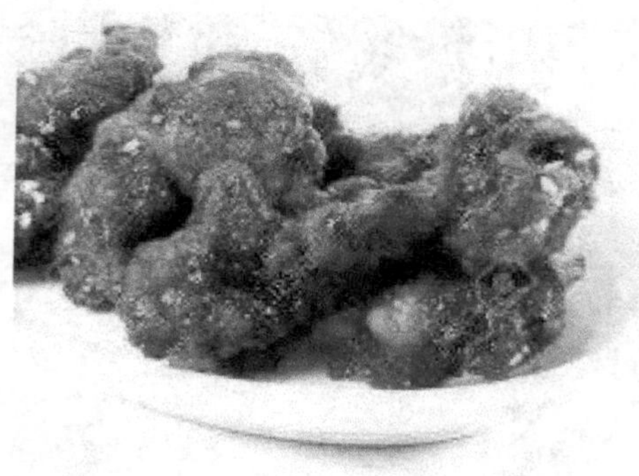

Cook Time: 10 minutes

Servings: 4

Ingredients:

1 cup cornstarch

½ teaspoon spice mix

¼ cup sweet and sour sauce

2 lbs. pork, chunked

3 tablespoons olive oil

2 large eggs, beaten

½ teaspoon sea salt

¼ teaspoon black pepper

Directions:

In a bowl, combine spice mix, cornstarch, pepper, and salt. In another bowl add beaten eggs. Coat pork chunks with cornstarch mixture then dip in eggs and again into cornstarch. Grease air fryer basket with olive oil and preheat to 340°Fahrenheit. Place the coated pork chunks into air fryer basket and cook for 10-minutes. Shake the basket halfway through the cook time. Place the air fried pork chunks on serving dish and drizzle with sweet and sour sauce.

Nutritional Values per serving: Calories: 282, Total Fat: 12.6g, Carbs: 11.5g, Protein: 17.3g

Panko-Crusted Tilapia

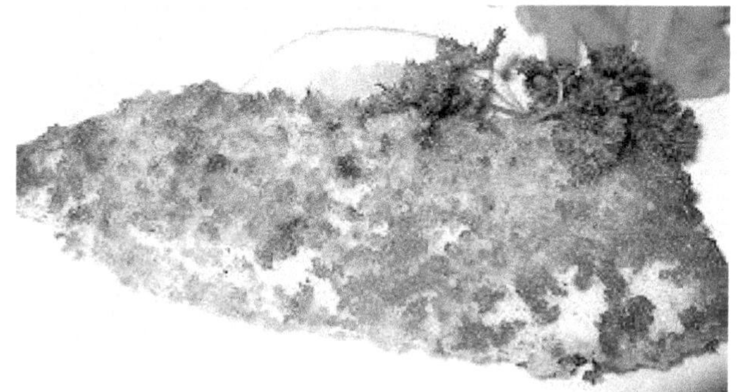

Cook Time: 5 minutes

Servings: 3

Ingredients:

2 tsp. Italian seasoning

2 tsp. lemon pepper

1/3 C. panko breadcrumbs

1/3 C. egg whites

1/3 C. almond flour

3 tilapia fillets

Olive oil

Directions:

Place panko, egg whites, and flour into separate bowls. Mix lemon pepper and Italian seasoning in with breadcrumbs.

Pat tilapia fillets dry. Dredge in flour, then egg, then breadcrumb mixture. Add to air fryer basket and spray lightly with olive oil.

Cook 10-11 minutes at 400 degrees, making sure to flip halfway through cooking.

Nutritional Values per serving: Calories: 256 Fat: 9g Protein: 39g Sugar: 5g

Air Fryer Pork Ribs

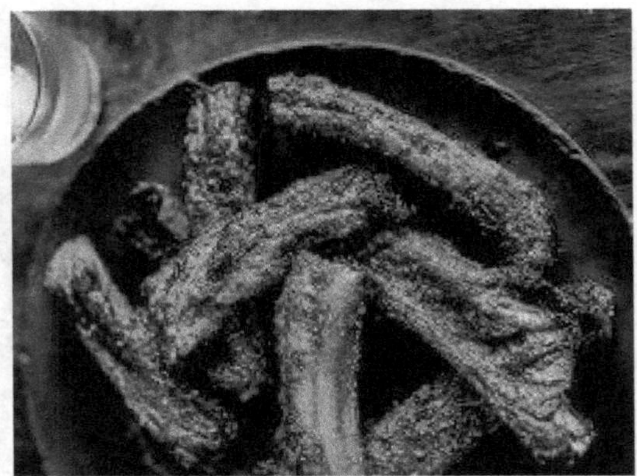

Cook Time: 27 minutes

Servings: 2

Ingredients:

1 lb. pork ribs

Salt and pepper to taste

½ cup BBQ sauce

1 teaspoon liquid Stevia

1 teaspoon spice mix

1 medium onion, chopped

1 tablespoon olive oil

Directions:

In a pan over medium heat, warm the oil. Add onion to pan and sautė for 2-minutes. Add spice mix, stevia, and BBQ sauce into pan and stir well. Remove pan from heat and set aside. Season pork ribs with salt and pepper and place inside of air fryer basket. Air fry the ribs at 320°Fahrenheit for 10-minutes. Brush BBQ sauce on both sides of pork. Air fry pork for an additional 15-minutes, cut into slices and serve.

Nutritional Values per serving: Calories: 284, Total Fat: 12.5g, Carbs: 11.2g, Protein: 16.5g

Vegetable Spring Rolls

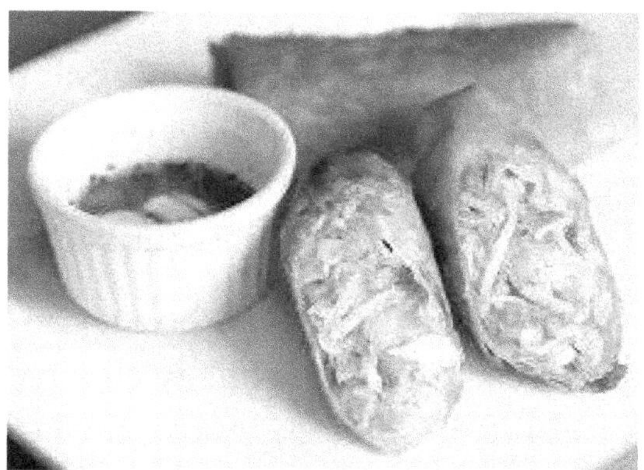

Cook Time: 23 minutes

Servings: 10

Ingredients:

10 spring roll wrappers

2 tablespoons cornstarch

Water

3 green onions, thinly sliced

1 tablespoon black pepper

1 teaspoon soy sauce

Pinches of salt

2 tablespoons cooking oil, plus more for brushing

8-cloves of garlic, minced

½ bell pepper, cut into thin matchsticks

2 large onions, cut into thin matchsticks

1 large carrot, cut into thin matchsticks

2 cups cabbage, shredded

2-inch piece of ginger, grated

Directions:

To prepare the filling: add to a large bowl the carrot, bell pepper, onion, cabbage, ginger, and garlic. Gently add two tablespoons of olive oil in a pan over high heat. Add the filling mixture and stir in salt and a dash of stevia sweetener if you like. Cook for 3-minutes. Add soy sauce, black pepper and mix well.

Add green onions, stir and set aside. In a small bowl, combine enough water and cornstarch to make a creamy paste. Fill the rolls with a tablespoon of filling in center of each wrapper and roll tightly, dampening the edges with cornstarch paste to ensure a good seal. Repeat until all wrappers and filling are used. Preheat your air fryer to 350°Fahrenheit. Brush the rolls with oil, and arrange them in the air fryer, and cook them until crisp and golden for about 20-minutes. Halfway through the cook time flip them over.

Nutritional Values per serving: Calories: 263, Total Fat: 11.2g, Carbs: 8.6g, Protein: 8.2g

Parsnip Fries

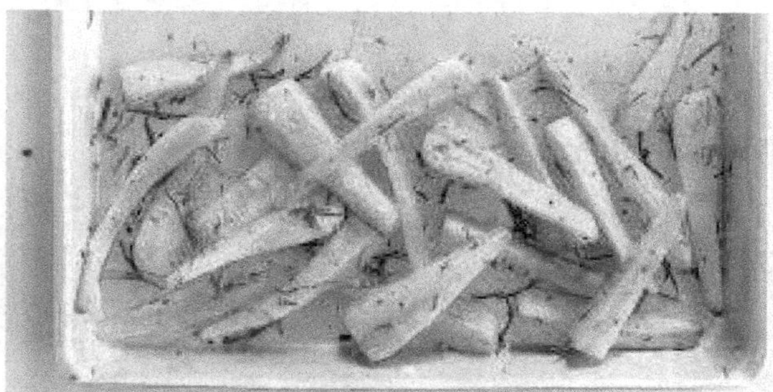

Cook Time: 12 minutes

Servings: 2

Ingredients:

2 tablespoons of olive oil

A pinch of sea salt

1 large bunch of parsnips

Directions:

Wash and peel the parsnips, then cut them into strips. Place the parsnips in a bowl with the olive oil and sea salt and coat well. Preheat your air fryer to 360°Fahrenheit. Place the parsnip and oil mixture into the air fryer basket. Cook for 12-minutes. Serve with sour cream or ketchup.

Nutritional Values per serving: Calories: 262g, Total Fat: 11.3g, Carbs: 10.4g, Protein: 7.2g

Bang Bang Panko Breaded Fried Shrimp

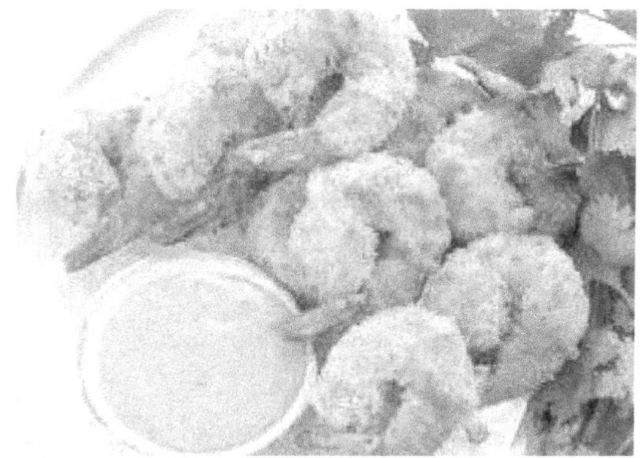

Cook Time: 15 minutes

Servings: 4

Ingredients:

1 tsp. paprika

Montreal chicken seasoning

¾ C. panko bread crumbs

½ C. almond flour

1 egg white

1 pound raw shrimp (peeled and deveined)

Bang Bang Sauce:

¼ C. sweet chili sauce

2 tbsp. sriracha sauce

1/3 C. plain Greek yogurt

Directions:

Ensure your air fryer is preheated to 400 degrees.
Season all shrimp with seasonings.

Add flour to one bowl, egg white in another, and breadcrumbs to a third.

Dip seasoned shrimp in flour, then egg whites, and then breadcrumbs.

Spray coated shrimp with olive oil and add to air fryer basket.

Cook 4 minutes, flip, and cook an additional 4 minutes.

To make the sauce, mix together all sauce ingredients until smooth.

Nutritional Values per serving: Calories: 212 Carbs: 12 Fat: 1g Protein: 37g Sugar: 0.5g

BBQ Pork Chops

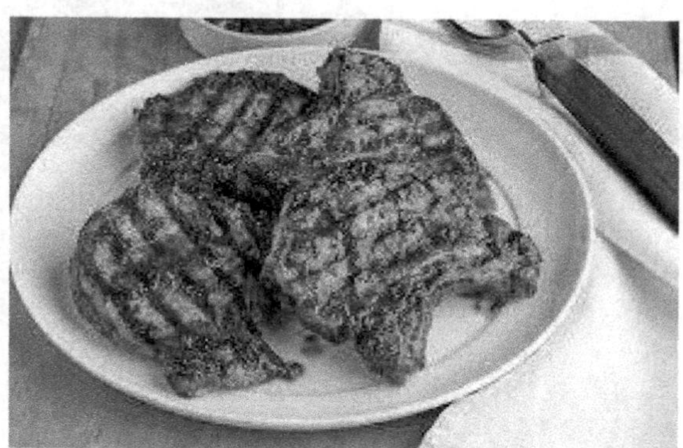

Cook Time: 10 minutes

Servings: 6

Ingredients:

6 pork loin chops

Pepper to taste

1 garlic clove

¼ teaspoon ground ginger

1 teaspoon balsamic vinegar

2 tablespoons soy sauce

2 tablespoons honey

Directions:

Preheat the air fryer to 350°Fahrenheit for 5-minutes. Season pork chops with pepper. In a mixing bowl, add soy sauce, honey, ground ginger, garlic, vinegar and mix well. Add seasoned pork chops to bowl and coat well. Place pork chops in fridge for 2 hours. Place marinated pork chops into air fryer basket and air fry for 10-minutes (5-minutes per side).

Nutritional Values per serving: Calories: 287, Total Fat: 12.4g, Carbs: 11.6g,

Ginger Garlic Pork Ribs

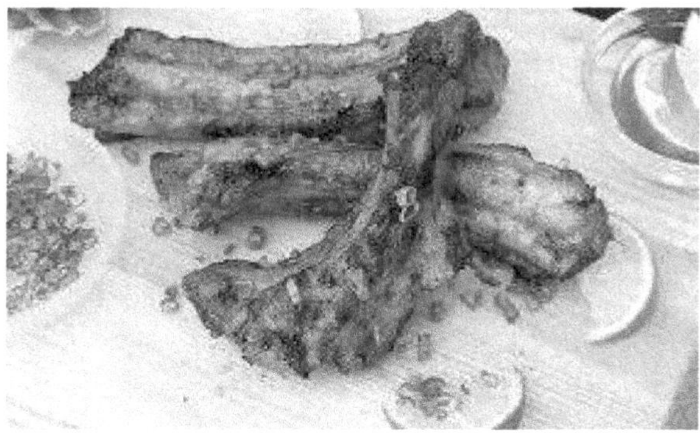

Cook Time: 40 minutes

Servings: 2

Ingredients:

1lb. baby pork ribs

1 tablespoon olive oil

1 tablespoon hoisin sauce

½ tablespoon honey

½ tablespoon soy sauce

3 garlic cloves, minced

Directions:

In a bowl, add the ingredients and mix well. Place the marinated ribs in fridge for 2-hours. Place marinated ribs in air fryer basket at 320°Fahrenheit for 40-minutes.

Nutritional Values per serving:, Calories: 287, Total Fat: 12.5g, Carbs: 11.5g, Protein: 16.2g

Bacon Wrapped Scallops

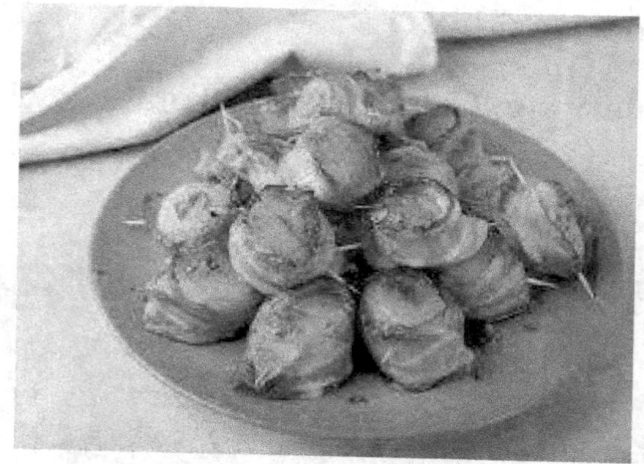

Cook Time: 10 minutes

Servings: 4

Ingredients:

1 tsp. paprika

1 tsp. lemon pepper

5 slices of center-cut bacon

20 raw sea scallops

Directions:

Rinse and drain scallops, placing on paper towels to soak up excess moisture.

Cut slices of bacon into 4 pieces.

Wrap each scallop with a piece of bacon, using toothpicks to secure. Sprinkle wrapped scallops with paprika and lemon pepper.

Spray air fryer basket with olive oil and add scallops.

Cook 5-6 minutes at 400 degrees, making sure to flip halfway through.

Nutritional Values per serving: Calories: 389 Fat: 17g Protein: 21g Sugar: 1g

Semolina Veggie Cutlets

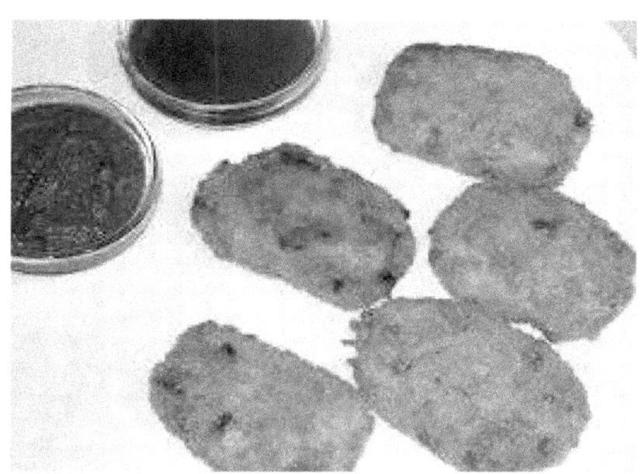

Cook Time: 23 minutes

Servings: 2

Ingredients:

1 cup semolina

Olive oil for frying

Salt and pepper to taste

1 ½ cups of your favorite veggies(suggestion: carrot, peas, green beans, bell pepper and cauliflower)

5 cups milk

Directions:

Stir and warm the milk in a saucepan over medium heat. Add vegetables when it becomes hot and cook until they are softened for about 3-minutes. Season with salt and pepper. Add the semolina to milk mixture and cook for another 10-minutes. Remove from heat and spread thin across a piece of parchment on a baking sheet, and chill for 4 hours in the fridge. Take out the baking sheet from the fridge, cut semolina mixture into cutlets. Preheat your air fryer to 350°Fahrenheit. Brush the cutlets with oil and bake for 10-minutes in your air fryer and serve with hot sauce!

Nutritional Value per serving: Calories: 252, Total Fat: 11.2g, Carbs: 10.3g, Protein: 7.3g

Perfect Cinnamon Toast

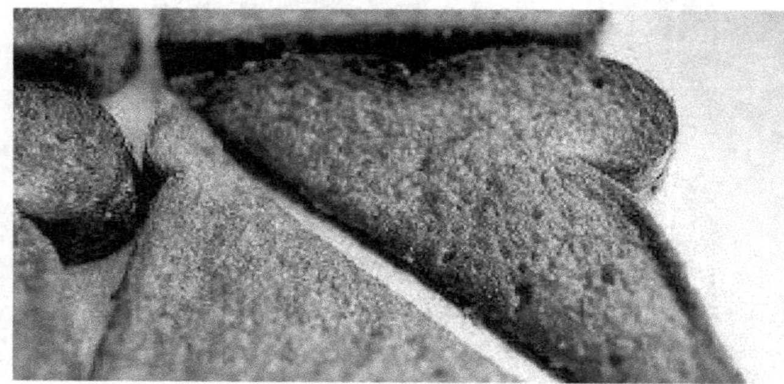

Cook Time: 5 minutes

Servings: 6

Ingredients:

2 tsp. pepper

1 ½ tsp. vanilla extract

1 ½ tsp. cinnamon

½ C. sweetener of choice

1 C. coconut oil

12 slices whole wheat bread

Directions:

Melt coconut oil and mix with sweetener until dissolved. Mix in remaining ingredients minus bread till incorporated.

Spread mixture onto bread, covering all area. Place coated pieces of bread in your air fryer.

Cook 5 minutes at 400 degrees.

Remove and cut diagonally. Enjoy!

Nutritional Values per serving: Calories: 124 Fat: 2g Protein: 0g Sugar: 4g

Chinese Pork Roast

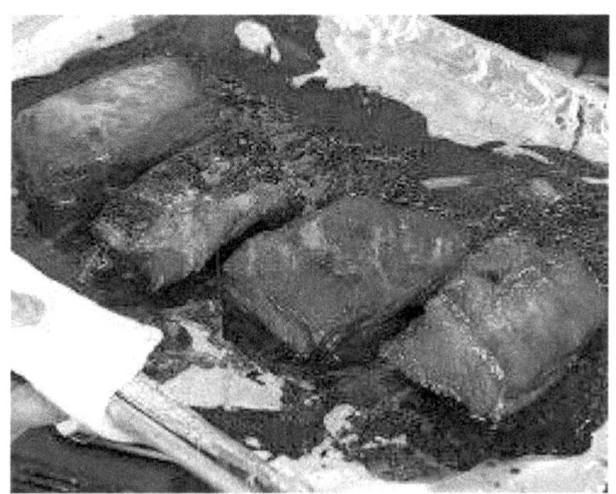

Cook Time: 15 minutes

Servings: 4

Ingredients:

2 lbs. pork shoulder, chopped

½ tablespoon salt

1/3 cup soy sauce

1 tablespoon honey

1 tablespoon liquid Stevia

Directions:

Place all the ingredients into a mixing bowl and combine well. Place marinated pork in fridge for 2-hours. Spray air fryer basket with cooking spray. Add marinated pork pieces into air fryer basket and cook at 350°Fahrenheit for 10-minutes. Now increase temperature to 400°Fahrenheit and cook for an additional 5-minutes.

Nutritional Values per serving: Calories: 283, Total Fat: 12.3g, Carbs: 11.5g, Protein: 16.7g

Air Fryer Salmon Patties

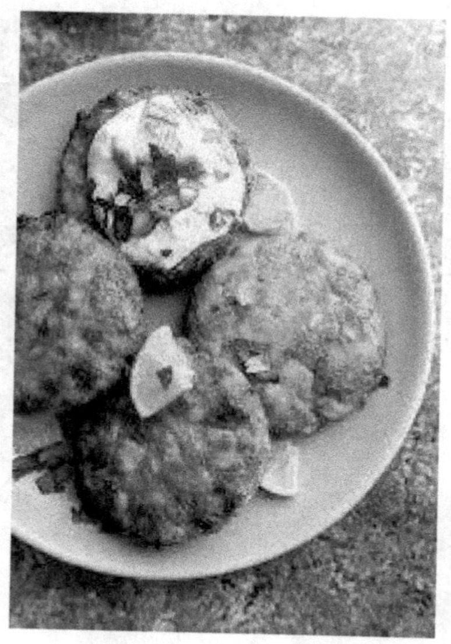

Cook Time: 15 minutes

Servings: 4

Ingredients:

1 tbsp. olive oil

1 tbsp. ghee

¼ tsp. salt

1/8 tsp. pepper

1 egg

1 C. almond flour

1 can wild Alaskan pink salmon

Directions:

Drain can of salmon into a bowl and keep liquid. Discard skin and bones.

Add salt, pepper, and egg to salmon, mixing well with hands to incorporate. Make patties.

Dredge in flour and remaining egg. If it seems dry, spoon reserved salmon liquid from the can onto patties.

Add patties to air fryer. Cook 7 minutes at 378 degrees till golden, making sure to flip once during cooking process.

Nutritional Values per serving: Calories: 437 Carbs: 55 Fat: 12g Protein: 24g Sugar: 2g

Fried Calamari

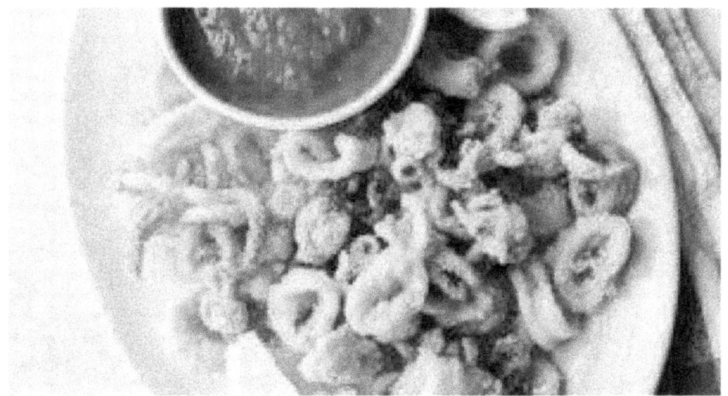

Cook Time: 15 minutes

Servings: 6-8

Ingredients:

½ tsp. salt

½ tsp. Old Bay seasoning

1/3 C. plain cornmeal

½ C. semolina flour

½ C. almond flour

5-6 C. olive oil

1 ½ pounds baby squid

Directions:

Rinse squid in cold water and slice tentacles, keeping just ¼-inch of the hood in one piece.

Combine 1-2 pinches of pepper, salt, Old Bay seasoning, cornmeal, and both flours together. Dredge squid pieces into flour mixture and place into air fryer. Spray liberally with olive oil.

Cook 15 minutes at 345 degrees till coating turns a golden brown.

Nutritional Values per serving: Calories: 211 Fat: 6g Protein: 21g Sugar: 1g

Crispy Air Fried Sushi Roll

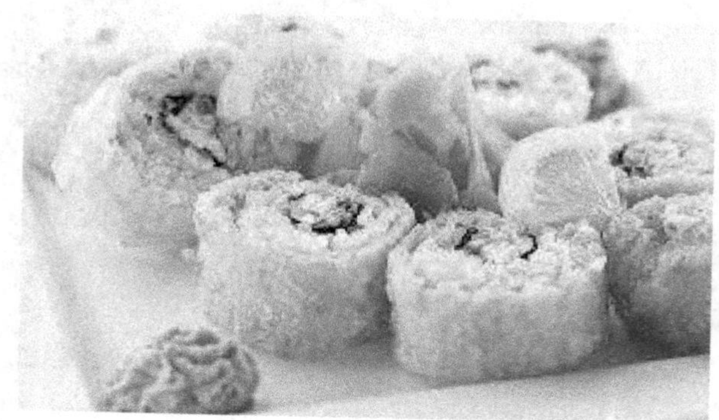

Cook Time: 15 minutes

Servings: 12

Ingredients:

Kale Salad:

1 tbsp. sesame seeds

¾ tsp. soy sauce

¼ tsp. ginger

1/8 tsp. garlic powder

¾ tsp. toasted sesame oil

½ tsp. rice vinegar

1 ½ C. chopped kale

Sriracha Mayo:

Sriracha sauce

¼ C. vegan mayo

Coating:

½ C. panko breadcrumbs

Sushi Rolls:

½ of a sliced avocado

3 sheets of sushi nori

1 batch cauliflower rice

Directions:

Combine all of kale salad ingredients together, tossing well. Set to the side.

Lay out a sheet of nori and spread a handful of rice on. Then place 2-3 tbsp. of kale salad over rice, followed by avocado. Roll up sushi.

To make mayo, whisk mayo ingredients together until smooth.

Add breadcrumbs to a bowl. Coat sushi rolls in crumbs till coated and add to air fryer.

Cook rolls 10 minutes at 390 degrees, shaking gently at 5 minutes.

Slice each roll into 6-8 pieces and enjoy!

Nutritional Values per serving: Calories: 267 Fat: 13g Protein: 6g Sugar: 3g

Air Fryer Fish Tacos

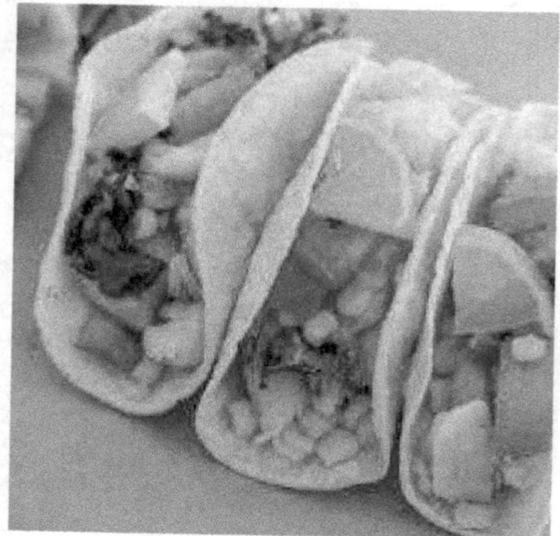

Cook Time: 5 minutes

Servings: 4

Ingredients:

1 pound cod

1 tbsp. cumin

½ tbsp. chili powder

1 ½ C. almond flour

1 ½ C. coconut flour

10 ounces Mexican beer

2 eggs

Directions:

Whisk beer and eggs together.

Whisk flours, pepper, salt, cumin, and chili powder together.
Slice cod into large pieces and coat in egg mixture then flour mixture.

Spray bottom of your air fryer basket with olive oil and add coated codpieces.

Cook 15 minutes at 375 degrees.

Serve on lettuce leaves topped with homemade salsa!

Nutritional Values per serving: Calories: 178 Fat: 10g Protein: 19g Sugar: 1g

Parmesan Shrimp

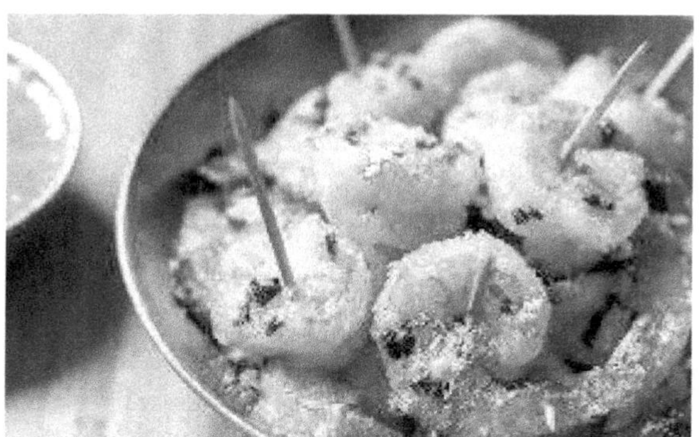

Cook Time: 10 minutes

Servings: 4-6

Ingredients:

2 tbsp. olive oil

1 tsp. onion powder

1 tsp. basil

½ tsp. oregano

1 tsp. pepper

2/3 C. grated parmesan cheese

4 minced garlic cloves

2 pounds of jumbo cooked shrimp (peeled/deveined)

Directions:

Mix all seasonings together and gently toss shrimp with mixture.

Spray olive oil into air fryer basket and add seasoned shrimp.

Cook 8-10 minutes at 350 degrees.

Squeeze lemon juice over shrimp right before devouring!

Nutritional Values per serving: Calories: 351 Fat: 11g Protein: 19g Sugar: 1g

Honey Glazed Salmon

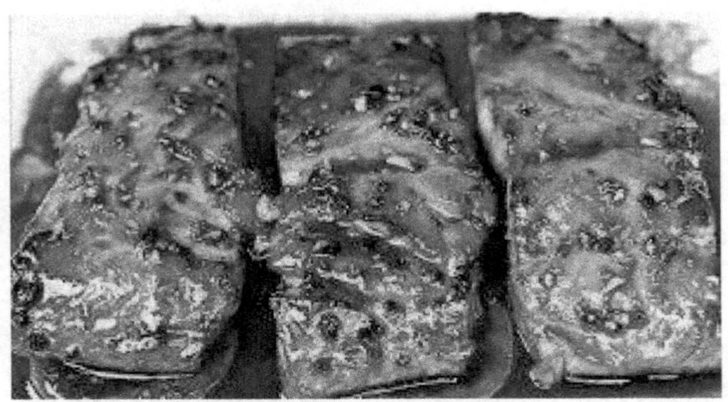

Cook Time: 5 minutes

Servings: 2

Ingredients:

1 tsp. water

3 tsp. rice wine vinegar

6 tbsp. low-sodium soy sauce

6 tbsp. raw honey

2 salmon fillets

Directions:

Combine water, vinegar, honey, and soy sauce together. Pour half of this mixture into a bowl.

Place salmon in one bowl of marinade and let chill 2 hours.

Ensure your air fryer is preheated to 356 degrees and add salmon.

Cook 8 minutes, flipping halfway through. Baste salmon with some of the remaining marinade mixture and cook another 5 minutes.

To make a sauce to serve salmon with, pour remaining marinade mixture into a saucepan, heating till simmering. Let simmer 2 minutes. Serve drizzled over salmon!

Nutritional Values per serving: Calories: 390 Fat: 8g Protein: 16g Sugar: 5g

Apple Dumplings

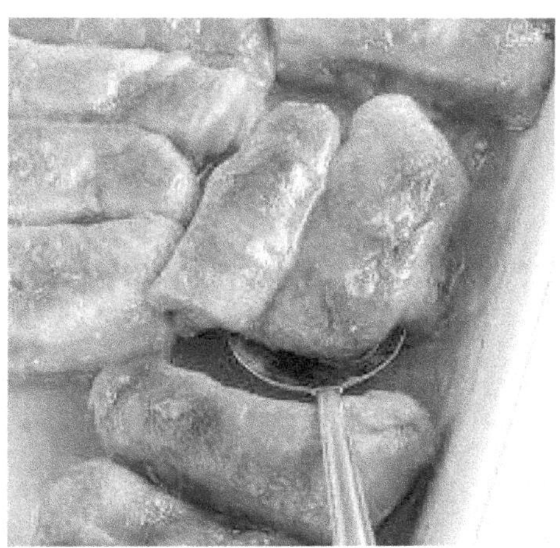

Cook Time: 15 minutes

Servings: 4

Ingredients:

2 tbsp. melted coconut oil

2 puff pastry sheets

1 tbsp. brown sugar

2 tbsp. raisins

2 small apples of choice

Directions:

Ensure your air fryer is preheated to 356 degrees.

Core and peel apples and mix with raisins and sugar.

Place a bit of apple mixture into puff pastry sheets and brush sides with melted coconut oil.

Place into air fryer. Cook 25 minutes, turning halfway through. Will be golden when done.

Nutritional Values per serving: Calories: 367 Fat: 7g Protein: 2g Sugar: 5g

Chapter 5: Dinner

Crumbed Pork & Semi-Dried Tomato Pesto

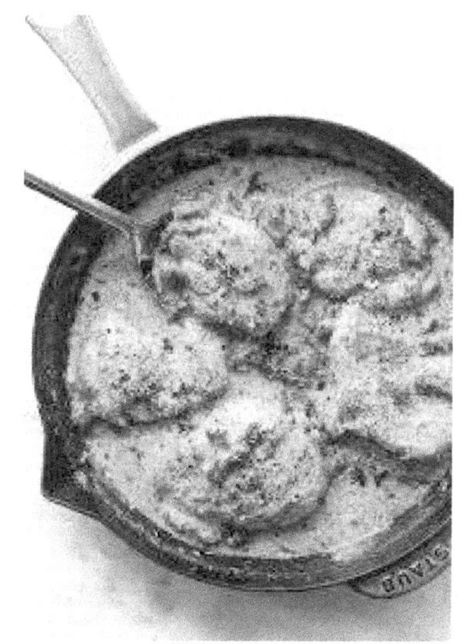

Cook Time: 20 minutes

Servings: 2

Ingredients:

½ cup milk

1 egg

1 cup breadcrumbs

1 tablespoon parmesan cheese, grated

¼ bunch of thyme, chopped

1 teaspoon pine nuts

¼ cup semi-dried tomatoes

½ cup almond flour

2 pork cutlets

1 lemon, zested

Sea salt and black pepper to taste

6 basil leaves

1 tablespoon olive oil

Directions:

Combine and whisk milk and egg in a bowl, then set aside. Mix in another bowl, breadcrumbs, parmesan, thyme, lemon zest, salt, and pepper. Add flour to another bowl. Dip pork cutlet in flour, then into egg and milk mixture, and finally into breadcrumb mixture. Preheat air fryer to 360°Fahrenheit. Spray basket with cooking spray. Set the air fryer timer to 20-minutes. Place pork inside of basket and cook until golden and crisp. Prepare the pesto: add the tomatoes, pine nuts, olive oil, and basil leaves into food processor. Blend for 20-seconds. When the pork is ready, serve with pesto and a salad of your choice.

Nutritional Values per serving: Calories: 264, Total Fat: 13.2g, Carbs: 11.7g, Protein: 16.3g

Pork Loin with Potatoes & Herbs

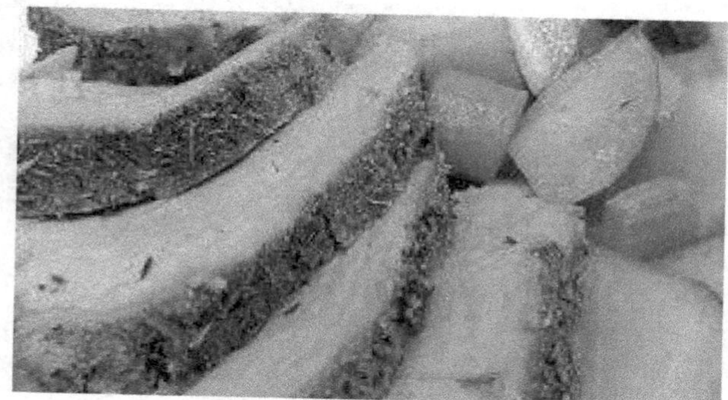

Cook Time: 25 minutes

Servings: 2

Ingredients:

2 lbs. pork loin

½ teaspoon garlic powder

½ teaspoon red pepper flakes

½ teaspoon black pepper

2 large potatoes, chunked

Directions:

Sprinkle the pork loin with garlic powder, red pepper flakes, parsley, salt, and pepper. Preheat your air fryer to 370°Fahrenheit and place pork loin and potatoes to one side in basket of air fryer. Cook for 25-minutes. Remove the pork loin and potatoes from air fryer. Allow pork loin to cool before slicing and enjoy!

Nutritional Values per serving: Calories: 268, Total Fat: 12.3g, Carbs: 11.6g, Protein: 16.2g

Tasty Beef Burgers

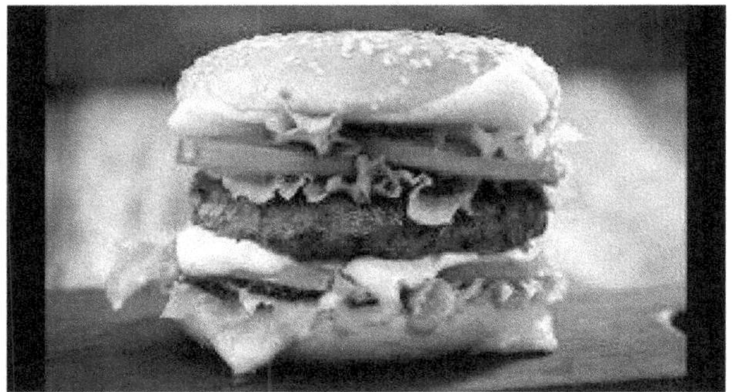

Cook Time: 18 minutes

Servings: 4

Ingredients:

1 ½ lbs. ground beef

1 tablespoon Montreal steak seasoning

1 cup cheddar cheese, shredded

1 tablespoon Worcestershire sauce

½ cup cheese sauce

Directions:

Preheat your air fryer to 370°Fahrenheit. Add the ground beef, Montreal steak seasoning, Worcestershire sauce in a bowl and mix well. Make four patties from mixture and place in preheated air fryer basket and cook for 15-minutes. Flip the patties halfway through. Combine the cheese sauce and cheddar cheese. Add cheese mixture to the top of patties and cook for an additional 3-minutes. Serve warm!

Nutritional Values per serving: Calories: 302, Total Fat: 12.3g, Carbs: 11.2g, Protein: 16.4g

Chinese Pork Ribs

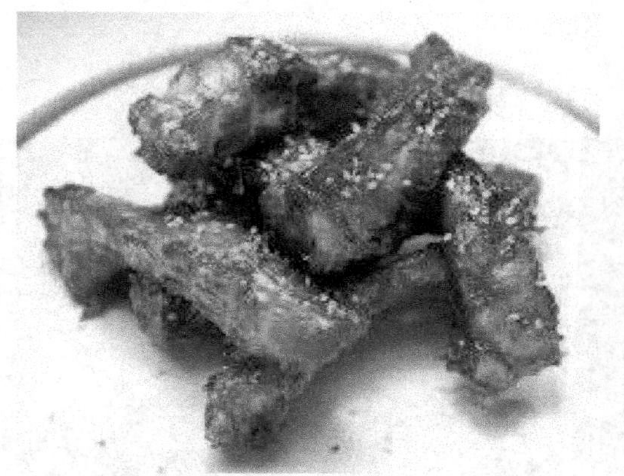

Cook Time: 40 minutes

Servings: 6

Ingredients:

4 garlic cloves, minced

1 tablespoon honey

2 lbs. pork ribs

2 tablespoons sesame oil

2 tablespoons ginger, minced

2 tablespoons hoisin sauce

2 tablespoons char Siu sauce

1 tablespoon soy sauce

Directions:

Place the ingredients in a bowl except for meat and combine well. Place the ribs in a bowl and pour the sauce over them and coat well. Place in the fridge for 4-hours. Place ribs into air fryer at 330°Fahrenheit for 40-minutes. Increase the temperature of air fryer to 350°Fahrenheit and cook for an additional 10-minutes. Serve warm.

Nutritional Values per serving: Calories: 287, Total Fat: 12.3g, Carbs: 10.6g, Protein: 16.2g

Turkey Sausage Patties

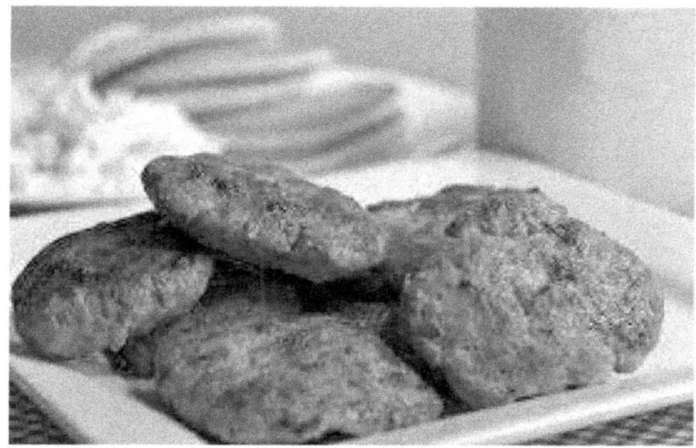

Cook Time: 4 minutes

Servings: 6

Ingredients:

1 teaspoon olive oil

1 small onion, diced

1 large garlic clove, chopped

Salt and pepper to taste

1 tablespoon vinegar

1 tablespoon chives, chopped

¾ teaspoon paprika

Pinch of nutmeg

1 lb. lean ground turkey

1 teaspoon fennel seeds

Directions:

Preheat your air fryer to 375°Fahrenheit. Add half of the oil along with onion and garlic to air fryer. Air fry for 1-minute then add fennel seeds then transfer to plate. In a mixing bowl, mix paprika, ground turkey, nutmeg, chives, vinegar, salt pepper, and onion. Mix well and form patties. Add the remaining oil to your air fryer and air fry patties for 3-minutes. Serve on buns.

Nutritional Values per serving: Calories: 302, Total Fat: 12.2g, Carbs: 10.2g, Protein: 16.3g

Pork Satay with Peanut Sauce

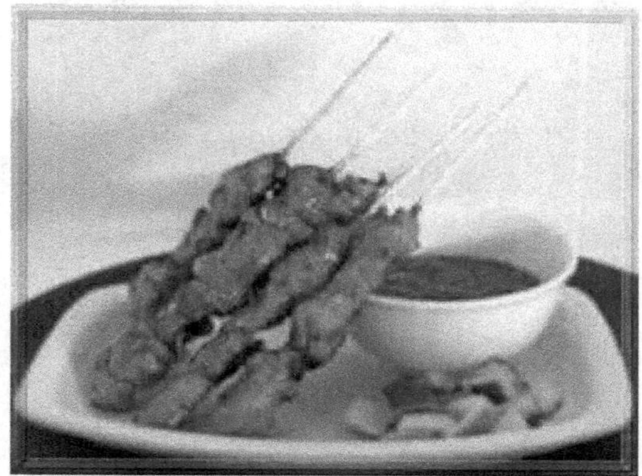

Cook Time: 21 minutes

Servings: 4

Ingredients:

1 teaspoon ground ginger

2 teaspoons hot pepper sauce

2 cloves garlic, crushed

3 tablespoons sweet soy sauce

3 ½ ounces unsalted peanuts, ground

¾ cup coconut milk

1 teaspoon ground coriander

2 tablespoons vegetable oil

14-ounces lean pork chops, in cubes of 1-inch

Directions:

In a large mixing bowl, combine hot sauce, ginger, half garlic, oil and soy sauce. Place the meat into the mixture and leave for 15-minutes to marinate. Place the meat into wire basket of your air fryer. Cook at 390°Fahrenheit for 12-minutes. Turn over halfway through cook time. For the peanut sauce, place the oil into a skillet and heat it up. Add the garlic and coriander and cook for 5-minutes, stirring often. Add the coconut milk, peanuts, hot pepper sauce and soy sauce to the pan and bring to boil. Stir often. Remove the pork from air fryer and pour sauce over it and serve warm.

Nutritional Values per serving: Calories: 262, Total Fat: 12.3g, Carbs: 11.4g, Protein: 17.3g

Onion Carrot Meatloaf

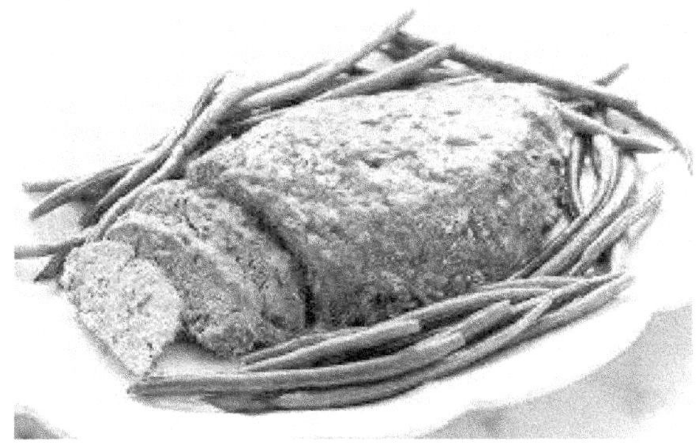

Cook Time: 25 minutes

Servings: 6

Ingredients:

1 lb. ground beef

Salt and pepper to taste

½ cup breadcrumbs

¼ cup milk

½ onion, shredded

2 carrots, shredded

1 egg

Directions:

Preheat your air fryer to 400˚Fahrenheit. Mix all your ingredients in a bowl. Add the meatloaf mixture to a loaf pan and place it in your air fryer basket. Cook in air fryer for 25-minutes and serve warm.

Nutritional Values per serving: Calories: 306, Total Fat: 12.7g, Carbs: 12.3g, Protein: 16.8g

Mozzarella Turkey Rolls

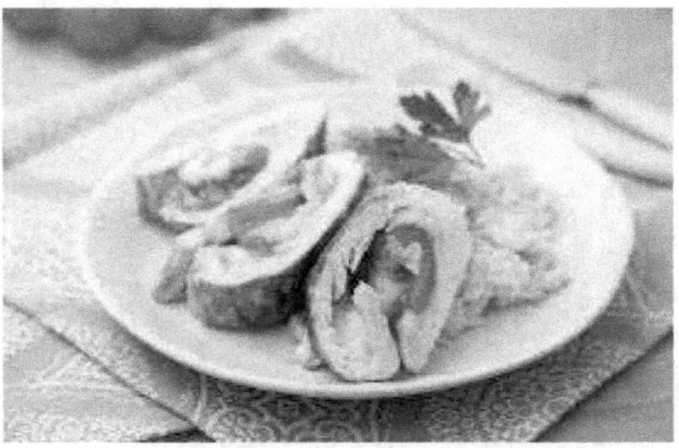

Cook Time: 10 minutes

Servings: 4

Ingredients:

4 slices turkey breast

4 chive shoots (for tying rolls)

1 tomato, sliced

½ cup basil, fresh, chopped

1 cup mozzarella, sliced

Directions:

Preheat your air fryer to 390°Fahrenheit. Place the slices of mozzarella cheese, tomato, and basil onto each slice of turkey. Roll up and tie with chive shoot. Place into air fryer and cook for 10-minutes. Serve warm.

Nutritional Values per serving: Calories: 296, Total Fat: 12.4g, Carbs: 10.2g, Protein: 16.2g

Turkey Balls Stuffed with Sage & Onion

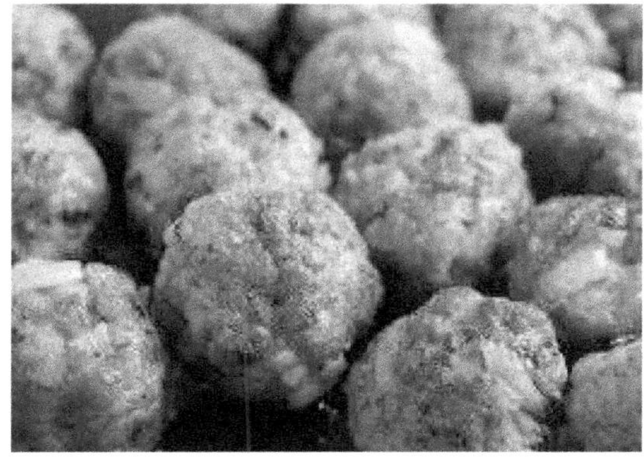

Cook Time: 15 minutes

Servings: 2

Ingredients:

3.5 ounces ground turkey

3 tablespoons breadcrumbs

Salt and pepper to taste

1 teaspoon sage

½ small onion, diced

1 egg

Directions:

Add all the ingredients into large mixing bowl and combine well. Form the mixture into small balls and put in air fryer and cook at 350°Fahrenheit for 15-minutes. Serve with tartar sauce and mashed potatoes.

Nutritional Values per serving: Calories: 268, Total Fat: 9.8g, Carbs: 8.6g, Protein: 11.9g

Chicken Schnitzel

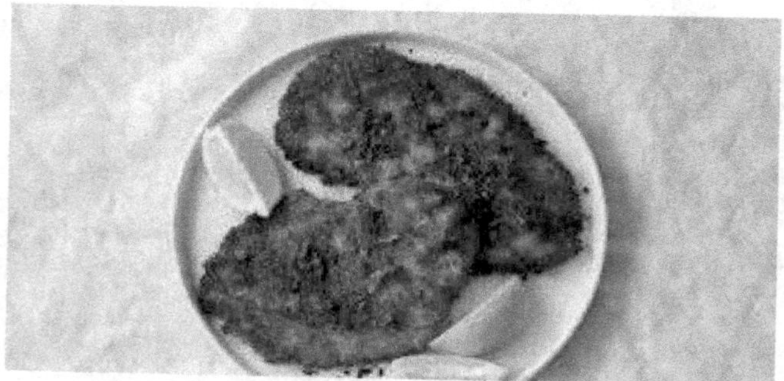

Cook Time: 12 minutes

Servings: 4

Ingredients:

2 chicken breasts

Salt and pepper to taste

Fresh parsley

2 tablespoons mustard powder

12 tablespoons gluten-free oats

2 free-range eggs

Directions:

Slice your chicken breasts into two lengthwise and use a rolling pin to roll them flat. Sprinkle with salt and pepper and then set aside. In a small bowl whisk the eggs and set aside. In your blender grind the oats with mustard, salt, pepper, and parsley. You want it to become like breadcrumbs. Place this mixture into a shallow dish. Dip chicken pieces into the egg and coat well. Next, dip them into the oats breadcrumb mixture. Place chicken pieces in your air fryer and cook for 12-minutes at 350°Fahrenheit. Flip over the chicken pieces halfway through the cook time.

Nutritional Values per serving: Calories: 282, Total Fat: 10.2g, Carbs: 8.7g, Protein: 14.8g

Turkey & Cheese Calzone

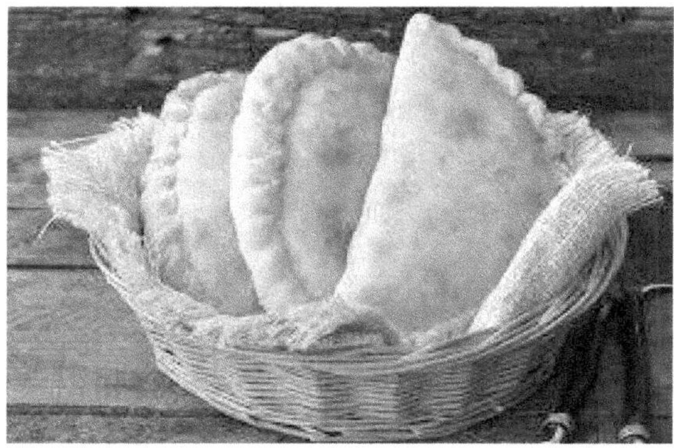

Cook Time: 10 minutes

Servings: 4

Ingredients:

1 free-range egg, beaten

¼ cup mozzarella cheese, grated

1 cup cheddar cheese, grated

1-ounce bacon, diced, cooked

Cooked turkey, shredded

4 tablespoons tomato sauce

Salt and pepper to taste

1 teaspoon thyme

1 teaspoon basil

1 teaspoon oregano

1 package frozen pizza dough

Directions:

Roll the pizza dough out into small circles, the same size as a small pizza. Add thyme, oregano, basil into a bowl with tomato sauce and mix well. Pour a small amount of sauce onto your pizza bases and spread across the surface. Add the turkey, bacon, and cheese. Brush the edge of dough with beaten egg, then fold over and pinch to seal. Brush the outside with more egg. Place into air fryer and cook at 350°Fahrenehit for 10-minutes. Serve warm.

Nutritional Values per serving: Calories: 289, Total Fat: 11.2g, Carbs: 10.3g, Protein: 11.4g

Country Style Ribs

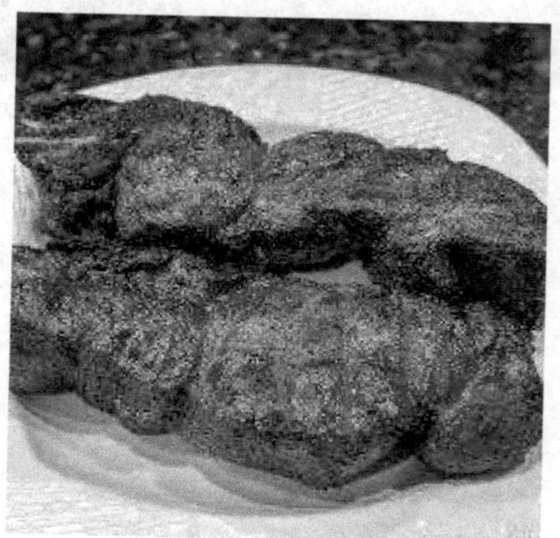

Cook Time: 12 minutes

Servings: 4

Ingredients:

4 country-style pork ribs, trimmed of excess fat

Salt and black pepper to taste

1 teaspoon dried marjoram

1 teaspoon garlic powder

1 teaspoon thyme

2 teaspoons dry mustard

3 tablespoons coconut oil

3 tablespoons cornstarch

Directions:

Preheat the air fryer to 400°Fahrenheit for 2 minutes. Place ingredients in a bowl, except pork ribs. Soak the ribs in the mixture and rub in. Place the ribs into air fryer for 12-minutes. Serve and enjoy!

Nutritional Value per serving: Calories: 265, Total Fat: 12.6g, Carbs: 12.2g, Protein: 16.5g

Air Fryer Classic Beef Pot Roast

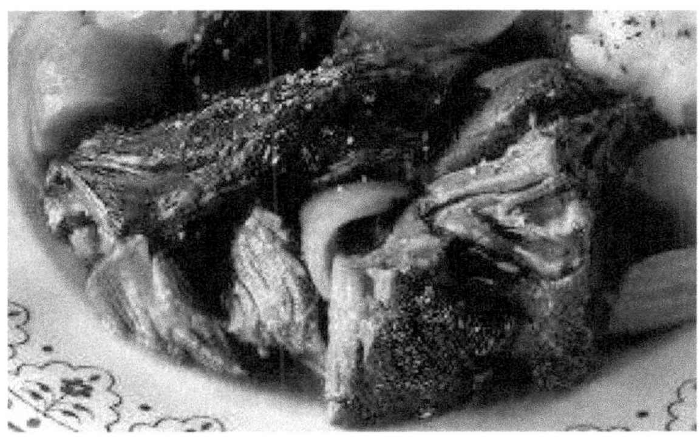

Cook Time: 60 minutes

Servings: 4

Ingredients:

1 lb. chuck roast

4 spring onions

2 cinnamon sticks

2 tablespoons of ginger garlic paste

2 tablespoons of olive oil

1 teaspoon paprika

2 cardamoms

1 cup of water

½ cup of fresh coriander, chopped

Salt and pepper to taste

1 bay leaf

Directions:

Preheat your air fryer to 400°Fahrenheit. Cut the chuck roast into medium-sized chunks. In a large bowl, add beef, onion, ginger garlic paste, salt, pepper, bay leaf, coriander, cardamoms, paprika, and water. Mix well and marinate for 1-hour. Add everything to casserole dish and roast in the air fryer for 1-hour. Remove bay leaf then serve hot!

Nutritional Values per serving: Calories: 303, Total Fat: 12.6g, Carbs: 11.3g, Protein: 16.4g

Sweet & Tangy Meatballs

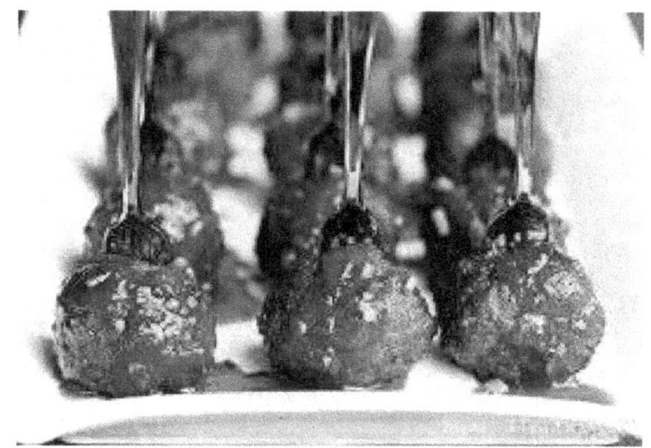

Cook Time: 15 minutes

Servings: 24

Ingredients:

1 lb. ground beef

1 tablespoon liquid stevia

½ teaspoon dry mustard

½ teaspoon ginger, ground

¾ cup tomato ketchup

1 tablespoon Tabasco sauce

1 tablespoon Worcestershire sauce

¼ cup vinegar

1 tablespoon lemon juice

Directions:

In a bowl, combine all the ingredients. Make small meatballs from the mixture and place them in air fryer basket. Air fry meatballs at 370°Fahrenheit for 15-minutes. Serve warm.

Nutritional Values per serving: Calories: 298, Total Fat: 12.2g, Carbs: 11.6g, Protein: 15.8g

Cheese Burgers

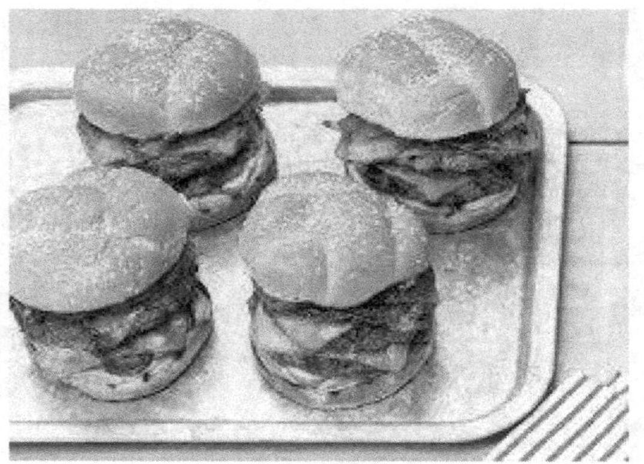

Cook Time: 11 minutes

Servings: 6

Ingredients:

1 lb. ground beef

6 slices cheddar cheese

Salt and pepper to taste

Directions:

Preheat the air fryer to 350°Fahrenheit. Season ground beef with pepper and salt. Make six patties from the mixture and place them into air fryer basket. Air fry patties for 10-minutes. After 10-minutes, place cheese slices over patties and cook for another minute. Serve warm.

Nutritional Values per serving: Calories: 302, Total Fat: 12.5g, Carbs: 12.2g, Protein: 16.2g

Air Fryer Beef Fajitas

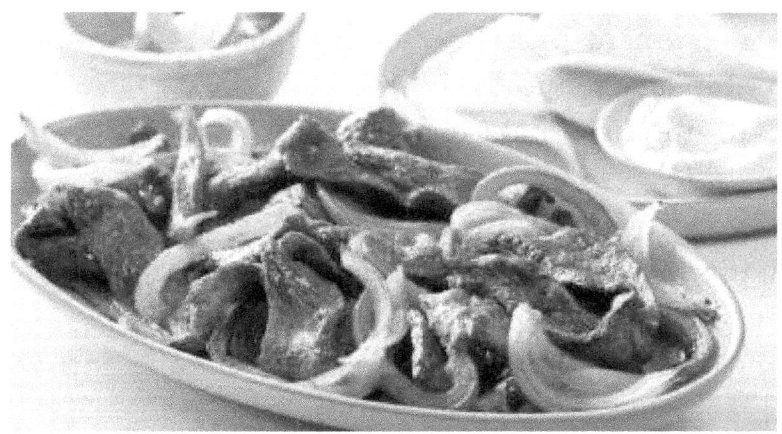

Calories: 412 Fat: 21g Protein: 13g Sugar: 1g

Cook Time: 5 minutes

Servings: 4-6

Ingredients:

Beef:

- 1/8 C. carne asada seasoning
- 2 pounds beef flap meat
- Diet 7-Up

Fajita veggies:

- 1 tsp. chili powder
- 1-2 tsp. pepper
- 1-2 tsp. salt
- 2 bell peppers, your choice of color
- 1 onion

Directions:

- Slice flap meat into manageable pieces and place into a bowl. Season meat with carne seasoning and pour diet soda over meat. Cover and chill overnight.
- Ensure your air fryer is preheated to 380 degrees.

- Place a parchment liner into air fryer basket and spray with olive oil. Place beef in layers into the basket.
- Cook 8-10 minutes, making sure to flip halfway through. Remove and set to the side.
- Slice up veggies and spray air fryer basket. Add veggies to the fryer and spray with olive oil. Cook 10 minutes at 400 degrees, shaking 1-2 times during cooking process.
- Serve meat and veggies on wheat tortillas and top with favorite keto fillings!

Turkey Breast with Maple Mustard Glaze

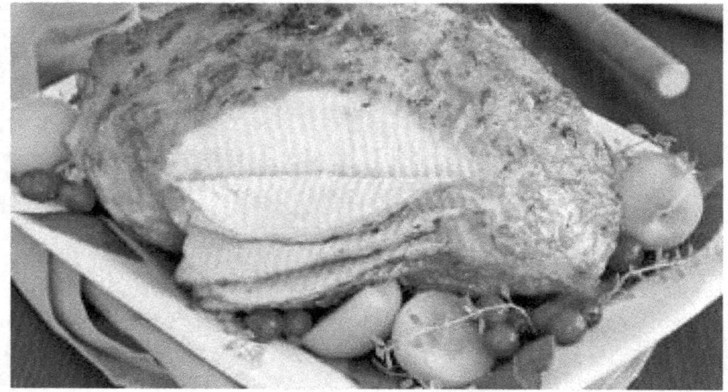

Cook Time: 49 minutes

Servings: 6

Ingredients:

5 lbs. turkey breast

1 tablespoon unsalted butter

2 tablespoons Dijon mustard

¼ cup sugar-free maple syrup

½ teaspoon black pepper

1 teaspoon sea salt

½ teaspoon paprika

1 teaspoon dried thyme

1 tablespoon olive oil

½ teaspoon sage

Directions:

Preheat your air fryer to 350°Fahrenheit. Prepare the turkey breast by brushing it with olive oil. Combine salt, pepper, paprika, sage, thyme in a bowl. Cover the turkey breast with this mixture. Place the turkey breast inside air fryer and cook for 25-minutes. Turn and cook for another 12-minutes. Turn once more and cook for an additional 12-minutes. Use a small saucepan to mix mustard, melted butter, and maple syrup, stir well. When turkey breast is done cooking, cover with sauce. Then air-fry for another 5-minutes. Take the turkey out of air fryer and set aside for at least 5-minutes, covering with aluminum foil. Slice turkey and serve.

Nutritional Values per serving: Calories: 268, Total Fat: 10.2g, Carbs: 8.5g, Protein: 14.3g

Beef Empanadas

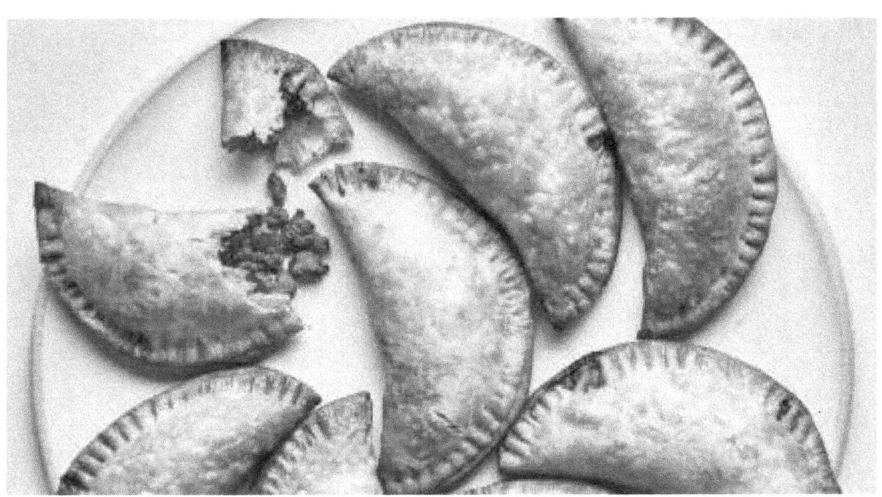

Calories: 183 Fat: 5g Protein: 11g Sugar: 2g

Cook Time: 15 minutes

Servings: 8

Ingredients:

- 1 tsp. water
- 1 egg white
- 1 C. picadillo
- 8 Goya empanada discs (thawed)

Directions:

- Ensure your air fryer is preheated to 325. Spray basket with olive oil.
- Place 2 tablespoons of picadillo into the center of each disc. Fold disc in half and use a fork to seal edges. Repeat with all ingredients.
- Whisk egg white with water and brush tops of empanadas with egg wash.
- Add 2-3 empanadas to air fryer, cooking 8 minutes until golden. Repeat till you cook all filled empanadas.

Air Fryer Burgers

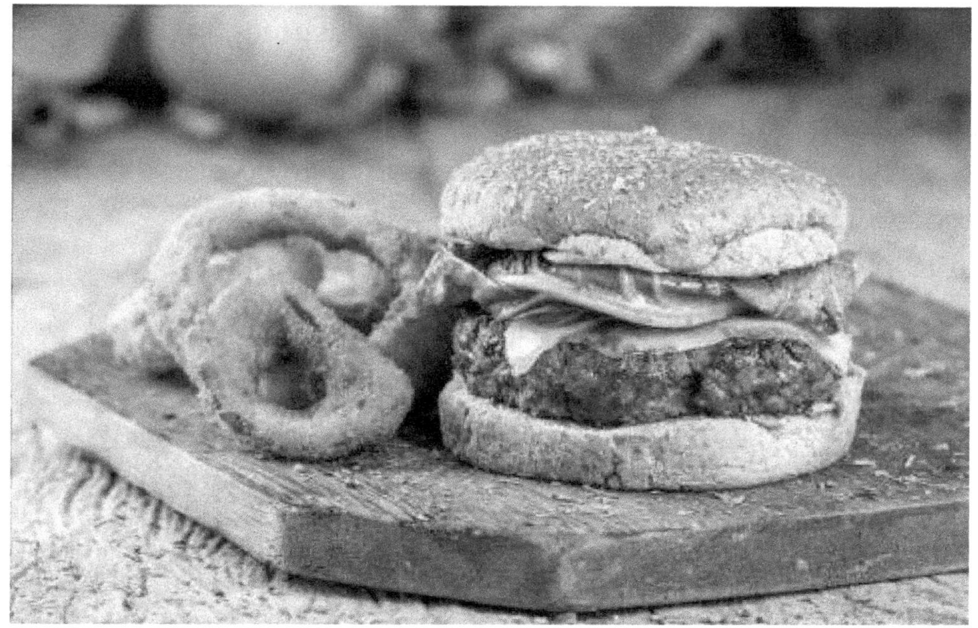

Calories: 148 Fat: 5g Protein: 24g Sugar: 1g

Cook Time: 10 minutes

Servings: 4

Ingredients:

- 1 pound lean ground beef
- ½ tsp. garlic powder
- ½ tsp. dried oregano
- ½ tsp. pepper
- ½ tsp. salt
- ½ tsp. onion powder
- Few drops of liquid smoke
- 1 tsp. Worcestershire sauce
- 1 tsp. dried parsley

Directions:

- Ensure your air fryer is preheated to 350 degrees.
- Mix all seasonings together till combined.
- Place beef in a bowl and add seasonings. Mix well, but do not overmix.
- Make 4 patties from the mixture and using your thumb, making an indent in the center of each patty.
- Add patties to air fryer basket and cook 10 minutes. No need to turn!

Roasted Stuffed Peppers

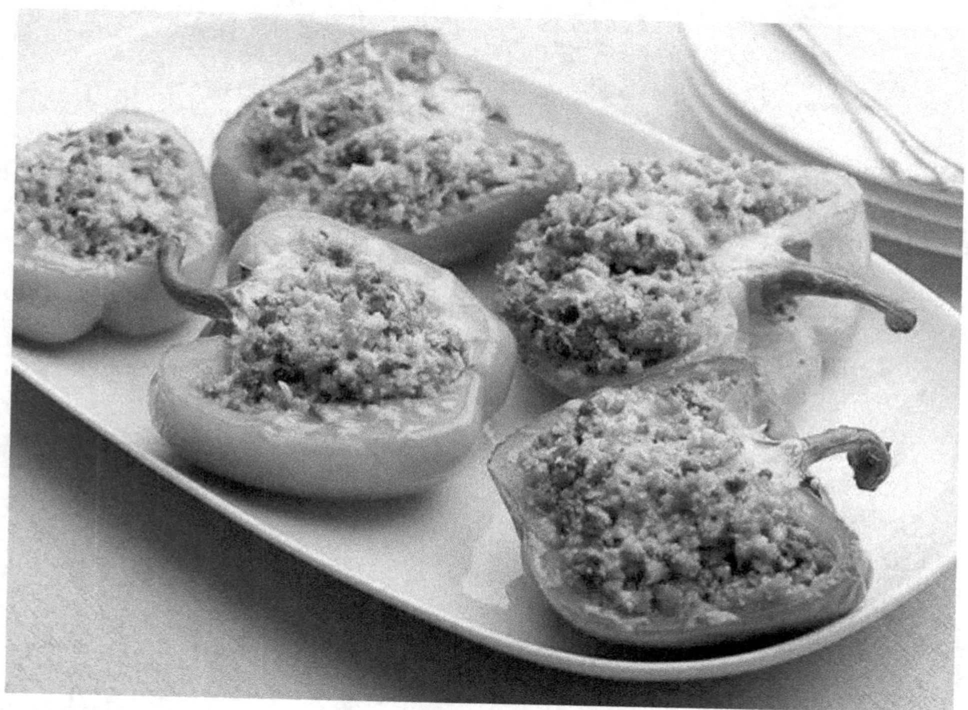

Calories: 295 Fat: 8g Protein: 23g Sugar: 2g

Cook Time: 5 minutes

Servings: 4

Ingredients:

- 4 ounces shredded cheddar cheese
- ½ tsp. pepper
- ½ tsp. salt
- 1 tsp. Worcestershire sauce
- ½ C. tomato sauce
- 8 ounces lean ground beef
- 1 tsp. olive oil
- 1 minced garlic clove
- ½ chopped onion
- 2 green peppers

Directions:

- Ensure your air fryer is preheated to 390 degrees. Spray with olive oil.
- Cut stems off bell peppers and remove seeds. Cook in boiling salted water for 3 minutes.
- Sauté garlic and onion together in a skillet until golden in color.
- Take skillet off the heat. Mix pepper, salt, Worcestershire sauce, ¼ cup of tomato sauce, half of cheese and beef together.
- Divide meat mixture into pepper halves. Top filled peppers with remaining cheese and tomato sauce.
- Place filled peppers in air fryer and bake 15-20 minutes.

Air Fryer Beef Steak

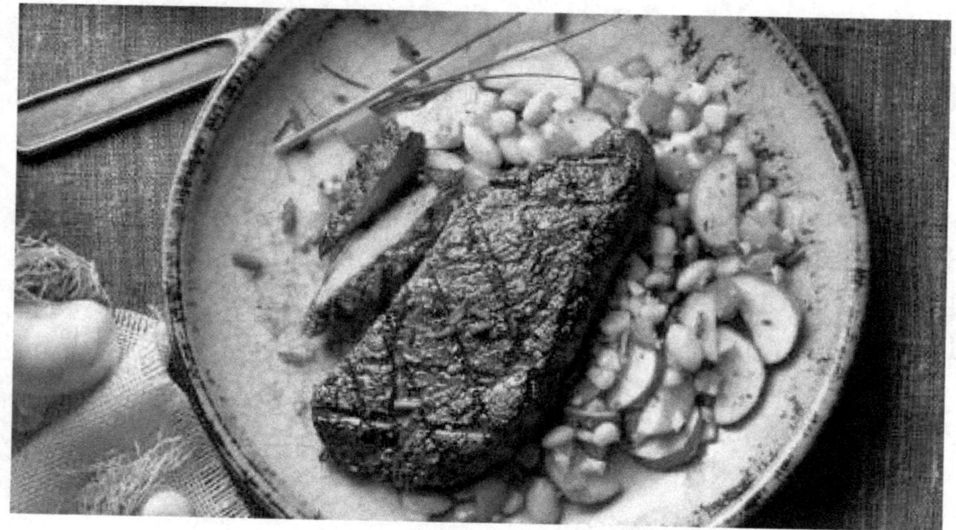

Calories: 233 Fat: 19g Protein: 16g Sugar: 0g

Cook Time: 17 minutes

Servings: 4

Ingredients:

- 1 tbsp. olive oil
- Pepper and salt
- 2 pounds of ribeye steak

Directions:

- Season meat on both sides with pepper and salt.
- Rub all sides of meat with olive oil.
- Preheat air fryer to 356 degrees and spritz with olive oil.
- Cook steak 7 minutes. Flip and cook an additional 6 minutes.
- Let meat sit 2-5 minutes to rest. Slice and serve with salad.

Beef and Broccoli

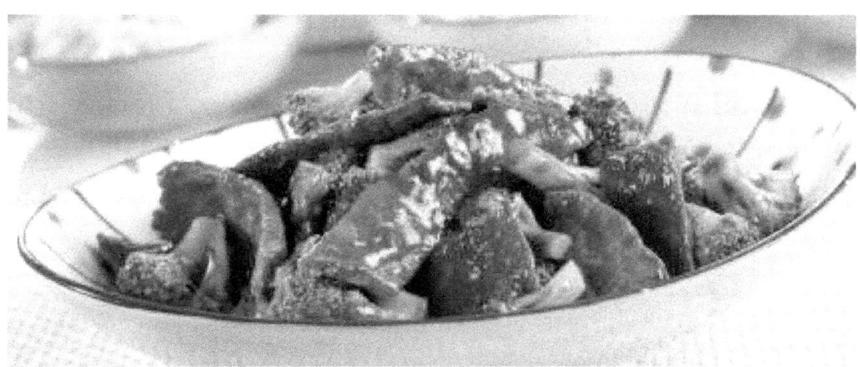

Calories: 384 Fat: 16g Protein: 19g Sugar: 4g

Cook Time: 10 minutes

Servings: 4

Ingredients:

- 1 minced garlic clove
- 1 sliced ginger root
- 1 tbsp. olive oil
- 1 tsp. almond flour
- 1 tsp. sweetener of choice
- 1 tsp. low-sodium soy sauce
- 1/3 C. sherry
- 2 tsp. sesame oil
- 1/3 C. oyster sauce
- 1 pounds of broccoli
- ¾ pound round steak

Directions:

- Remove stems from broccoli and slice into florets. Slice steak into thin strips.
- Combine sweetener, soy sauce, sherry, almond flour, sesame oil, and oyster sauce together, stirring till sweetener dissolves.
- Put strips of steak into the mixture and allow to marinate 45 minutes to 2 hours.
- Add broccoli and marinated steak to air fryer. Place garlic, ginger, and olive oil on top.
- Cook 12 minutes at 400 degrees. Serve with cauliflower rice!

Coconut Shrimp

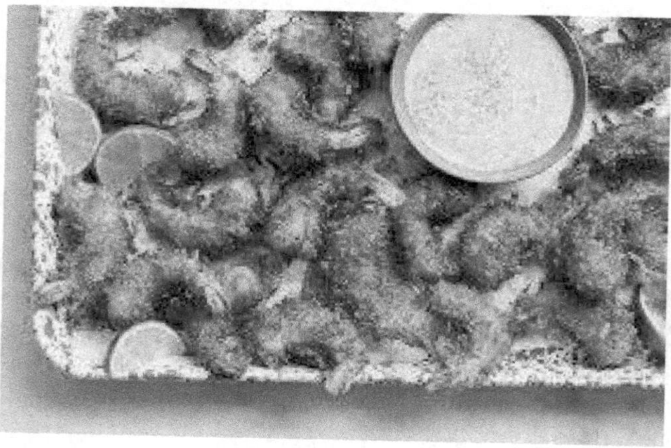

Calories: 213 Fat: 8g Protein: 15g Sugar: 3g

Cook Time: 5 minutes

Servings: 3

Ingredients:

- 1 C. almond flour
- 1 C. panko breadcrumbs
- 1 tbsp. coconut flour
- 1 C. unsweetened, dried coconut

- 1 egg white
- 12 raw large shrimp

Directions:

- Put shrimp on paper towels to drain.
- Mix coconut and panko breadcrumbs together. Then mix in coconut flour and almond flour in a different bowl. Set to the side.
- Dip shrimp into flour mixture, then into egg white, and then into coconut mixture.
- Place into air fryer basket. Repeat with remaining shrimp.
- Cook 10 minutes at 350 degrees. Turn halfway through cooking process.

Air Fryer Salmon

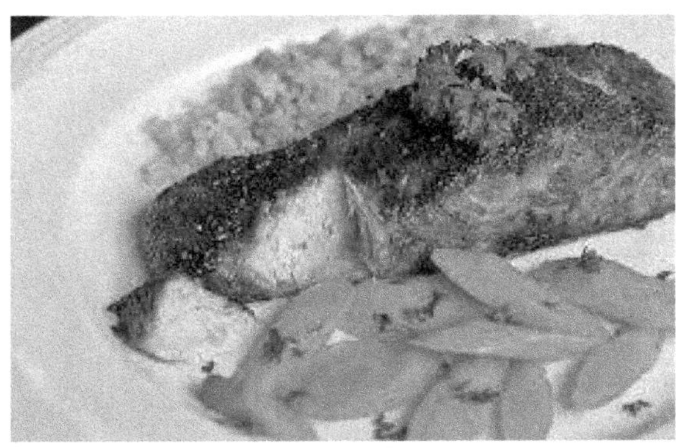

Calories: 185 Fat: 11g Protein: 21g Sugar: 0g

Cook Time: 5 minutes

Servings: 2

Ingredients:

- ½ tsp. salt
- ½ tsp. garlic powder
- ½ tsp. smoked paprika
- Salmon

Directions:

- Mix spices together and sprinkle onto salmon.
- Place seasoned salmon into air fryer.
- Cook 8-10 minutes at 400 degrees.

Healthy Fish and Chips

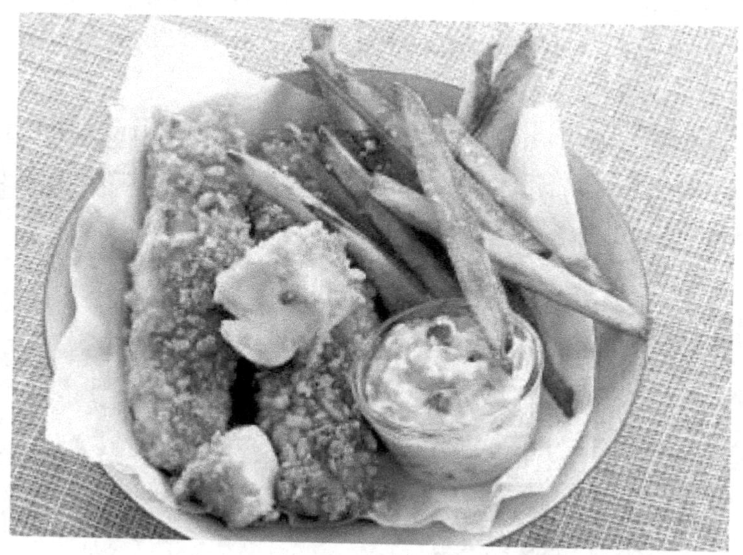

Calories: 219 Carbs: 18 Fat: 5g Protein: 25g Sugar: 1g

Cook Time: 15 minutes

Servings: 3

Ingredients:

- Old Bay seasoning
- ½ C. panko breadcrumbs
- 1 egg
- 2 tbsp. almond flour
- 2 4-6 ounce tilapia fillets
- Frozen crinkle cut fries

Directions:

- Add almond flour to one bowl, beat egg in another bowl, and add panko breadcrumbs to the third bowl, mixed with Old Bay seasoning.
- Dredge tilapia in flour, then egg, and then breadcrumbs.
- Place coated fish in air fryer along with fries.
- Cook 15 minutes at 390 degrees.

Chapter 6: Appetizers & Side Dishes

Spanish Style Spiced Potatoes

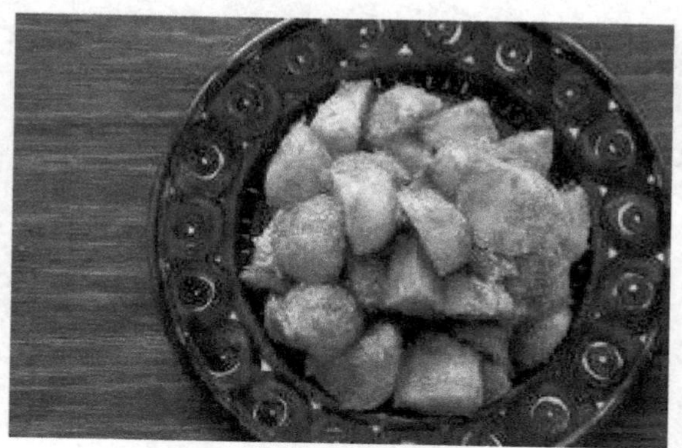

Cook Time: 23 minutes

Servings: 4

Ingredients:

3 potatoes, peeled and chopped into chips

1 onion, diced

½ cup tomato sauce

1 tomato, thinly sliced

1 tablespoon red wine vinegar

2 tablespoons olive oil

1 teaspoon paprika

1 teaspoon chili powder

Salt and pepper to taste

1 teaspoon rosemary

1 teaspoon oregano

1 teaspoon mixed spice

2 teaspoons coriander

Directions:

Toss the chips in the olive oil and cook in your air fryer for 15-minutes at 360°Fahrenheit. Mix remaining ingredients in a baking dish. Place the sauce in air fryer for 8-minutes. Toss the potatoes in the sauce and serve warm!

Nutritional Values per serving: Calories: 265, Total Fat: 7,3g, Carbs: 6.2g, Protein: 5.2g

Bell Peppers with Potato Stuffing

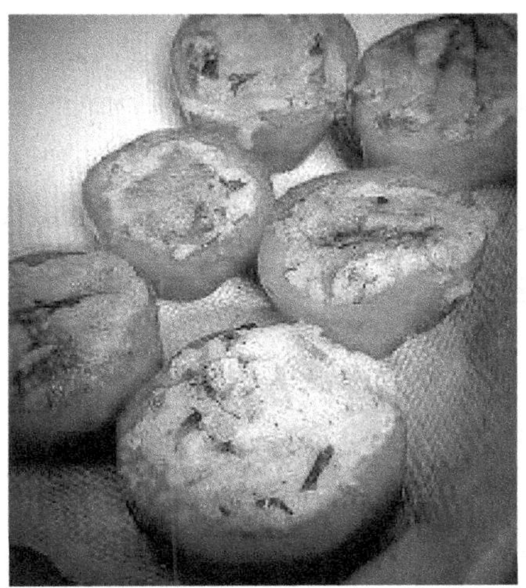

Cook Time: 20 minutes

Servings: 4

Ingredients:

4 green bell peppers, top cut and deseeded

4 potatoes, boiled, peeled and mashed

2 onions, finely chopped

1 teaspoon lemon juice

2 tablespoons coriander leaves, chopped

2 green chilies, finely chopped

Olive oil as needed

Salt to taste

¼ teaspoon Garam Masala

½ teaspoon chili powder

¼ teaspoon turmeric powder

1 teaspoon cumin seeds

Directions:

Heat the oil in a pan and sautė the onion, chilies and cumin seeds. Add the rest of the ingredients except the bell peppers and mix well. Preheat your air fryer to 390°Fahrenheit for 10-minutes. Brush your bell peppers with olive oil, inside and out and stuff each pepper with potato mixture. Place in air fryer basket and grill for 10-minutes. Check and grill for an additional 5-minutes.

Nutritional Values per serving: Calories: 282, Total Fat: 9.2g, Carbs: 7.1g, Protein: 4.2g

Chopped Liver with Eggs

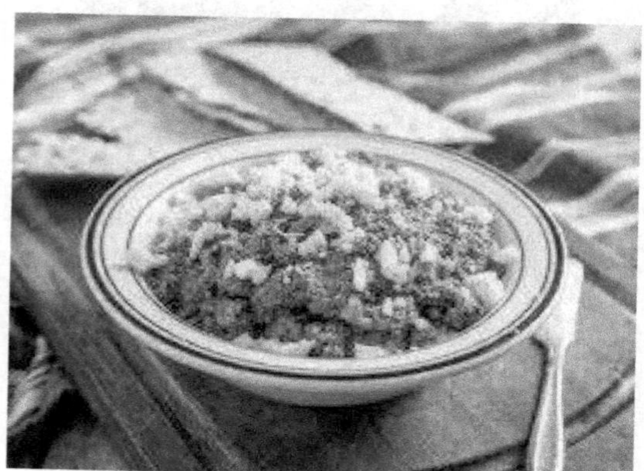

Cook Time: 12 minutes

Servings: 2

Ingredients:

2 large eggs

1 lb. sliced liver

Salt and pepper to taste

1 tablespoon cream

½ tablespoon black truffle oil

1 tablespoon butter

Directions:

Preheat your air fryer to 340°Fahrenheit. Cut liver into thin slices and place in the fridge. Separate the whites from the yolks of the eggs and put each yolk in a cup. In another bowl, add the cream, the black truffle oil, salt, pepper and beat to combine. Take the liver and arrange half of the mixture in a small ramekin. Pour the white of the egg and divide equally between two ramekins. Put the yolks on top. Surround the yolks with the liver and cook for 12-minutes. Serve cool.

Nutritional Values per serving: Calories: 374, Total Fat: 10g, Carbs: 8.5g, Protein: 59g

Bacon & Veggie Mash

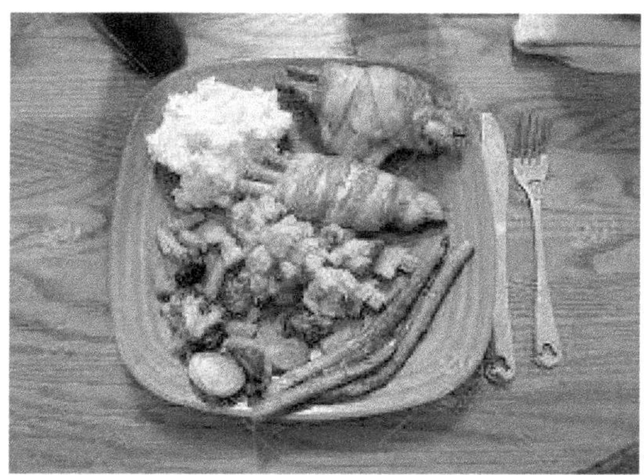

Cook Time: 1 hour and 15 minutes

Servings: 8

Ingredients:

4 strips of bacon, chopped into pieces

1 tablespoon butter

¾ cup Yellow onion, diced

½ cup red bell pepper, diced

¼ cup celery, diced

2 teaspoons garlic, minced

¾ teaspoon fresh thyme leaves

1 ½ cups whole milk

3 eggs

½ cup heavy cream

1 teaspoon sea salt

¼ teaspoon cayenne pepper

3 cups day-old bread, cubed

3 tablespoons parmesan cheese, grated

1 cup Monterey Jack cheese grated

Seasoning:

2 ½ teaspoons paprika

2 teaspoons salt

2 teaspoons garlic powder

1 teaspoon black pepper

1 teaspoon onion powder

1 teaspoon cayenne pepper

1 teaspoon oregano, dried

1 teaspoon thyme, dried

Directions:

Grease a casserole dish with the butter. Cook bacon in small frying pan until crisp, then place aside. Cook the corn in the pan until caramelized for about 10-minutes, then add in celery, onion, bell pepper and cook for an additional 5-minutes. Mix in the thyme and garlic and remove from heat. Stir in the eggs, milk, and cream, whisking well to combine. Add in salt, cayenne pepper, bread and Monterey Jack cheese. Transfer to casserole dish and place in air fryer basket. Cook for 30-minutes at 320°Fahrenheit. Sprinkle with parmesan cheese and cook for another 30-minutes.

Nutritional Values per serving: Calories: 42, Total Fat: 8.3g, Carbs: 9.5g, Protein: 16.2g

Spicy Cheesy Breaded Mushrooms

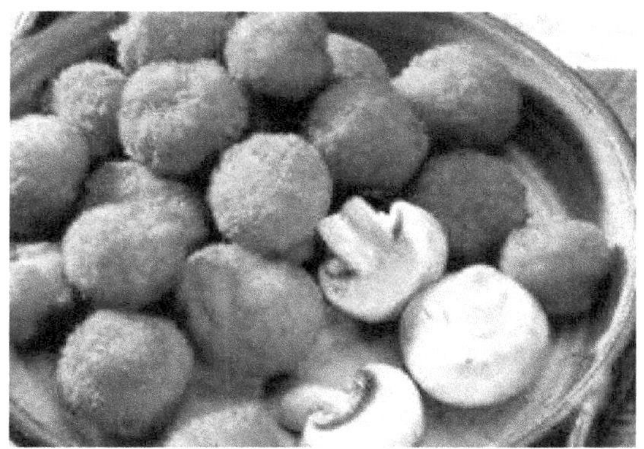

Cook Time: 7 minutes

Servings: 2

Ingredients:

8-ounces of Button mushrooms (pat dried)

1 egg

Almond flour as required

3-ounces parmesan cheese, freshly grated

Breadcrumbs as needed

Salt and pepper to taste

1 teaspoon paprika

Directions:

Mix the cheese and the breadcrumbs and paprika in a mixing bowl. Whisk the egg in another bowl. Dredge the Button mushrooms in the flour, dip in egg then coat them in breadcrumb mix. Cook for 7-minutes in your air fryer at 360° Fahrenheit, tossing once halfway through cook time.

Nutritional Values per serving: Calories: 203, Total Fat: 4.2g, Carbs: 3.2g, Protein: 3.6g

Chickpea & Zucchini Burgers

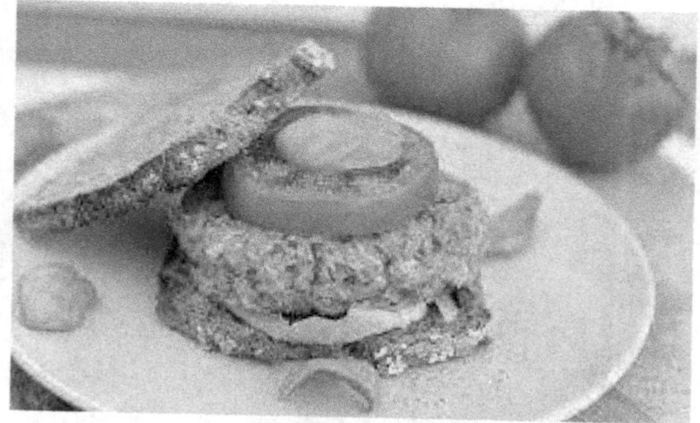

Cook Time: 10 minutes

Servings: 4

Ingredients:

1 can of chickpeas, strained

1 red onion, diced

2 eggs, beaten

1-ounce almond flour

3 tablespoons coriander

1 teaspoon garlic puree

1-ounce cheddar cheese, shredded

1 Courgette, spiralized

1 teaspoon chili powder

Salt and pepper to taste

1 teaspoon mixed spice

Directions:

Add your ingredients to a bowl and mix well. Shape portions of the mixture into burgers. Place in the air fryer for 15-minutes until cooked.

Nutritional Values per serving: Calories: 263, Total Fat: 11.2g, Carbs: 8.3g, Protein: 6.3g

Turmeric & Garlic Roasted Carrots

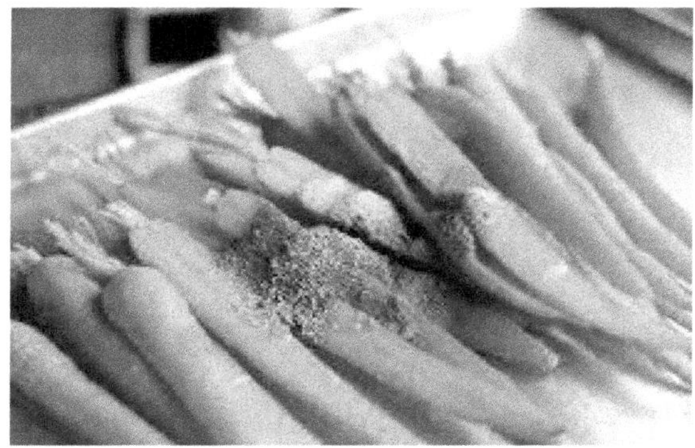

Cook Time: 20 minutes

Servings: 4

Ingredients:

21-ounces of carrots, peeled

1 handful of fresh coriander

1 teaspoon turmeric

1 tablespoon olive oil

1 teaspoon garlic, minced

Directions:

Lightly drizzle the olive oil over the carrots and sprinkle the turmeric and garlic over them. Place in pan in air fryer and cook for 20-minutes at 290°Fahrenheit. Toss once during cook time. Serve carrots garnished with fresh coriander.

Nutritional Values per serving: Calories: 60, Total Fat: 0.35g, Carbs: 10.2g, Protein: 0.48g

Vegetable Fries

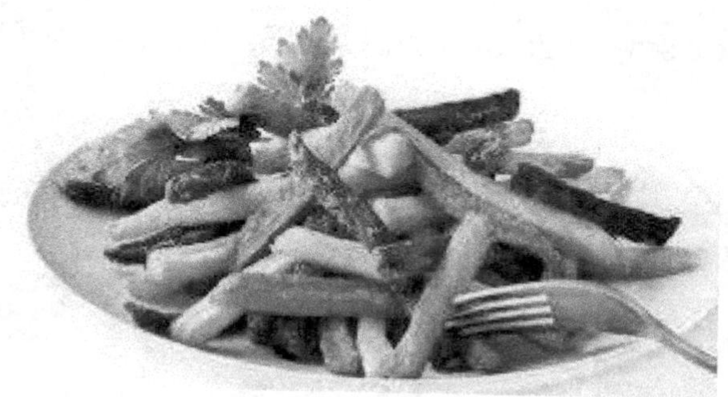

Cook Time: 18 minutes

Servings: 4

Ingredients:

5-ounces sweet potatoes, peeled and chopped as chips

5-ounces Courgette, peeled and chopped as chips

5-ounces carrots, peeled and chopped as chips

2 tablespoons olive oil

Salt and pepper to taste

Pinch of basil

Pinch of mixed spice

Directions:

Toss the veggies in olive oil and place in an air fryer preheated to 360˚Fahrenehit for 18-minutes. Toss twice during cook time. Season with salt, pepper, and other seasonings.

Nutritional Values per serving: Calories: 42, Total Fat: 1.3g, Carbs: 2.1g, Protein: 1.4g

Spicy Mango Okra

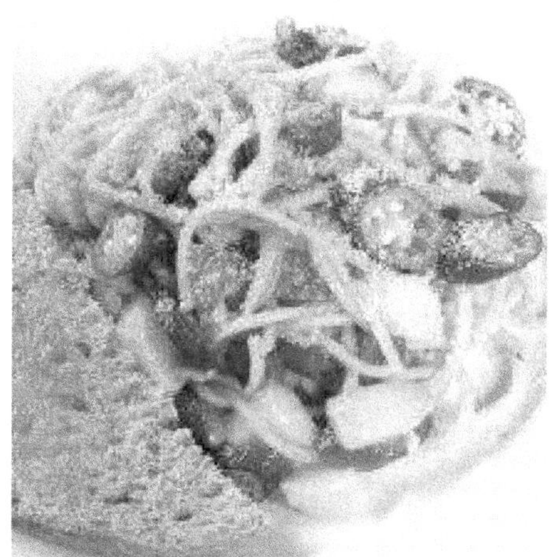

Cook Time: 25 minutes

Servings: 5

Ingredients:

35-ounces Okra, washed, drained and wiped dry

1 teaspoon red chili powder

2 tablespoons coriander powder

2 tablespoons almond flour

1 ½ tablespoons olive oil

Pinch of caraway seeds

Pinch of Fenugreek seeds

Pinch of Asafoetida

½ teaspoon turmeric

2 green chilies

4 teaspoons dry mango powder

Salt to taste

Directions:

Slit the okra lengthwise into half. Brush some olive oil on okra then fry in the air fryer. Heat some oil in a pan and add the asafetida, heating it for 10-seconds. Add the fenugreek and caraway seeds, fry them for 10-seconds. Stir in the almond flour and cook for 10-minutes. Mix in the air fried okra and sprinkle the spices on top. Cook for 10-minutes, adding the green chilies cook for an additional 2-minutes.

Nutritional Values per serving: Calories: 35, Total Fat: 0.11g, Carbs: 7.7g, Protein: 2.27g

Honey Roasted Carrots

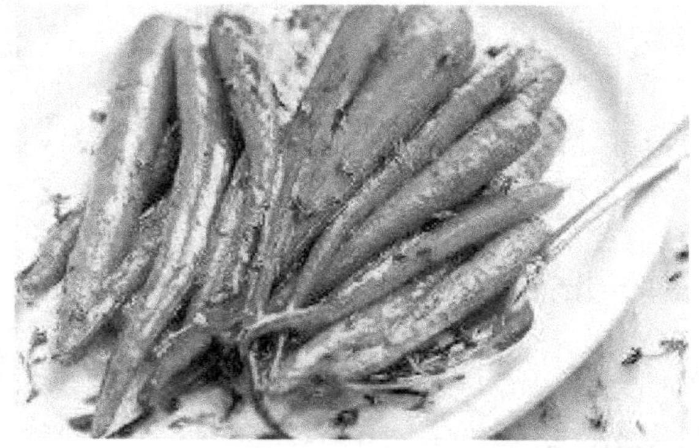

Cook Time: 25 minutes

Servings: 4

Ingredients:

3 cups baby carrots

1 tablespoon olive oil

1 tablespoon honey

Salt and pepper to taste

Directions:

Toss all the ingredients in a bowl. Cook for 12-minutes in an air fryer at 390°Fahrenheit.

Nutritional Values per serving: Calories: 82, Total Fat: 3.2g, Carbs: 2.1g, Protein: 1.0g

Hot Pepper Pin Wheel

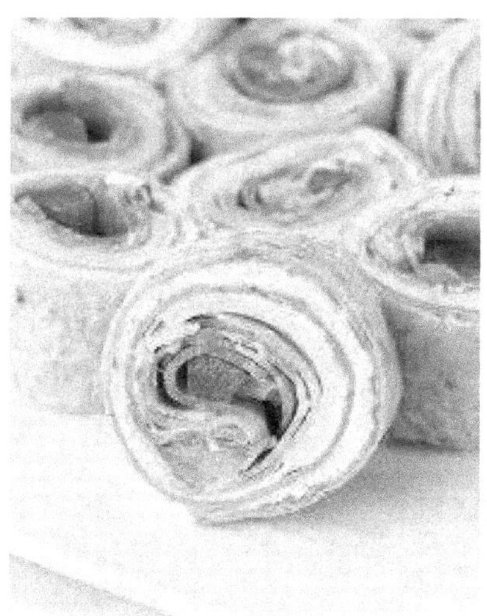

Cook Time: 6 minutes

Servings: 3

Ingredients:

2 lbs. dill pickles

3 almond tortillas

Salt and pepper to taste

3-ounces sliced ham

1 lb. softened cream

1 hot pepper, finely diced

Directions:

Mix diced hot pepper in with cheese. On one side of the tortilla spread cheese over it. Place the ham slice over it. Spread a layer of cheese on top of ham slice. Roll 1 pickle up in the tortilla. Preheat the air fryer to 340°Fahrenheit. Place the rolls in air fryer basket and cook for 6-minutes.

Nutritional Values per serving: Calories: 67, Total Fat: 2.1g, Carbs: 0.11g, Protein: 3.2g

Lemon Courgette Caviar

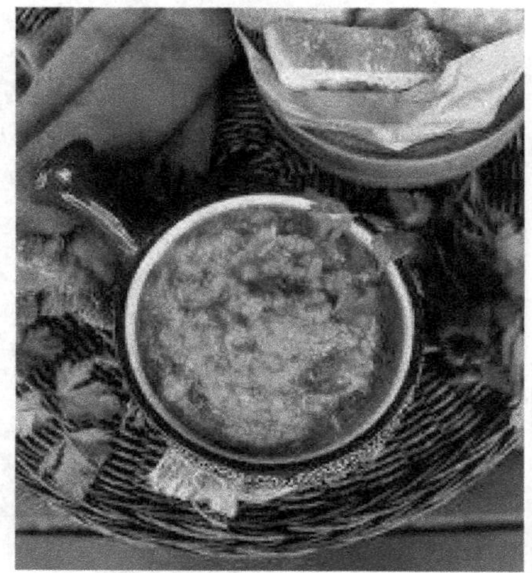

Cook Time: 20 minutes

Servings: 3

Ingredients:

2 medium Courgettes

1 tablespoon olive oil

1 ½ tablespoons balsamic vinegar

½ red onion

Juice of one lemon

Directions:

Preheat your air fryer. Wash, then dry courgettes. Add lemon juice to over courgettes. Arrange courgettes in a baking dish, then bake them in the air fryer for 20-minutes. Remove the courgettes from the oven and allow them to cool. Blend the onion in a blender. Slice the courgettes in half, lengthwise, then remove their insides using a spoon. Place courgettes into mixer and process everything. Add the vinegar, the olive oil and a little bit of salt, then blend again. Serve cool with tomato sauce.

Nutritional Values per serving: Calories: 76, Total Fat: 0.3g, Carbs: 18g, Protein: 3g

Parmesan Asparagus Fries

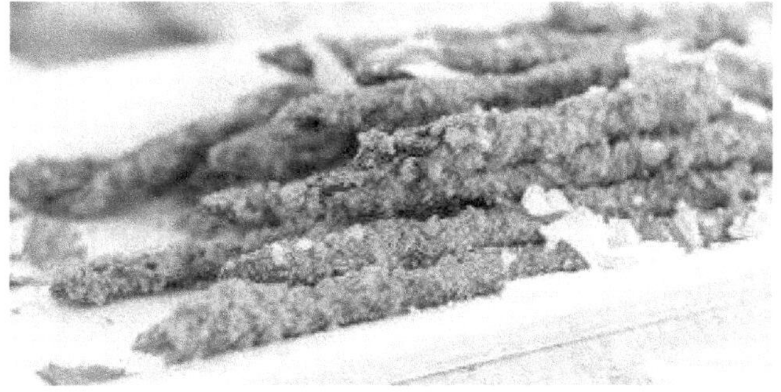

Cook Time: 10 minutes

Servings: 5

Ingredients:

1 lb. asparagus spears

¼ cup almond flour

Salt and pepper to taste

2 eggs, beaten

½ cup Parmesan cheese, grated

1 cup pork rinds

Directions:

Preheat your air fryer to 380°Fahrenheit. Combine pork rinds and parmesan cheese in a small bowl. Season with salt and pepper. Line baking sheet with parchment paper. First, dip half the asparagus spears into flour, then into eggs, and finally into pork rind mixture. Place asparagus spears on the baking sheet and bake for 10-minutes. Repeat with remaining spears.

Nutritional Values per serving: Calories: 20, Total Fat: 0.1g, Carbs: 3.9g, Protein: 2.2g

Garlic & Parsley Roasted Mushrooms

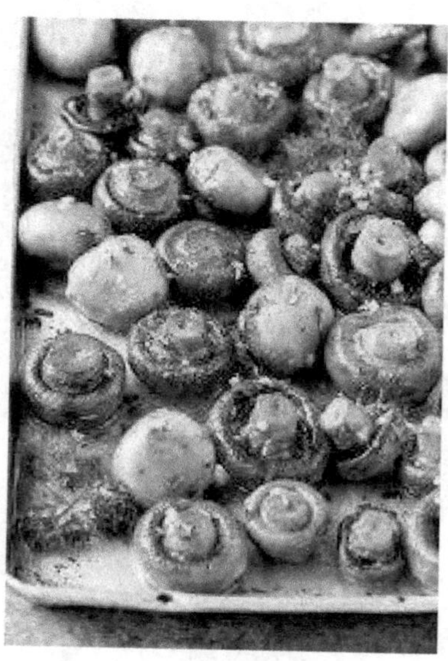

Cook Time: 30 minutes

Servings: 4

Ingredients:

2 lbs. mushrooms, washed, quartered, dried

1 tablespoon duck fat

½ teaspoon garlic powder

2 teaspoons Herbes de Provence

2 tablespoons white vermouth

1 teaspoon parsley, fresh, finely chopped

Directions:

Place the duck fat, garlic powder, Herbes de Provence in an air fryer pan and heat for 2-minutes. Stir in the mushrooms. Cook for 25-minutes at 300°Fahrenheit. Mix in the vermouth and cook for an additional 5-minutes. Sprinkle mushrooms with parsley for garnish.

Nutritional Values per serving: Calories: 92, Total Fat: 0.23g, Carbs: 0.52g, Protein: 1.2g

Grilled Pineapple with Cinnamon

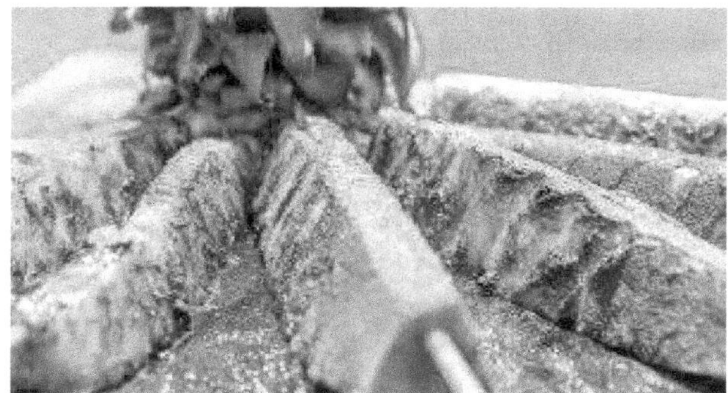

Cook Time: 20 minutes

Servings: 2

Ingredients:

4 pineapple slices

2 tablespoons Truvia

1 teaspoon cinnamon

Directions:

Add the cinnamon and Truvia into a Ziploc bag and shake well. Add the pineapple slices to it and shake and coat. Leave to marinate in the fridge for 20-minutes. Preheat your air fryer for 5-minutes at 360°Fahrenheit. Place the pineapple pieces on the air fryer rack and grill them for 10-minutes. Flip and grill them for an additional 10-minutes.

Nutritional Values per serving: Calories: 276, Total Fat: 5.3g, Carbs: 4.2g, Protein: 4.6g

Ginger & Honey Cauliflower Bites

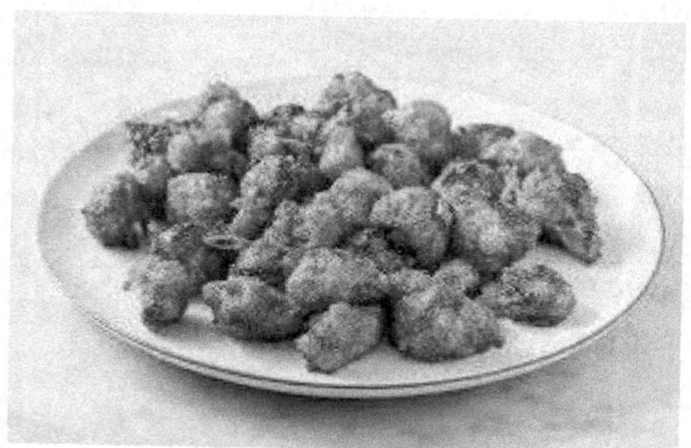

Cook Time: 20 minutes

Servings: 4

Ingredients:

1 head of cauliflower, cut into florets

1/3 cup oats

1/3 cup almond flour

1 egg, beaten

1 teaspoon mixed spice

2 tablespoons soy sauce

2 tablespoons honey

Salt and pepper to taste

½ teaspoon mustard powder

1 teaspoon mixed herbs

1/3 cup desiccated coconut

1 teaspoon ginger powder

Directions:

Preheat your air fryer to 360°Fahrenheit. In a bowl, combine flour, oats, ginger powder and coconut. Season it with salt and pepper. Add egg into another bowl. Season the cauliflower florets with the mixed herbs, salt, and pepper. Dip florets into the egg and then dredge in coconut mix. Cook in your air fryer for 15-minutes at 315°Fahrenheit. Mix remaining ingredients in a bowl. Dip the cauliflower in the honey mixture and cook for an additional 5-minutes in air fryer.

Nutritional Values per serving: Calories: 42, Total Fat: 2.3g, Carbs: 3.1g, Protein: 3.2g

Baked Tomato & Egg

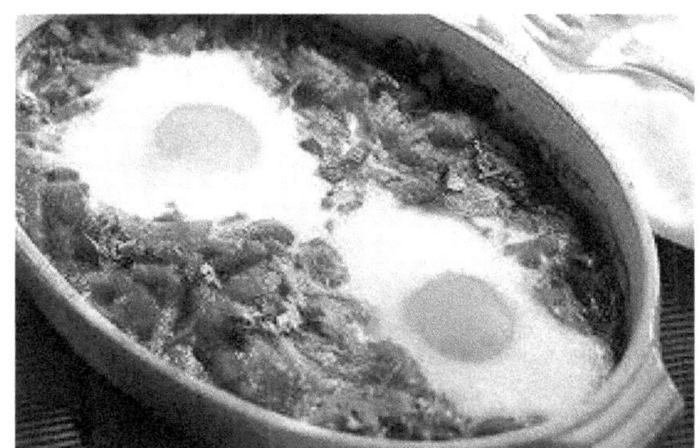

Cook Time: 20 minutes

Servings: 2

Ingredients:

2 tomatoes

4 eggs

1 cup mozzarella cheese, shredded

Salt and pepper to taste

1 tablespoon olive oil

A few basil leaves

Directions:

Preheat your air fryer to 360°Fahrenheit. Cut each tomato into two halves and place them in a bowl. Season with salt and pepper. Place cheese around the bottom of the tomatoes and add the basil leaves. Break one egg into each tomato slice. Garnish with cheese and drizzle with olive oil. Set the temperature to 360°Fahrenheit and bake for 20-minutes.

Nutritional Values per serving: Calories: 28.9, Total Fat: 2.4g, Carbs: 2.0g, Protein: 0.4g

Paprika Chips

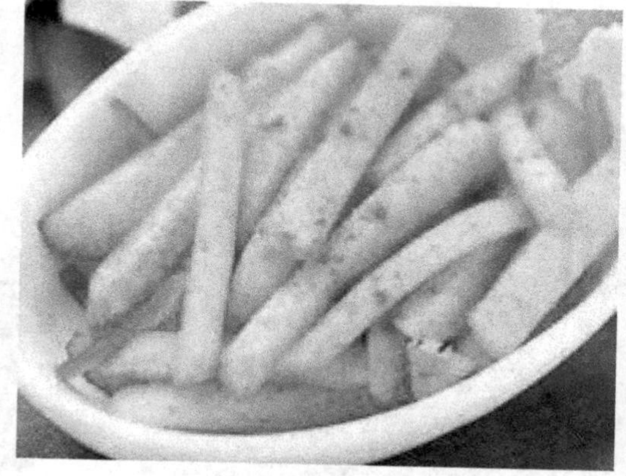

Cook Time: 40 minutes

Servings: 4

Ingredients:

31-ounces of sweet potatoes, peeled and cut into chips

½ teaspoon salt

2 tablespoons olive oil

½ tablespoon paprika

Directions:

Toss all the ingredients together in a bowl. Place in a pan inside your air fryer and cook for 40-minutes at 300°Fahrenheit.

Nutritional Values per serving: Calories: 62, Total Fat: 6.5g, Carbs: 41.5g, Protein: 5.3g

French Beans with Walnuts & Almonds

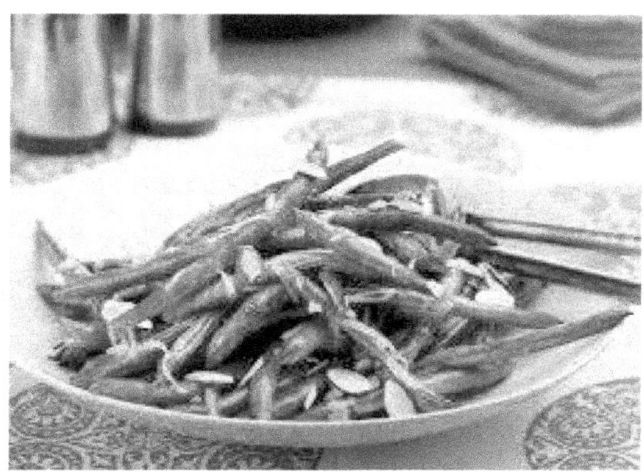

Cook Time: 27 minutes

Servings: 6

Ingredients:

1 ½ lbs. of French green beans

(stems removed)

¼ cup slivered almonds (lightly toasted)

¼ cup walnuts, finely chopped

½ teaspoon ground white pepper

½ lb. shallots, peeled and quartered

1 teaspoon sea salt

2 tablespoons olive oil

Directions:

Boil some water in a pan, adding the green beans to it. Cook beans for 2-minutes with salt. Drain the beans. Place the green beans into a bowl and toss with the rest of the ingredients except the walnuts and almonds. Mix nuts together in small bowl and set aside. Place into air fryer basket and cook for 25-minutes at 400°Fahrenheit. Toss twice during cook time. Serve garnished with mixed nuts.

Nutritional Values per serving: Calories: 213, Total Fat: 5.2g, Carbs: 3.4g, Protein: 4.3g

Crab & Cheese Soufflé

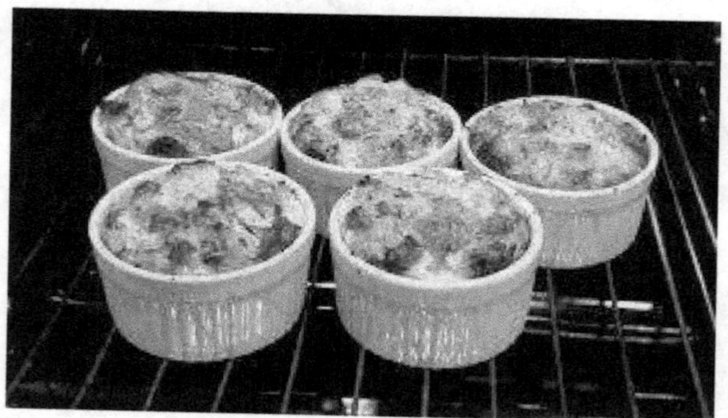

Cook Time: 18 minutes

Servings: 2

Ingredients:

1 lb. cooked crab meat

1 capsicum

1 small onion, diced

1 cup cream

1 cup milk

4-ounces Brie

Brandy to cover crab meat

3 eggs

5 drops liquid stevia

3-ounces cheddar cheese, grated

4 cups bread, cubed

Directions:

Soak the cram meat in brandy and 4-parts water. Loosen the meat in brandy. Sautė onion and bread. Grate cheddar cheese and mix ingredients. In the same pan, add some of the butter and stir for a minute. Add the crab to pan. Add ½ of the milk and 1 tablespoon of brandy and cook for 2-minutes. Add the bread cubes to frying pan and mix well. Sprinkle with cheese and pepper. Put the stuffing in 5 ramekins, without brushing them with oil. Distribute the brie evenly. In a bowl, combine ½ cup of cream with stevia. Heat the cream in a pan and add remaining milk. Pour mixture into ramekins. Preheat your air fryer to 350°Fahreneheit add dish and cook for 20-minutes.

Broccoli with Cheese & Olives

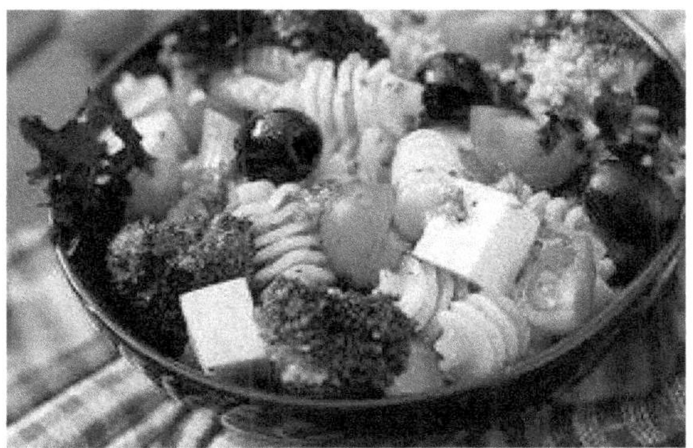

Cook Time: 15 minutes

Servings: 4

Ingredients:

2lbs. broccoli florets

¼ cup parmesan cheese, shaved

2 teaspoons lemon zest, grated

1/3 cup Kalamata olives, halved, pitted

½ teaspoon ground black pepper

1 teaspoon sea salt

2 tablespoons olive oil

Directions:

Boil the water in a pan and cook the broccoli for 4-minutes. Drain broccoli. Toss the broccoli with oil, salt, and pepper. Place broccoli in your air fryer basket and cook for 15-minutes at 400°Fahrenheit. Toss twice during cook time. Move to a serving bowl and toss in lemon zest, olives, and cheese.

Nutritional Values per serving: Calories: 242, Total Fat: 7.2g, Carbs: 3.2g, Protein: 5.6g

Spicy Mozzarella Stick

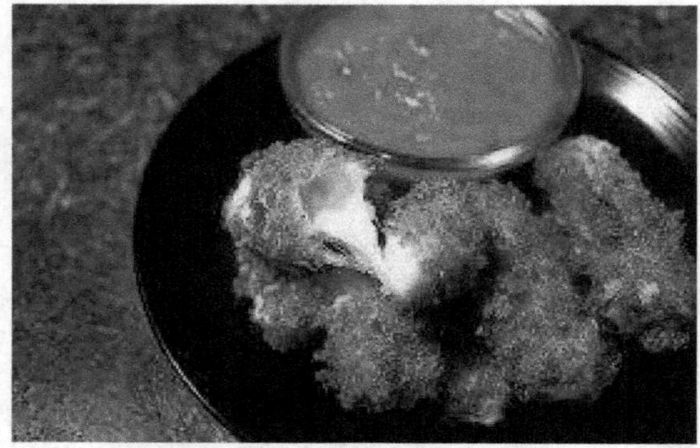

Cook Time: 5 minutes

Servings: 3

Ingredients:

8-ounces mozzarella cheese, cut into strips

2 tablespoons olive oil

½ teaspoon salt

1 cup pork rinds

1 egg

1 teaspoon garlic powder

1 teaspoon paprika

Directions:

Cut the mozzarella into 6 strips. Whisk the egg along with salt, paprika, and garlic powder. Dip the mozzarella strips into egg mixture first, then into pork rinds. Arrange them on a baking platter and place in the fridge for 30-minutes. Preheat your air fryer to 360°Fahrenheit. Drizzle olive oil into the air fryer. Arrange the mozzarella sticks in the air fryer and cook for about 5-minutes. Make sure to turn them at least twice, to ensure they will become golden on all sides.

Nutritional Values per serving: Calories: 156, Total Fat: 9.6g, Carbs: 1.89g, Protein: 16g

Fried Zucchini, Squash, & Carrot Mix

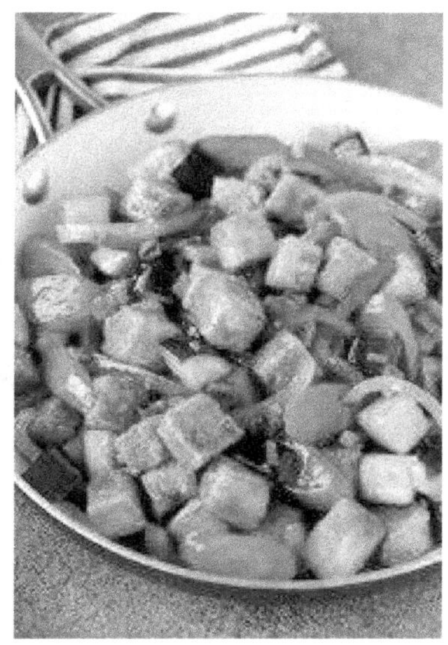

Cook Time: 35 minutes

Servings: 4

Ingredients:

½ lb. carrots, peeled and cubed

6 teaspoons olive oil

1 lb. zucchini, chopped into half-moons

1 lb. yellow squash, chopped in half-moons

1 teaspoon sea salt

½ teaspoon white pepper

1 tablespoon Tarragon leaves, chopped

Directions:

Toss carrots in a bowl with 2 teaspoons of olive oil, then place them into air fryer basket. Cook for 5-minutes at 400°Fahrenheit. Toss the zucchini and squash in the rest of the oil, salt and pepper and place into air fryer. Cook for 30-minutes, tossing three times during cook time. Toss with tarragon and serve.

Nutritional Values per serving: Calories: 217, Total Fat: 4.2g, Carbs: 3.9g, Protein: 6.2g

Parsley & Garlic Flavored Potatoes

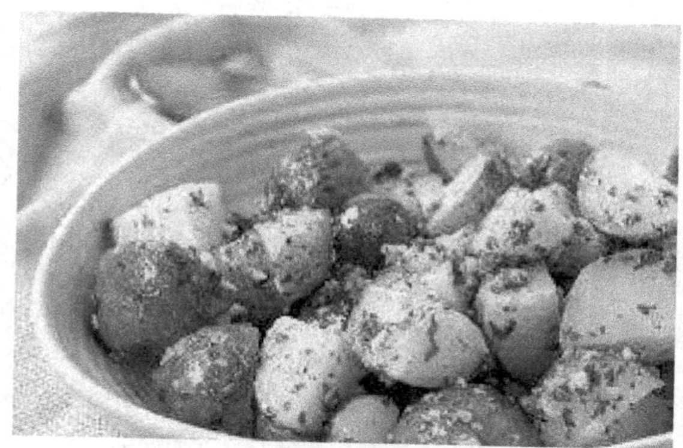

Cook Time: 40 minutes

Servings: 4

Ingredients:

3 Idaho baking potatoes (pricked with a fork)

2 tablespoons olive oil

1 teaspoon parsley

1 tablespoon garlic, minced

Salt to taste

Directions:

Stir ingredients together in a bowl. Rub the potatoes with the mix. Place them into air fryer basket and cook for 40-minutes at 390°Fahrenheit. Toss twice during cook time.

Nutritional Values per serving: Calories: 97, Total Fat: 0.64g, Carbs: 25.2g, Protein: 10.2g

Hot Spicy Thyme Cherry Tomatoes

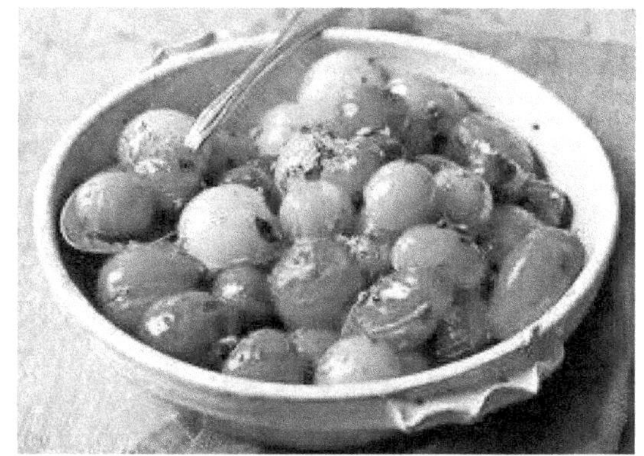

Cook Time: 25 minutes

Servings: 4

Ingredients:

1 dozen cherry tomatoes

1 tablespoon olive oil

½ teaspoon thyme, dried

Salt and pepper to taste

1 garlic clove, minced

1 teaspoon paprika

Directions:

Chop the tomatoes in half and discard the seeds. Toss the tomatoes with the rest of the ingredients in a bowl. Place in the air fryer at 390°Fahrenheit for 15-minutes.

Nutritional Values per serving: Calories: 232, Total Fat: 5.2g, Carbs: 4.3g, Protein: 5.1g

Conclusion

I hope that your air fryer is giving you lots of joy, time and most importantly, tasty dishes. Please feel free to adjust and alter these recipes, or simply use them as a springboard of inspiration for your own creations!

Putting together interesting and unexpected ingredients is so much fun and can be really rewarding, so get creative in your kitchen.

Always remember to clean your air fryer and accessories according to the instructions and safety precautions after each cooking adventure.

Like every appliance, maintenance is needed to get what you would like in the device. Any tool employed for preparing food must be stored spotlessly clean. Don't let dirt develop and clean the environment fryer frequently so you get great results any time you make use of the air fryer. You have to make certain you retain it keep clean and maintain it for results efficiently along with a taken care of appliance always lasts longer. We provides you with some cleanings tips, however it is not difficult. The outdoors and inside parts could be cleaned fairly easily and ought to be done frequently. Within the situation from the heating coil, get it done a couple of occasions annually only.

The Healthy Air Fryer Cookbook with Pictures

70+ Fried Tasty Recipes to Kill Hunger, Be Super Energetic and Make Your Day Brighter

Haile Banister

Table of Contents:

Introduction

An air fryer is a little kitchen appliance which imitates the outcomes of deep frying foods with the excess grease. As opposed to submerging food in order to fry it, the more food is put within the fryer together with a rather tiny quantity of oil. The food is subsequently "fried" having just hot air cooking. Food is cooked fast Because of the high heat and, because of the small quantity of oil onto the exterior of the meals, the outside will be emptied, like it was fried!

So, here we have discussed 70 best and healthy recipes for you that you can try at home and enjoy cooking using an air fryer.

Chapter 1: Air fryer Basics and 20 Recipes

Type of air fryer:

There're some air fryers that are over $300 and the one I used was less than a hundred. I didn't want you to splurge on the expensive one immediately because I was like what if I don't even use this thing? I want you to know that I'm going to use it first so I bought this for less than $100. This one is perfectly fine. It's big, it cooks a lot and it works just as good if not better than the more expensive models.

I'm going to bring you many air fryer recipes that are super easy. Even though it takes up quite a bit of counter space, it does a good job getting things crispy and delicious. Let's start with four recipes i.e. Bacon, Brussels sprouts, chicken wings and chicken breasts. So, let's get started.

1. Air fryer Bacon Recipe

I'm going to use four slices of bacon and I'm going to cut them in half on the cutting board.

So, here's the air fryer that I have:

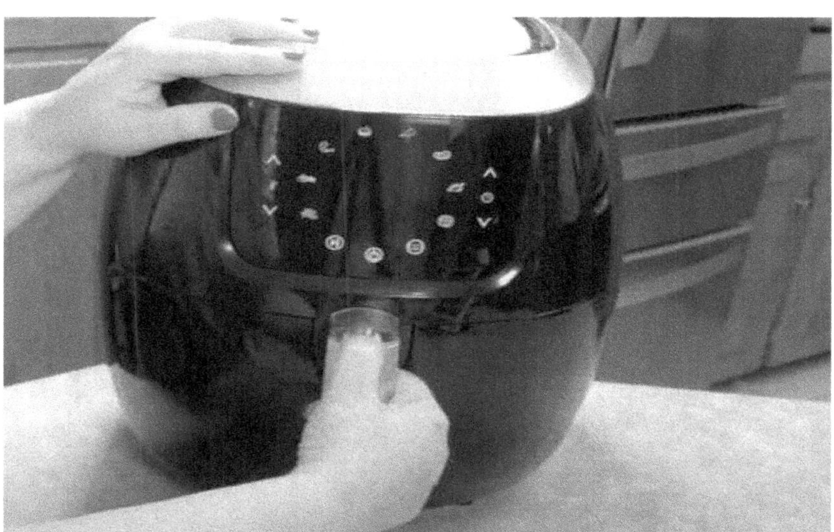

It is a 5.7 quart which is a pretty large air fryer. You take out the drawer and then we're going to lay the bacon inside of the air fryer, as it all fits. You want it to be a single layer so that they get evenly cooked. We're going to put this back in so we set the temperature for 350 degrees and they will cook for about nine minutes. We will also check them a couple of times just to make sure they're not getting too overdone. That's all there is to it, so our air fryer bacon is already and let's pull it out.

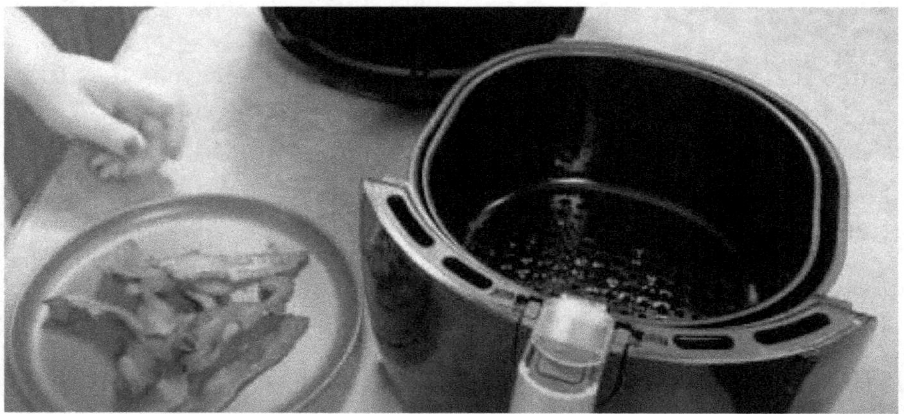

If you wanted it a little crispy, you could leave it in for probably just one more minute but I like it like this.

2. Air Fryer Apple Pie Chips

Let us be honest: If you are craving super-crispy, crunchy apple chips, then baking them in the oven is not good for you. The air fryer, on the other hand, is best.

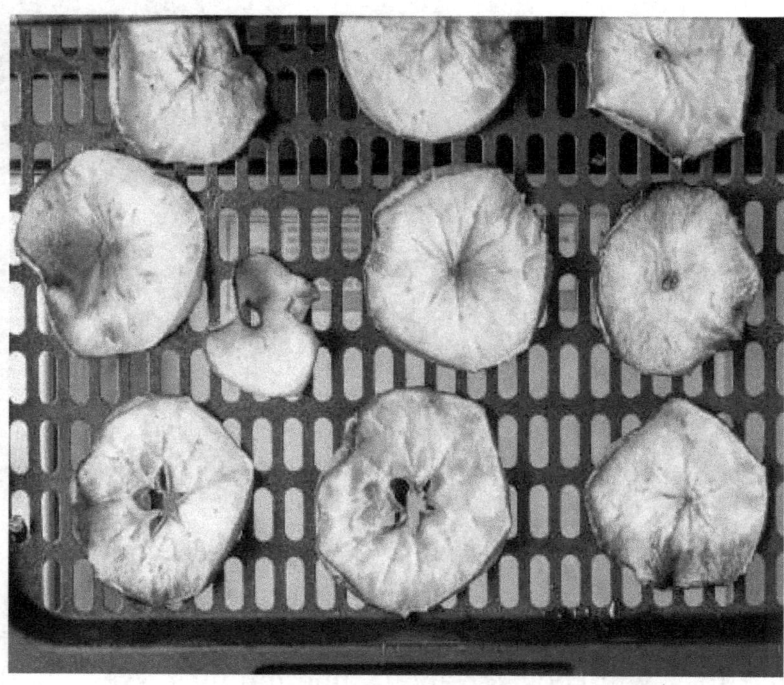

You'll begin by slicing an apple (any variety will probably work, although a red apple generates extra-pretty processors), and in case you've got a mandolin, utilize it as the thinner the slice, the crispier the processor. Toss the pieces with cinnamon and nutmeg, put an even coating into a preheated air fryer, coat with cooking spray, and stir fry until golden. You will have a tasty snack in under 10 minutes. For maximum crunchiness, let cool completely before eating.

Ingredients

- Moderate red apple
- 1/4 tsp ground nutmeg
- 1/2 tsp ground cinnamon
- Cooking spray

Instructions

- ❑ Thinly slice the apple into 1/8-inch-thick slices using a knife or rather on a mandoline.
- ❑ Toss the apple slices with 1/2 teaspoon ground cinnamon along with 1/4 teaspoon ground nutmeg.
- ❑ Preheat in an air fryer into 375°F and place for 17 minutes. Coat the fryer basket with cooking spray. Put just one layer of apple pieces into a basket and then spray with cooking spray.
- ❑ Air fry until golden-brown, rotating the trays halfway through to keep the apples at level, about 7 minutes total.
- ❑ Allow the chips to cool entirely too crisp.
- ❑ Repeat with the air fryer for the remaining apple pieces.

3. Air-fryer Chicken Wings

We will get started on the chicken wings.

Ingredients:

- 12 Chicken wings

- Salt
- Pepper

Method:

I'm going to put them in the air fryer basket and then I'm going to season them with salt and pepper. I've got these all in a single layer and they're kind of snug in there which is fine because they're going to shrink as they cook.

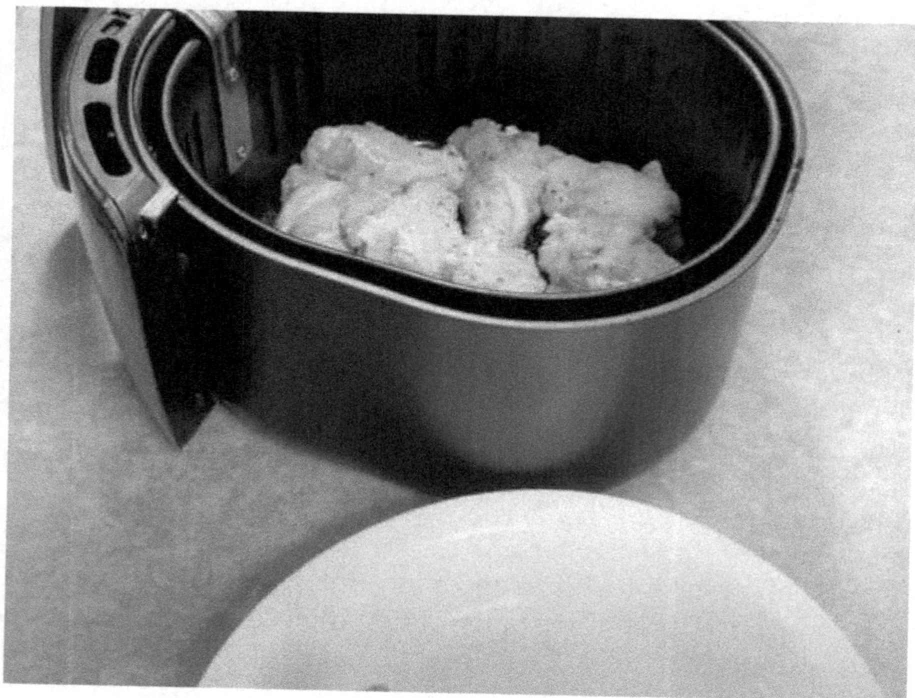

I put in about 12 chicken wings fit in my air fryer basket and now we're going to cook them for 25 minutes at 380 degrees. What that's going to do is it really get them cooked and then we're going to bump up the temperature and we will get them crispy. The first cook on our wings is done and now we are going to put it back in the air fryer at 400 degrees for about three to five minutes to get them nice and crispy. With this recipe and most air fryer recipes, whenever you're cooking things for longer than I would say five minutes, you may want to pull the basket out and shake what's inside. It is to make sure that it gets evenly cooked and I like to do that about every five minutes. Our wings are done. Look at how good they look in there nice and crispy.

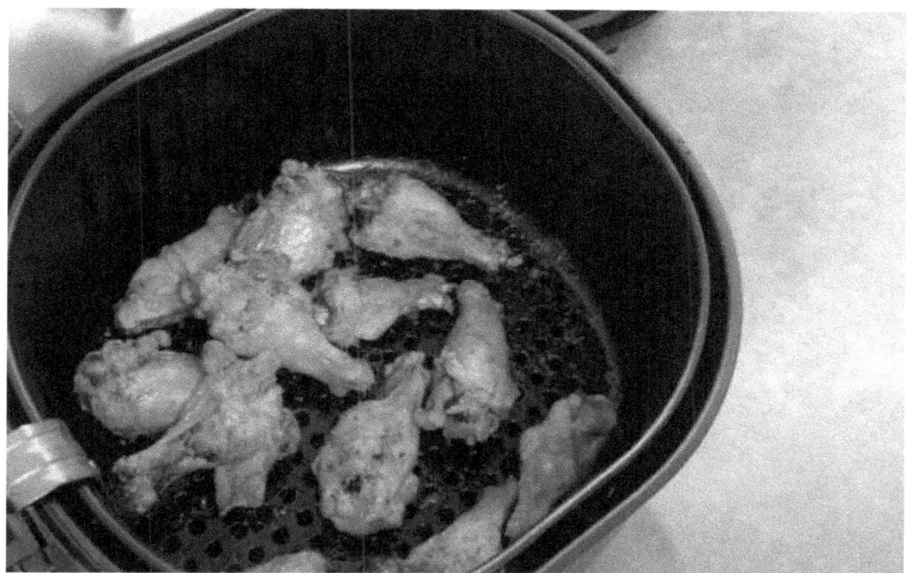

This took about three minutes as I didn't have to do the full five minutes for these.

4. **Air Fryer Mini Breakfast Burritos**

All these air-fried miniature burritos are fantastic to get a catch's go breakfast or perhaps to get a midday snack. Leave the serrano Chile pepper for a spicy version.

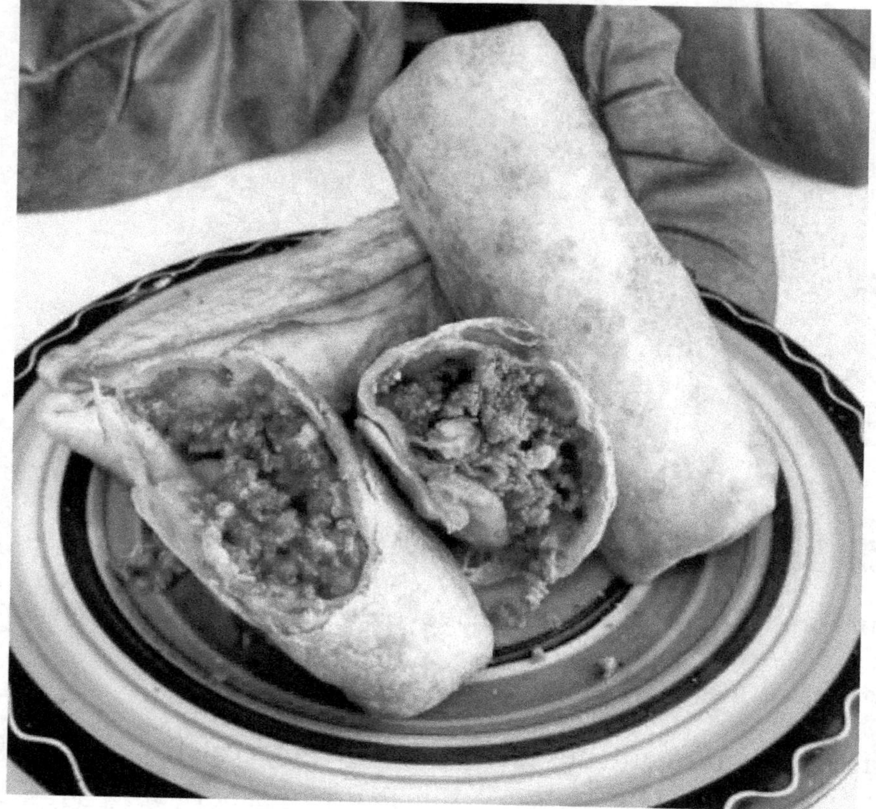

Ingredients

- 1 tablespoon bacon grease
- 1/4 cup Mexican-style chorizo
- 2 tbsp. sliced onion
- 1 serrano pepper, chopped
- salt and ground black pepper to taste
- 4 (8 inch) flour tortillas
- 1/2 cup diced potatoes
- 2 large eggs
- avocado oil cooking spray

Instructions

- ❖ Cook chorizo in an air fryer over medium-high heat, stirring often, until sausage operates into a dark crimson, 6 to 8 minutes.
- ❖ Melt bacon grease in precisely the exact way over medium-high warmth.
- ❖ Add onion and serrano pepper and continue stirring and cooking until berries are fork-tender, onion is translucent, and serrano pepper is tender in 2 to 6 minutes.
- ❖ Add eggs and chorizo; stir fry till cooked and fully integrated into curry mixture in about 5 minutes. Season with pepper and salt.
- ❖ Meanwhile, heat tortillas directly onto the grates of a gasoline stove until pliable and soft.
- ❖ Put 1/3 cup chorizo mixture down the middle of each tortilla.
- ❖ Fold top and bottom of tortillas over the filling, then roll into a burrito form. Mist with cooking spray and put in the basket of a fryer.
- ❖ Flip each burrito above, peppermint with cooking spray, and fry until lightly browned, 2 to 4 minutes longer.

5. Herb Chicken Breast

Now let's get to the herb chicken breast.

Ingredients

- Salt
- Pepper
- Chicken Breast
- Smoked Paprika
- Butter

Method:

We've got two chicken breasts. We've got butter, Italian seasoning salt, pepper and smoked paprika. We're going to mix all of that into the butter to give it a quick mix. Now we've got our two chicken breasts here and we're going to spread the mixture over each chicken breast to give it a nice flavorful crust.

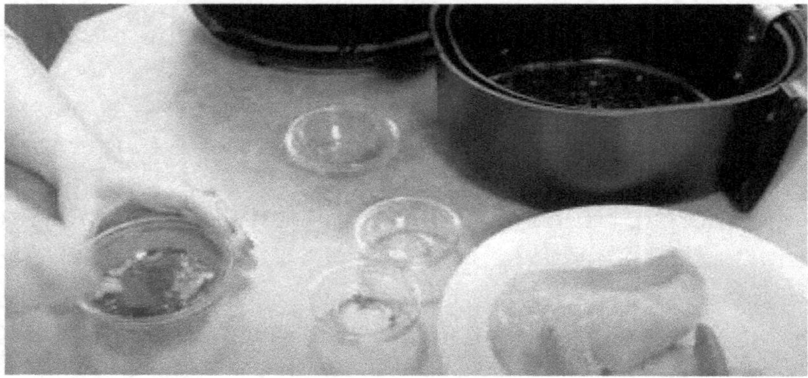

Put these in the air fryer with some tongs. We're ready to cook these in the air fryer.

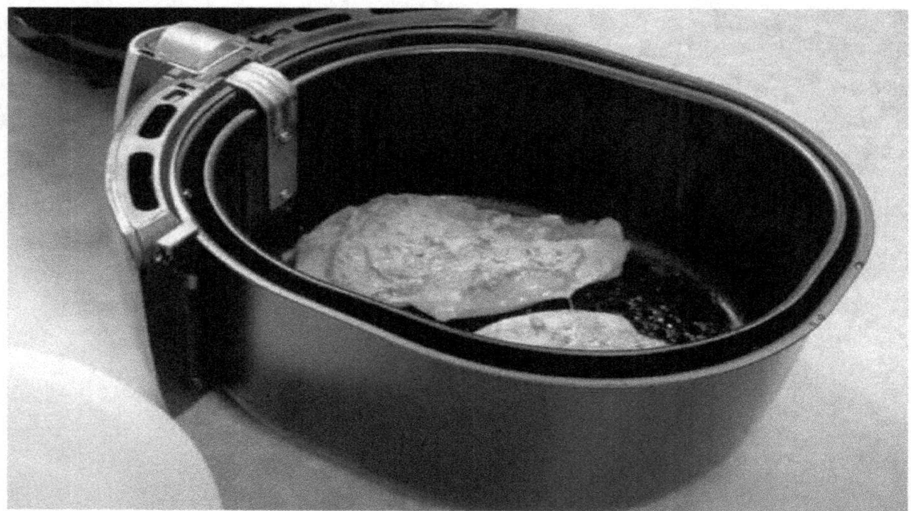

Cook them at 370 degrees for about 10 to 15 minutes and then check it with a meat thermometer to make sure that they're perfectly cooked. Because we don't want them to be overcooked, then they'll be dry and we definitely don't want them to be undercooked.

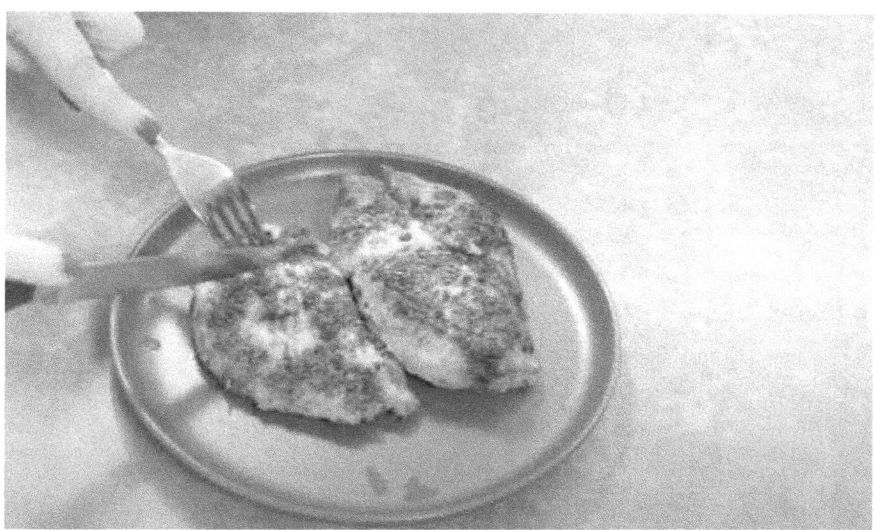

Okay, we pulled our chicken out of the air fryer. We had one chicken breast that was smaller so it came out a little bit earlier and now we have this one that's ready and its right at 165. So, we know that our chickens are not going to be dry. Let's cut into one of these. Those are perfectly cooked and juicy

6. **Three Cheese Omelet**

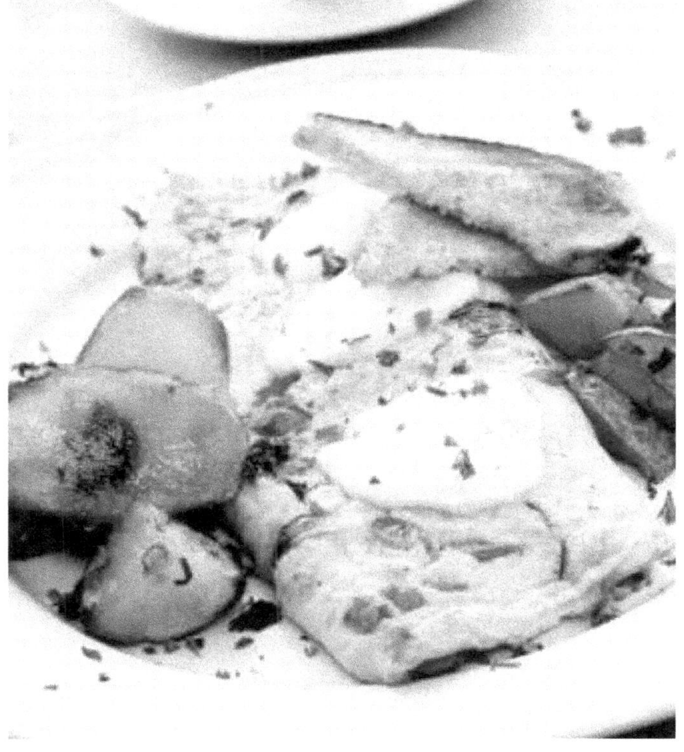

Ingredients

- 3 Tbsp. heavy whipping cream
- ½ tsp salt
- 4 eggs
- ¼ cup cheddar cheese, grated
- ¼ cup provolone cheese
- ¼ tsp ground black pepper
- ¼ cup feta cheese

Method:

- ❖ Preheat your air fryer to 350 degrees F and line a baking pan using parchment paper. Be sure the pan will fit on your fryer- normally a seven inch round pan will do the job flawlessly.
- ❖ In a small bowl, whisk together the eggs, cream, pepper and salt
- ❖ Pour the mixture into the prepared baking pan then place the pan on your preheated air fryer.
- ❖ Cook for approximately ten minutes or till the eggs are completely set.
- ❖ Sprinkle the cheeses round the boiled eggs and then return the pan into the air fryer for one more moment to melt the cheese.

7. Patty Pan Frittata

I had a gorgeous patty pan squash sitting on my counter tops and was wondering exactly what to do with this was fresh and yummy for my loved ones. I had not made breakfast however so a summer squash frittata appeared in order! Comparable to zucchini, patty pan squash leant itself well to my fundamental frittata recipe. Serve with your favorite brunch sides or independently. You could also cool and serve cold within 24 hours.

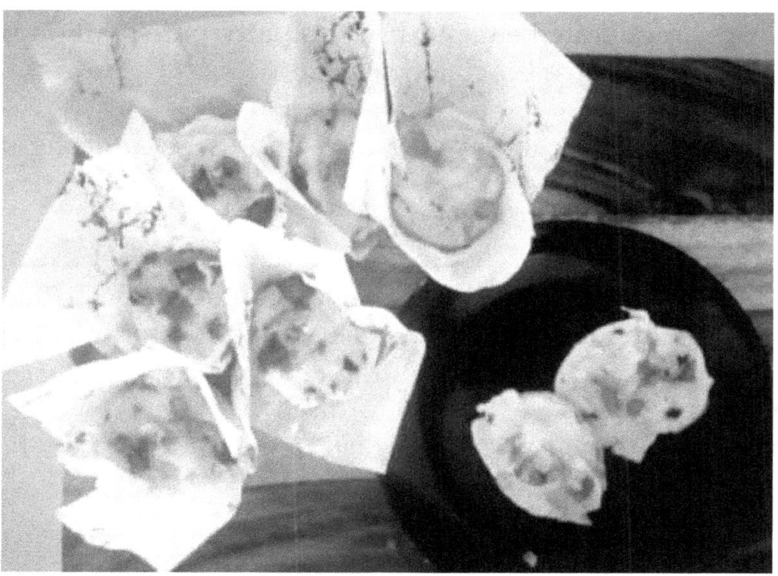

Ingredients

- 1 patty pan squash
- 1 tbsp. unsalted butter
- 4 large eggs
- 1/4 cup crumbled goat cheese
- 1/4 cup grated Parmesan cheese
- salt and ground black pepper to taste
- 1/4 cup
- 2 medium scallions, chopped, green and white parts split
- 1 tsp garlic, minced
- 1 small tomato, seeded and diced
- 1 tsp hot sauce, or to flavor

Instructions

- ❖ Press 5-inch squares of parchment paper to 8 cups of a muffin tin, creasing where essential.

- ❖ Heat butter over moderate heat; stir fry into patty pan, scallion whites, salt, garlic, and pepper. Transfer into a bowl and set aside.
- ❖ Add sausage in the identical way and cook until heated through, about 3 minutes. Add sausage into patty pan mix.
- ❖ Fold in goat milk, Parmesan cheese, and tomato. Add hot sauce and season with pepper and salt. Twist in patty pan-sausage mix. Put frittata mixture to the prepared muffin cups, filling to the peak of every cup and then overfilling only when the parchment paper may encourage the mix.
- ❖ Put muffin tin in addition to a cookie sheet in the middle of the toaster.

8. Bacon and Cheese Frittata

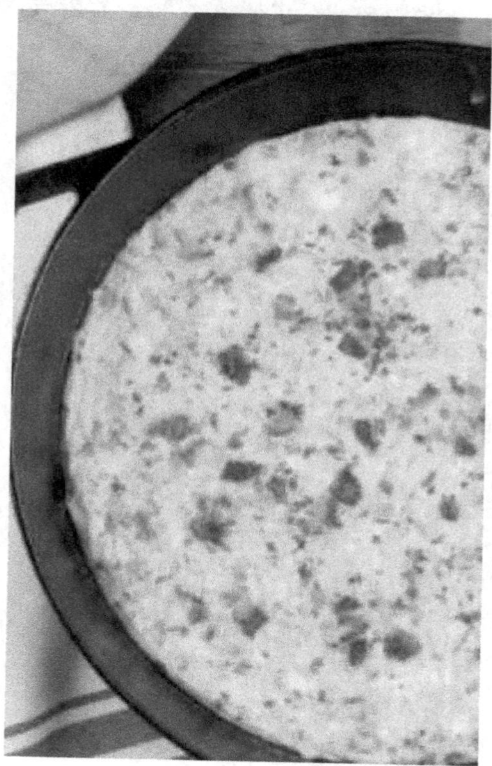

Ingredients

- ½ cup cheddar cheese, grated
- 4 eggs
- ½ cup chopped, cooked bacon

- ½ tsp salt
- 3 Tbsp. heavy whipping cream
- ¼ tsp ground black pepper

Method:

- ❖ Preheat your air fryer to 350 degrees F and line a baking pan using parchment paper. Be sure the pan will fit on your fryer- normally a seven inch round pan will do the job flawlessly.
- ❖ In a small bowl, whisk together the eggs, cream, pepper and salt
- ❖ Stir in the cheese and bacon into the bowl.
- ❖ Pour the mixture into the prepared baking pan then place the pan on your preheated air fryer.
- ❖ Cook for approximately 15 minutes or till the eggs are completely set.

9. Meat Lovers Omelet

Ingredients:

- ¼ cup cheddar cheese, grated
- ¼ cup cooked, crumbled bacon
- ½ tsp salt
- 4 eggs
- ¼ cup cooked, crumbled sausage
- 3 Tbsp. heavy whipping cream
- ¼ tsp ground black pepper

Method:

- ❑ Preheat your air fryer to 350 degrees F and line a baking pan using parchment paper. Be sure the pan will fit on your fryer- normally a seven inch round pan will do the job flawlessly.

- ❑ In a small bowl whisk together the eggs, cream, pepper and salt.
- ❑ Pour the mixture into the prepared baking pan then place the pan on your preheated air fryer.
- ❑ Cook for approximately ten minutes or till the eggs are completely set.
- ❑ Sprinkle the cheeses round the boiled eggs and then return the pan into the fryer for another two minutes to melt the cheese.

10. Crispy Brussels sprouts

Next on our list is air fryer crispy Brussels sprouts.

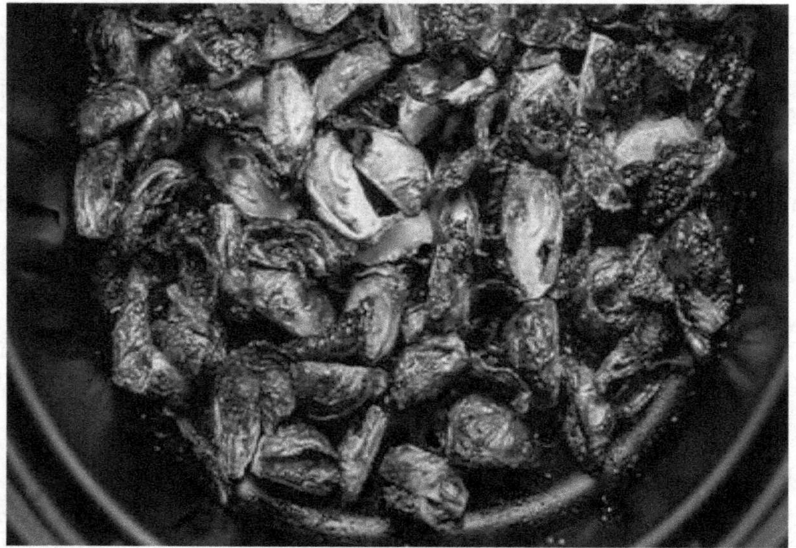

Ingredients:

- Brussels sprouts
- Salt
- Pepper

Method:

Let's get started with these Brussels sprouts. Use fresh Brussels sprouts and we could also use frozen ones. I've got a bag of frozen Brussels sprouts and actually they're still broke. I'm going to season them with some salt and some pepper.

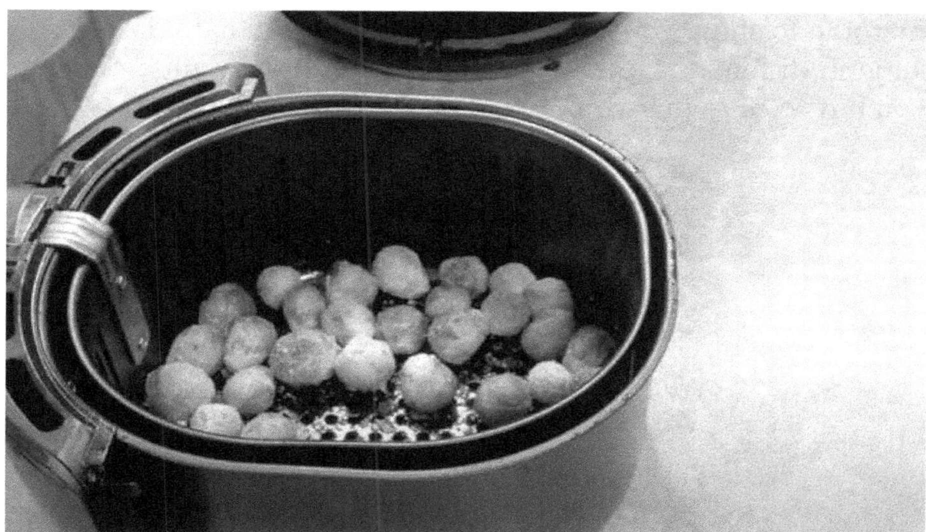

Shake them up and now I'm going to cook them at 400 or I'm going to start with 10 minutes. Let's see how it goes. I think you're going to be surprised because they're crispy. Can you believe that? I think these are better than fresh ones.

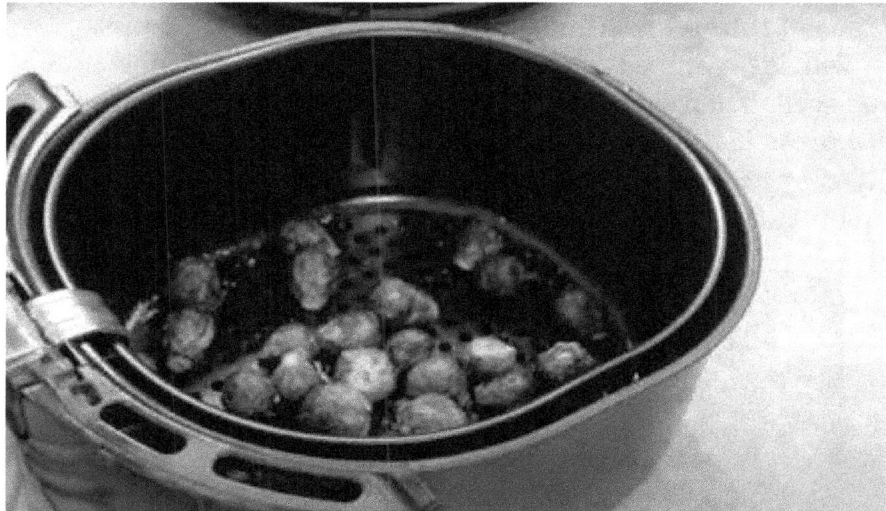

Use frozen if you want to make air fryer Brussels sprouts because the fresh ones take forever to get soft on the inside. You got to cut them into quarters, you've got to trim the leaves off these. They're frozen. I just threw them in the air fryer for 15minutes and they're good to go.

Now what I'm going to show you are actually dessert ideas that you can cook in your air fryer. They come in different sizes and one and a half liter is quite common too, so just check when you buy your own if you do that.

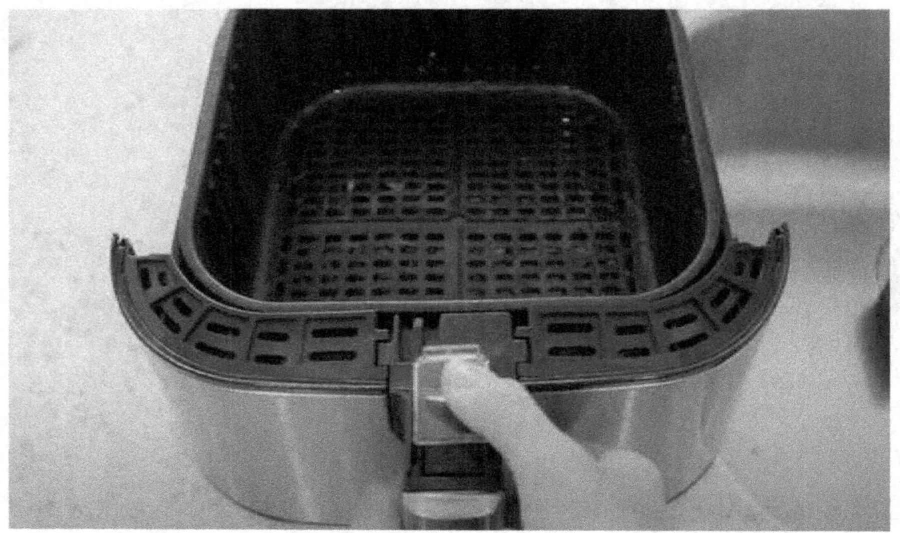

It is a bigger liter air fryer because I promise you, you're going to want to cook everything in this. What I love about this style of air fryer is that it's so simple on the front. You will see that you have got different settings but if you want to cook chips, prawns, fish, steak and muffins as well, it's really easy to adjust the temperature up and down. Also the time up and down as well. Then once you put your tray back in, all you need to do is select your setting and press the play button and the air fryer does everything else for you. It is also really really easy to clean. All you need to do is remove your tray from your air fryer, press the button on at the handle and detach your basket from the tray.

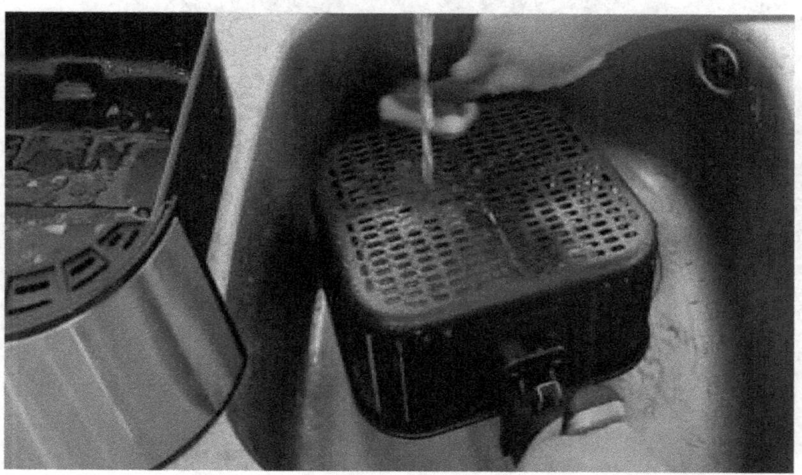

I then use a handheld scrubbing brush which dispenses washing-up liquid and I just go over my basket and my outer tray as well which is where all the fats from your food drip. I just go in with some warm water and my washing up liquid washes it all away. It's got a really nice TEFL coating so everything just wipes off. It's nonstick, then I just leave it on the side, let it dry and then pop it back in my air fryer. At once it is dry, so with all that said I'm just going to jump straight on into the recipes.

11. **Hard Boiled Eggs**

Ingredients:

- 4 eggs

Method:

➢ Preheat your air fryer to 250 degrees F.

➢ Place a wire rack in the fryer and set the eggs in addition to the rack.

➢ Cook for 17 minutes then remove the eggs and put them into an

➢ Ice water bath to cool and then stop the cooking procedure.

➢ Peel the eggs and love!

1. **Spinach Parmesan Baked Eggs**

Ingredients:

- 1 Tbsp. frozen, chopped spinach, thawed
- 1 Tbsp. grated parmesan cheese
- 2 eggs
- 1 Tbsp. heavy cream
- ¼ tsp salt
- 1/8 tsp ground black pepper

Method:

❑ Preheat your air fryer to 330 degrees F.

- ❑ Spray a silicone muffin cup or a little ramekin with cooking spray.
- ❑ In a small bowl, whisk together all of the components
- ❑ Pour the eggs into the ready ramekin and bake for 2 minutes.
- ❑ Enjoy directly from the skillet!

12. Fried hushpuppies.

Inside my home, stuffing is consistently the very popular Thanksgiving dish on the table. Because of this, we create double the amount we all actually need just so we can eat leftovers for a week! And while remaining stuffing alone is yummy, turning it into hushpuppies? Now that is only pure wizardry. Here is the way to use your air fryer to produce near-instant two-ingredient fried hushpuppies.

Ingredients:

- large egg
- cold stuffing
- Cooking spray

Directions:

- ★ Put 1 large egg in a large bowl and gently beat. Add 3 cups leftover stuffing and stir till blended.
- ★ Preheat in an air fryer into 355ºF and place it for 12 minutes. Put one layer of hushpuppies on the racks and then spray the tops with cooking spray.
- ★ Repeat with the remaining mixture.

13. Keto Breakfast Pizza

An egg, sausage, and pork rind "crust" holds sauce, cheese, and other savory toppings within this keto-friendly breakfast pizza recipe.

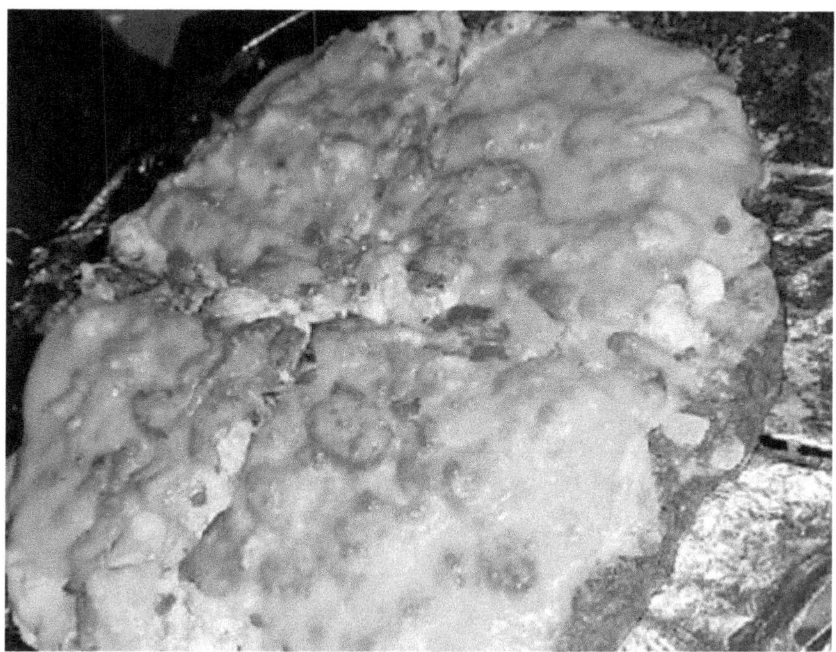

Ingredients

- 3 large eggs, split
- 2 tbsp. Italian seasoning
- 1 cup ready country-style sauce
- 10 tbsp. bacon pieces
- 1 pound bulk breakfast sausage
- cooking spray
- 1/3 cup crushed pork rinds
- 2 tbsp. chopped yellow onion
- 2 tbsp. diced jalapeno pepper
- 1 cup shredded Cheddar cheese

Instructions

★ Grease a rimmed pizza sheet.

- ★ Spread mixture out on the pizza sheet at a big, thin circle.
- ★ Meanwhile, spray a large air fryer with cooking spray and heat over medium-high heat. Whisk remaining eggs together in a bowl and then pour into it.
- ★ Place an oven rack about 6 inches from the heat source and then turn on the oven's broiler.
- ★ Spread sausage evenly over the beef "crust", sprinkle scrambled eggs. Sprinkle with bacon pieces, onion, and jalapeno.
- ★ Broil pizza in the preheated oven till cheese is melted, bubbling, and lightly browned, 3 to 5 minutes. Let cool and cut into fourths prior to serving.

14. Mozzarella stick

Ready for the simplest mozzarella stick recipe? These air fryer mozzarella sticks are created completely from pantry and refrigerator staples (cheese sticks and breadcrumbs), which means that you can dig to the crispy-coated, nostalgic bite anytime you would like.

INGREDIENTS:

- ➢ 1 (12-ounce) bundle mayonnaise
- ➢ 1 large egg
- ➢ 1/2 tsp garlic powder
- ➢ all-purpose flour
- ➢ 1/2 tsp onion powder

Method:

- ★ Before frying pan, set the halved cheese sticks onto a rimmed baking sheet lined with parchment paper. Freeze for half an hour. Meanwhile, construct the breading and get outside the air fryer.
- ★ Whisk the egg and lettuce together in a skillet. Put the flour, breadcrumbs, onion, and garlic powder in a large bowl and whisk to mix.

★ Working in batches of 6, then roll the suspended cheese sticks at the mayo-egg mix to coat, and then in the flour mixture.

★ Pour the coated cheese sticks into the parchment-lined baking sheet. Pour the baking sheet into the freezer for 10 minutes.

★ Heat the fryer to 370°F. Fry 6 the mozzarella sticks for 5 minutes -- it's important not to overcrowd the fryer.

★ Repeat with the rest of the sticks and serve hot with the marinara for dipping.

15. Raspberry Muffins

Ingredients:

- ¼ cup whole milk
- 1 egg
- 1 Tbsp. powdered stevia
- ¼ tsp salt
- ¼ tsp ground cinnamon
- 1 ½ tsp baking powder
- 1 cup almond flour
- ½ cup frozen or fresh raspberries

Steps:

I. Preheat your air fryer to 350 degrees F.

II. In a large bowl, stir together the almond milk, stevia, salt, cinnamon, and baking powder.

III. Add the milk and eggs and then stir well.

IV. Split the muffin batter involving each muffin cup, filling roughly 3/4 of this way complete.

V. Set the muffins to the fryer basket and cook for 14 minutes or till a toothpick comes out when inserted to the middle.

VI. Eliminate from the fryer and let cool.

16. Sausage Tray Bake

I have just chopped up some new potatoes and then I've got some chipolata sausages so I'm going to make a tray bake.

Ingredients:

- Potatoes
- Chipolata Sausage
- corvette
- Onion
- Garlic

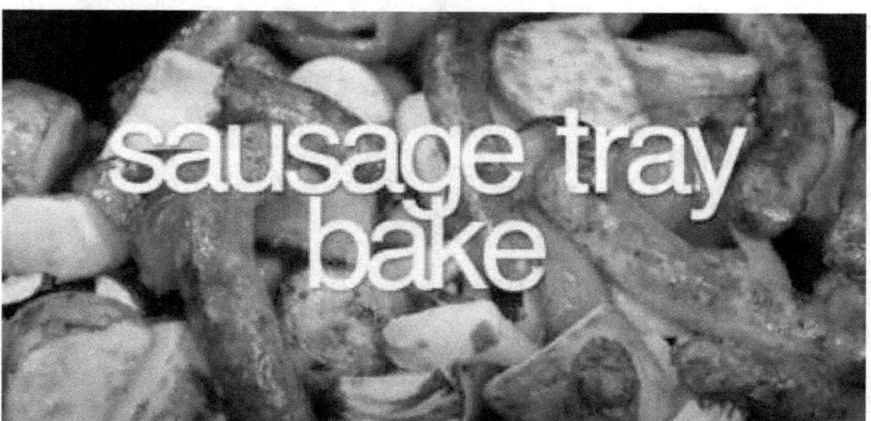

Method:

I would put potato and chipotle sausage into the air fryer for about 20 minutes at first before I add in my other veggies.

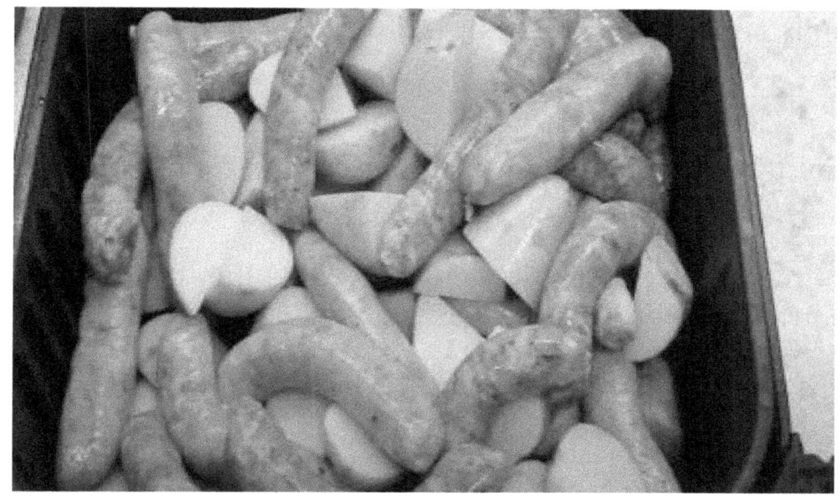

Once these have been in for 20 minutes or so, I will then add in two papers of corvette, an onion and some garlic to go in as well. Cook them for a further 10 minutes and then dinner should be ready.

17. Strawberry Muffins

Ingredients:

- ¼ cup whole milk
- 1 ½ tsp baking powder
- ½ cup chopped strawberries
- 1 egg
- ¼ tsp salt
- ¼ tsp ground cinnamon
- 1 cup almond flour
- 1 Tbsp. powdered stevia

Steps:

1. Preheat your air fryer to 350 degrees F.
2. In a large bowl, stir together the almond milk, stevia, salt, cinnamon, and baking powder.

3. Add the milk and eggs and then stir well.
4. Fold in the berries.
5. Split the muffin batter involving each muffin cup, filling roughly 3/4 of this way complete.
6. Set the muffins to the fryer basket and cook for 14 minutes or till a toothpick comes out when inserted to the middle.
7. Eliminate from the fryer and let cool.

18. Bacon and Eggs for a single

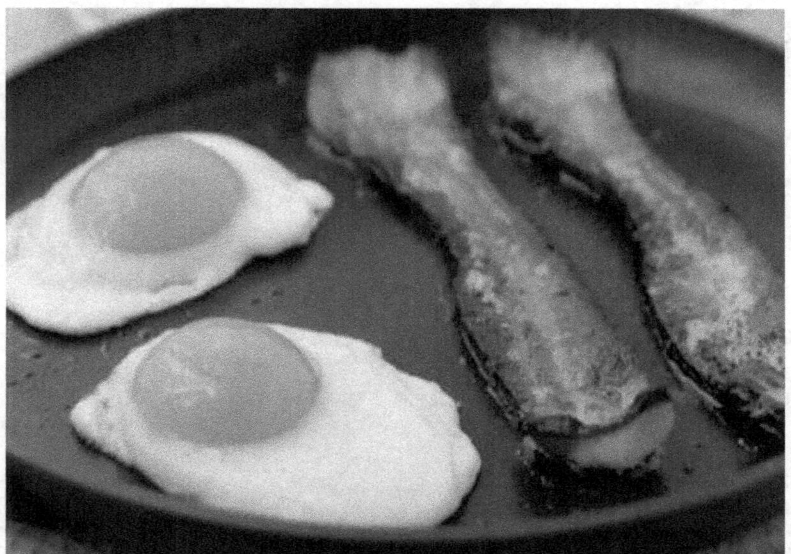

Ingredients:

- 1 Tbsp. heavy cream
- two Tbsp. cooked, crumbled bacon
- 1/4 tsp salt
- 2 eggs
- 1/8 tsp ground black pepper

Directions

- ❑ Preheat your air fryer to 330 degrees F.
- ❑ Spray a silicone muffin cup or a little ramekin with cooking spray.
- ❑ In a small bowl, whisk together all of the components
- ❑ Pour the eggs into the ready ramekin and bake for 2 minutes.
- ❑ Enjoy directly from the skillet!

19. Mini Sausage Pancake Skewers with Spicy Syrup

These small savory skewers are fantastic for breakfast or a fantastic addition to your brunch buffet. The hot maple syrup garnish kicks up the flavor and adds some zest to sandwiches and sausage.

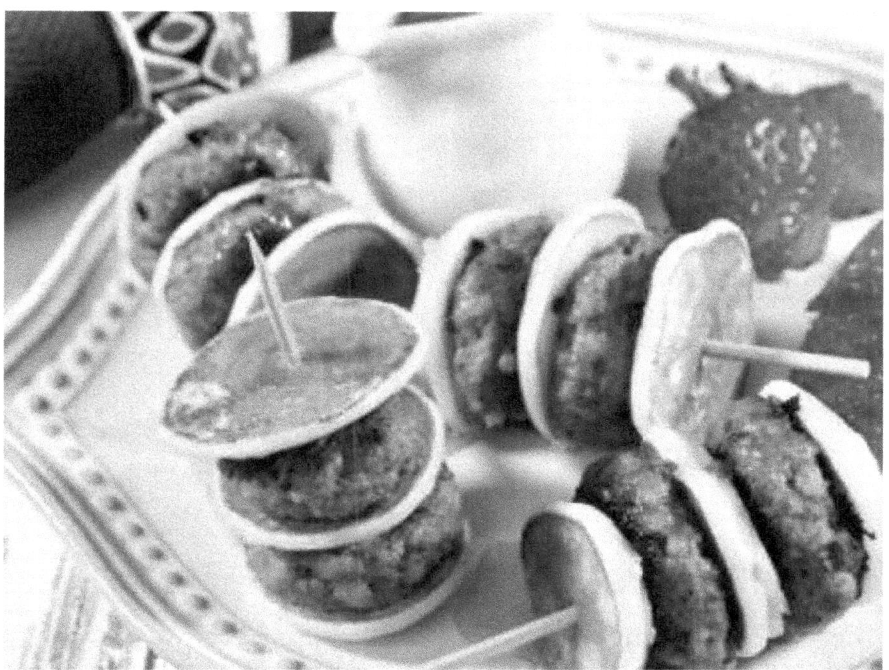

Ingredients

Syrup:

- 4 tbsp. unsalted butter
- 1/2 tsp salt

- 1/2 cup maple syrup
- 1 tsp red pepper flakes, or to taste

Pancake

- 1 cup buttermilk
- 2 tbsp. unsalted butter, melted
- 1 cup all-purpose flour
- 1 large egg
- 1 tbsp. olive oil
- 1 lb. ounce standard pork sausage (like Jimmy Dean®)
- 13 4-inch bamboo skewers
- 2 tablespoons sour cream
- 1/2 tbsp. brown sugar
- 1/4 tsp baking powder
- 1/4 tsp salt
- 2 tsp maple syrup

Instructions

- ❑ Bring to a boil and cook for 3 to 4 minutes.
- ❑ Meanwhile, prepare pancakes: whisk flour, sugar, baking powder, and salt in a huge bowl. Whisk buttermilk, egg, sour cream, melted butter and maple syrup together in another bowl. Pour the wet ingredients into the flour mixture. Stir lightly until just blended but slightly lumpy; don't overmix. Let sit for 10 minutes.
- ❑ Heat in an air fryer over moderate heat. Drop teaspoonfuls of batter onto them to make 1-inch diameter sandwiches.

- ❑ Cook for approximately 1 to 2 minutes, then reverse, and keep cooking until golden brown, about 1 minute. Transfer cooked pancakes into a plate and repeat with remaining batter.
- ❑ Heat olive oil at precisely the exact same fryer over moderate heat. Form table-spoonfuls of sausage to 1-inch patties, exactly the exact same size as the miniature pancakes.
- ❑ Cook until patties are cooked through, about 3 minutes each side. Transfer to a newspaper towel-lined plate.
- ❑ Blend 3 pancakes and two sausage patties onto each skewer, beginning and end with a pancake.
- ❑ Repeat to create staying skewers. Serve drizzled with hot syrup.

20. Avocado Baked Eggs

Ingredients:

- 1 Tbsp. heavy cream
- ¼ tsp salt
- ¼ avocado, diced
- 1 Tbsp. grated cheddar cheese
- 2 eggs
- 1/8 tsp ground black pepper

Method:

- ❑ Preheat your air fryer to 330 degrees F.
- ❑ Spray a silicone muffin cup or a little ramekin with cooking spray.
- ❑ In a small bowl, whisk together the eggs, cream, cheddar cheese, salt, and pepper.
- ❑ Stir in the avocado and pour the eggs into the ready ramekin and bake for 2 minutes.

- ❑ Enjoy directly from the skillet!

Chapter 2: Air Fryer 50 more Recipes for You!

21. Sausage and Cheese Omelet

Ingredients:

- ¼ cup cheddar cheese, grated
- ½ cup cooked, crumbled sausage
- 4 eggs
- 3 Tbsp. heavy whipping cream
- ½ tsp salt
- ¼ tsp ground black pepper

Method

01. Preheat your air fryer to 320 degrees F and line a baking pan using parchment paper. Be sure the pan will fit on your fryer- normally a seven inch round pan will do the job flawlessly.

02. In a small bowl, whisk together the eggs, cream, pepper and salt.

03. Pour the mixture into the prepared baking pan then place the pan on your preheated air fryer.

04. Cook for approximately ten minutes or till the eggs are completely set.

05. Sprinkle the cheeses round the boiled eggs and then return the pan into the fryer for another two minutes to melt the cheese.

22. Pita bread Pizza

I am making some pita bread pizzas now.

Ingredients:

- Bread
- Tomato puree

- Passat

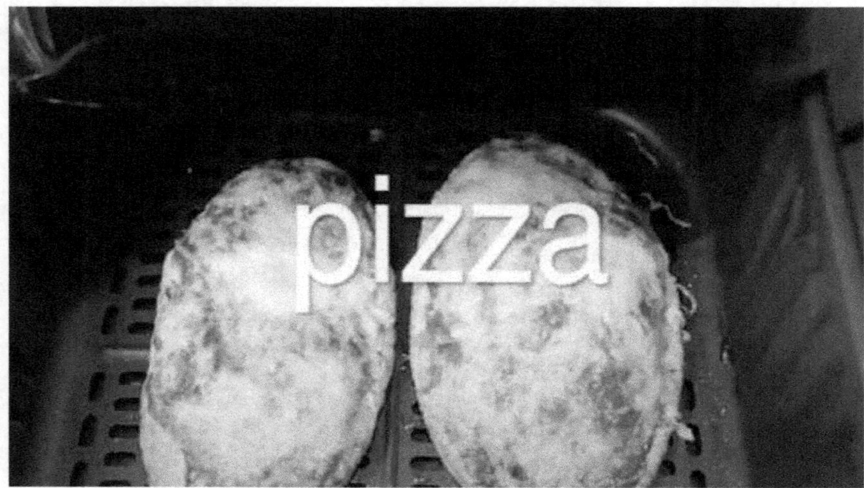

Method:

I usually would make these in the oven and I would put them in there for about 10 to 15 minutes. I'm just going to put some ketchup on top of the pizza bread base.

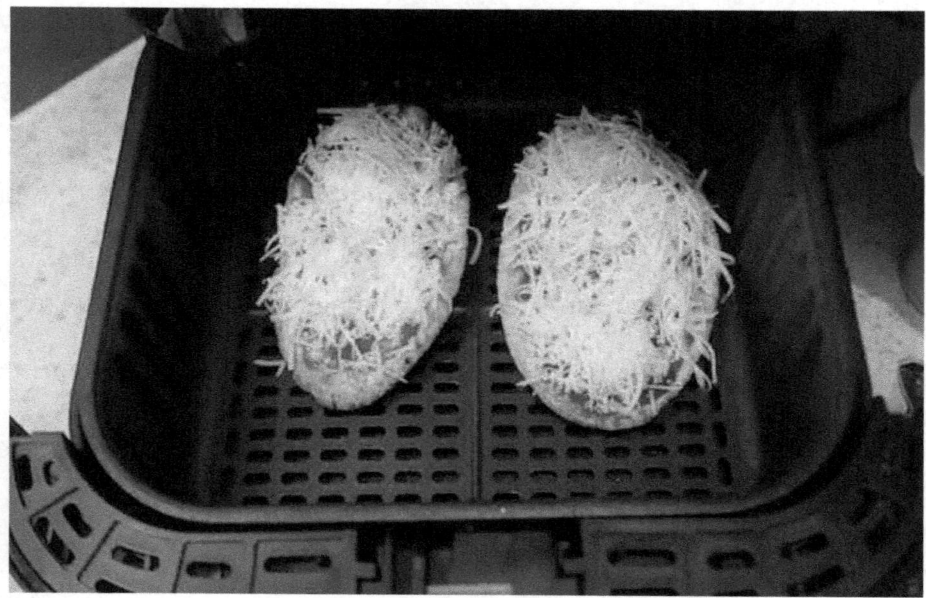

Or you can put tomato puree on there or some pasta whatever you've got. Then I'm just going to put some cheese on really nice and simple. I'm going to pop them on the pizza setting in the air fryer so that's eight minutes when I do my pizzas in the oven the base isn't really nice and crispy. So, I am really pleased with how they've turned out in the air fryer. Pizzas are done, crispy delicious, ready to eat.

23. Air Fryer Hanukkah Latkes

If you have never needed a latke, it is about time we change this. Traditionally served throughout Hanukkah, these crispy fritters -- frequently made with grated potatoes, lettuce, onion, and matzo meal -- are kind of impossible to not love.

Traditionally latkes are fried in oil (or poultry schmaltz!)) , however I wanted to see if I could create them using the popular air fryer. Since the fryer is a high-heat convection oven, the large fan speed and focused warmth yields a crispy potato pancake that is also soft at the middle.

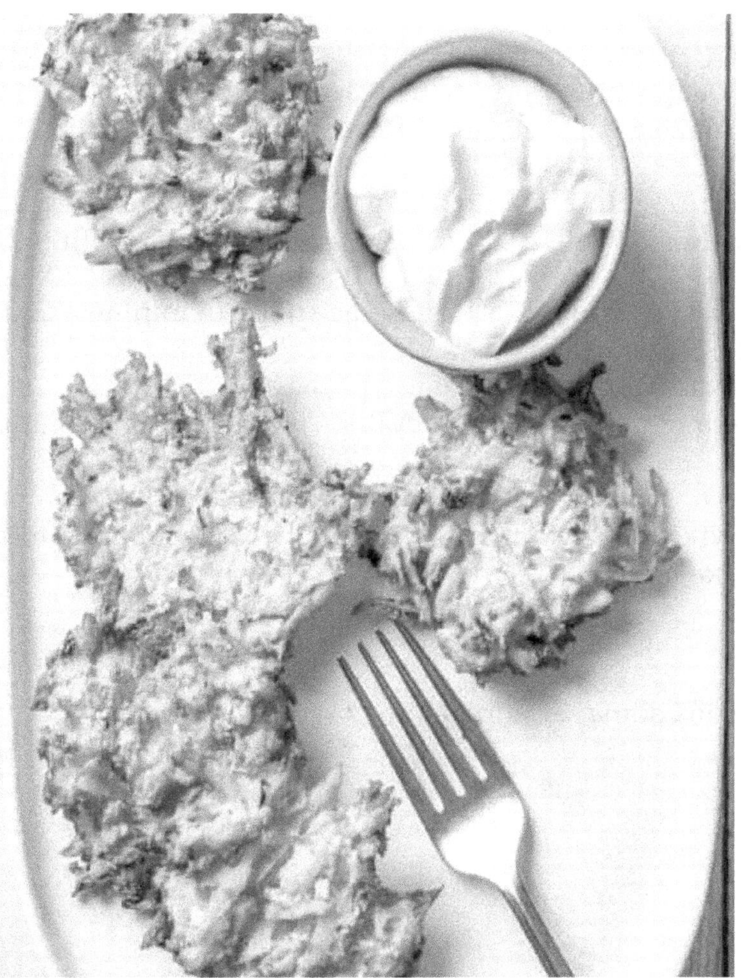

INGREDIENTS

- 1 1/2 Pounds Russet potatoes (2 to 3 tbsp.)
- ½ medium yellow onion

- 1/2 tsp freshly ground black pepper
- Cooking spray
- Two large eggs
- matzo meal
- 2 tsp kosher salt

Description:

- ❖ Peel 1 1/2 lbs. russet potatoes. Grate the potatoes and 1/2 yellow onion onto the large holes of a box grater. Put with a clean kitchen towel, then pull up the sides of the towel to make a package, and squeeze out excess moisture.
- ❖ Transfer the curry mixture into a large bowl. Add two large eggs, 1/4 cup matzo meal, two tsp kosher salt, and 1/2 tsp black pepper, and stir to blend.
- ❖ Preheat the Air Fryer into 375°F and place it for 16 minutes. Coat the air fryer racks together with cooking spray.
- ❖ Dip the latke mix in 2-tablespoon dollops to the fryer, flattening the shirts to make a patty.
- ❖ Air fry, rotating the trays halfway through, for 2 minutes total. Repeat with the rest of the latke mix.

24. Salmon Fillet

Now, I'm going to cook some salmon in it.

Ingredients:

- Salmon

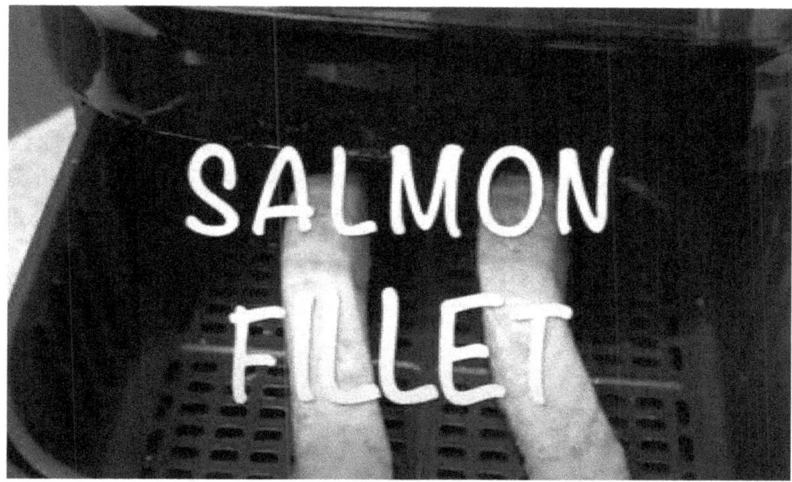

Method:

I put my salmon in, with nothing on top of it, just a salmon filet. I pop it in on the fish sitting for ten minutes and when it comes out it has got the crispy skin ever. The salmon was in for ten minutes and I wanted to show you how crispy the skin is.

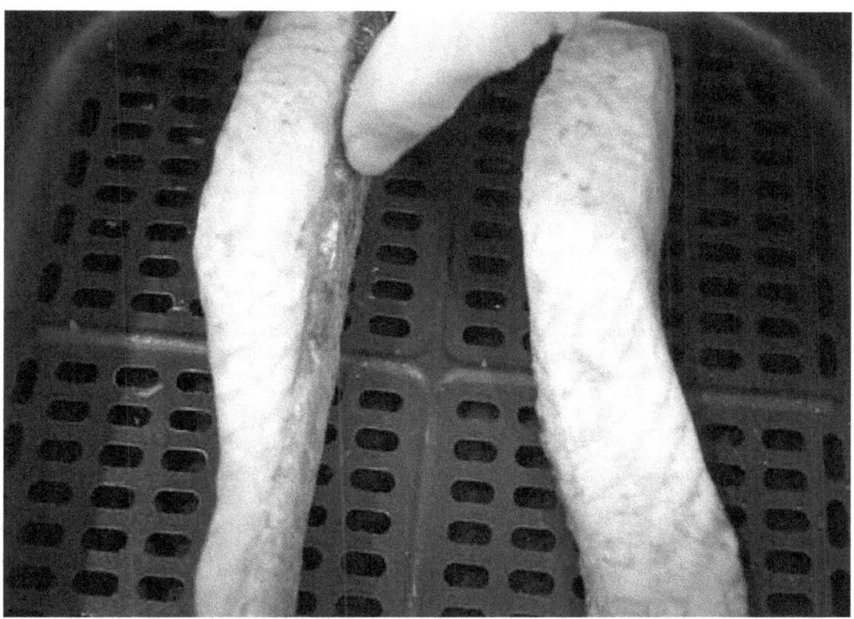

I'm someone who loves eating salmon skin and that is just perfectly done right.

25. Air Fryer Mini Calzones

Among the greatest approaches to utilize an air fryer is a miniature oven that will not heat up your entire kitchen for party snacks. It's possible to turn out batch after batch of wings, mozzarella sticks, and also, yes, miniature calzones which are hot, crispy, and superbly nostalgic by one air fryer.

These mini calzones utilize ready pizza dough to produce delicious pockets full of gooey cheese, piquant tomato sauce, and hot pepperoni that are fantastic for celebrations, after-school snacks, or even for satisfying your craving to get your dessert rolls of your childhood.

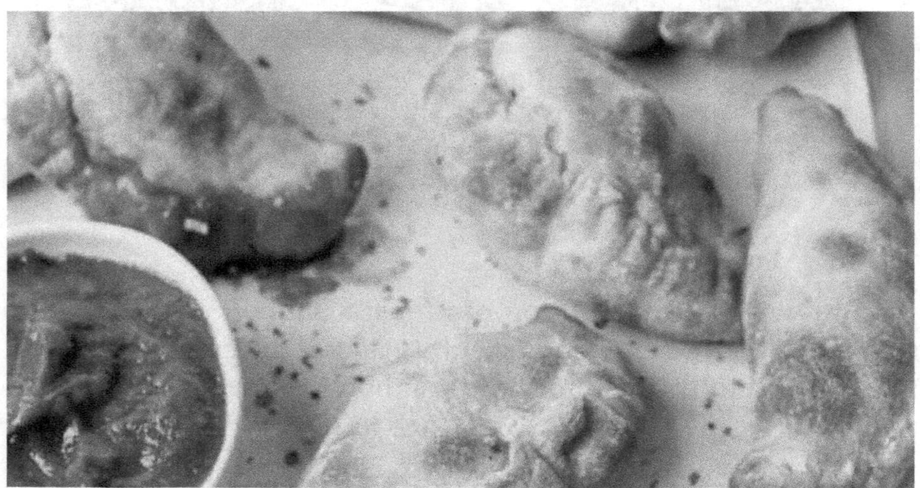

Ingredients:

- All-purpose flour, for rolling the dough out
- Pizza sauce, and more for dipping
- Thinly sliced pepperoni
- miniature pepperoni, chopped

Directions:

- ❖ Utilize a 3-inch round cutter or a large glass to cut 8 to 10 rounds of bread.
- ❖ Transfer the rounds into some parchment paper-lined baking sheet. Gather up the dough scraps, then reroll and replicate cutting rounds out until you've got 16.
- ❖ Top each round with two tsp of sauce, 1 tablespoon of cheese, and one tsp of pepperoni.

- ❖ Working with a single dough around at a time, fold in half an hour, then pinch the edges together to seal. When every calzone is sealed, then use a fork to crimp the borders shut to additional seal.

- ❖ Heat the air fryer into 375°F. Working in batches of 4, air fry the calzones until golden brown and crispy, about 8 minutes. Serve with extra pizza sauce for dipping, if desired.

26. Fajitas

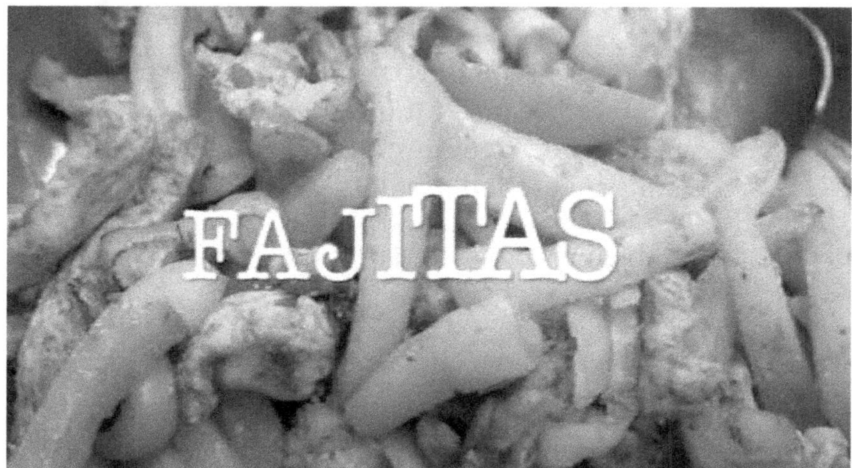

Ingredients:

- Turkey Strips
- Yellow Pepper
- Onion
- Orange Pepper

Method:

It's a night that we are going to be having for heaters. So, here, I've chopped up yellow and orange pepper and also half an onion. I have got some turkey strips.

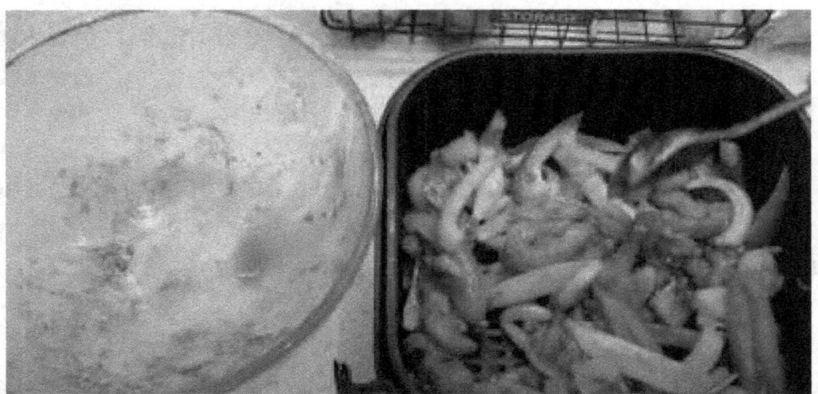

I'll pass it over heat as it makes barbecue flavor onto all of this. So, I'm just going to pop these all into the air fryer together because I think they'll actually cook through at a very similar rate. Then I am going to pop them on the chicken setting and let the air fryer get cooking alright. This is the fajita mix in ten minutes.

I put on the chicken setting which is actually 20 minutes but I was just checking it.

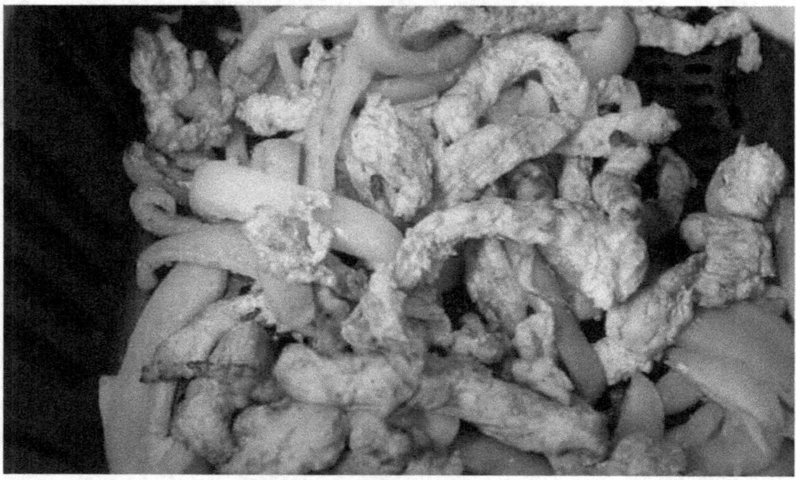

I cut a piece of the turkey and it's perfect all the way through, I cut it like one of the biggest pieces up as well. So, it's absolutely perfect so all this needs is ten minutes in the air fryer and it's done right.

27. Pot Sweet Potato Chips

Replace the humble sweet potato to a freshly-fried bite, and it is sure to be yummy. Sweet potato chips, sweet potato tater tots -- you name it, we will take it. The comparison between the sweetness of the curry and the saltiness of this bite is really impossible to not love.

These air fryer sweet potato chips provide everything you adore about these deep-fried snacks. That is the great thing about the air fryer that it requires less oil, after all -- you have to bypass the hassle and clutter of heating a massive pot of oil to the stove -- but the "fried" cure comes out evenly as yummy. And unlike a store-bought bag of chips, you have to personalize the seasonings. Here, we are using dried herbs and a pinch of cayenne for an earthy, somewhat spicy beverage.

Ingredients:

- medium sweet potato
- 1 tbsp. canola oil
- 1/2 tsp freshly ground black pepper
- 1/4 tsp paprika
- 1 tsp kosher salt
- 3/4 tsp dried thyme leaves
- Cooking spray

Directions:

- ❑ Wash 1 sweet potato and dry nicely. Thinly slice 1/8-inch thick using a knife or rather on a mandolin. Set in a bowl, then cover with cool water, and then soak at room temperature for 20 minutes to remove the excess starch.
- ❑ Drain the pieces and pat very dry with towels. Put into a large bowl, then add 1 tbsp. canola oil, 1 tsp kosher salt, 3/4 tsp dried thyme leaves, 1/2 tsp black pepper, 1/4 tsp paprika, and a pinch cayenne pepper if using, and toss to blend.
- ❑ Gently coat in an air fryer rotisserie basket with cooking spray.
- ❑ Air fry in batches: put one layer of sweet potato pieces from the rotisserie basket. Put the rotisserie basket at the fryer and press on.
- ❑ Preheat the fryer into 340°F and place for 22 minutes, until the sweet potatoes are golden brown and the edges are crispy, 19 to 22 minutes.
- ❑ Transfer the chips into a newspaper towel-lined plate to cool completely

- They will crisp as they cool. Repeat with the remaining sweet potato pieces.

28. Easy Baked Eggs

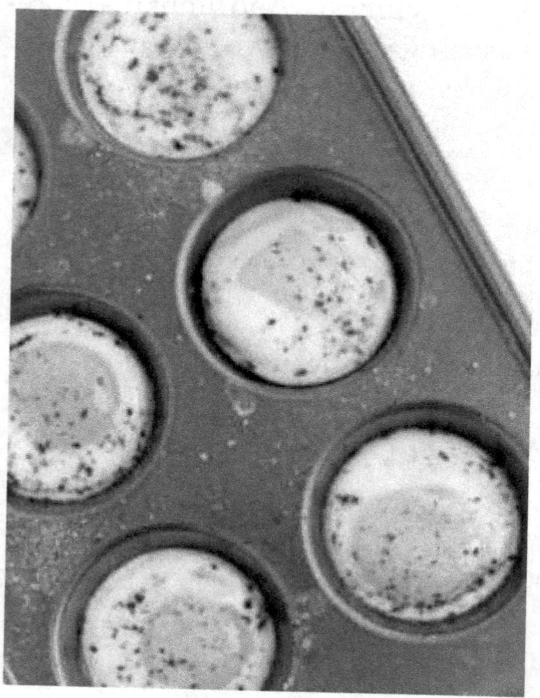

Ingredients:

- 1 Tbsp. heavy cream
- ¼ tsp salt
- 2 eggs
- 1/8 tsp ground black pepper

Method:

- Preheat your fryer to 330 degrees F.
- Spray a silicone muffin cup or a little ramekin with cooking spray.
- In a small bowl, whisk together all of the components
- Pour the eggs into the ready ramekin and bake for 6 minutes.

➢ Enjoy directly from the skillet!

29. Air Fryer Buttermilk Fried Chicken

I went to school in the South, so I have had my fair share of crispy, succulent, finger-licking fried chicken. As you might imagine, I had been skeptical about creating a much healthier version from the air fryer.

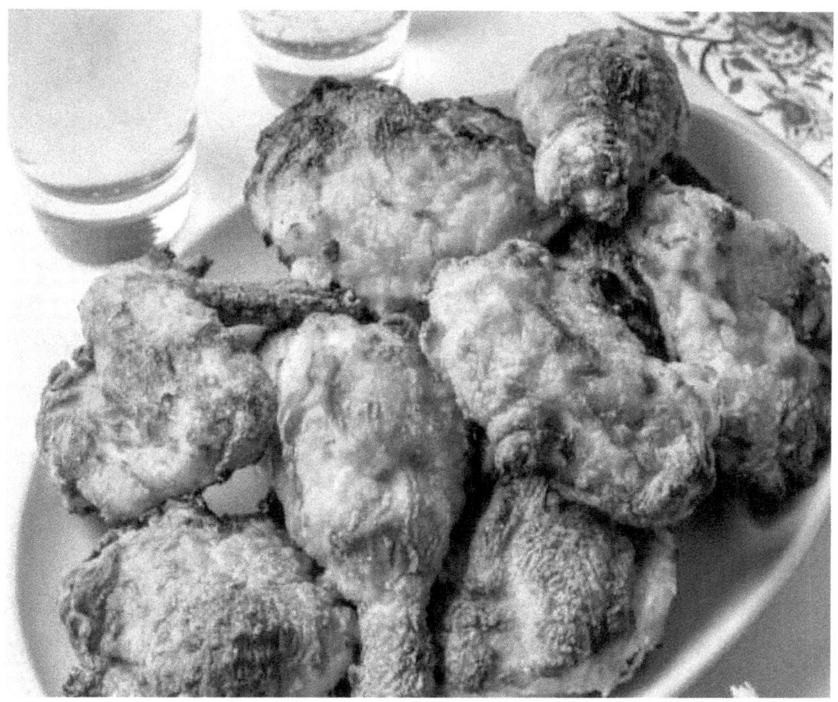

The second I pulled out my first batch, but my worries disappeared. The epidermis was crispy, the coat was cracker-crisp (as it ought to be), and also, above all, the chicken itself was tender and succulent -- the indication of a perfect piece of fried chicken.

Air fryer fried chicken is lighter, quicker, than and not as cluttered as deep-fried chicken. Here is the way to get it done.

Ingredients

- 1 tsp Freshly ground black pepper, divided
- Buttermilk
- 1 tsp Cayenne pepper
- 1 tbsp. Garlic powder

- 2 tbsp. paprika
- 1 tbsp. onion powder
- 1 tsp kosher salt, divided
- all-purpose flour
- 1 tbsp. ground mustard
- Cooking spray

Directions

- ❑ Put all ingredients into a large bowl and season with 1 teaspoon of the kosher salt and 1/2 tsp of honey.
- ❑ Add 2 cups buttermilk and simmer for 1 hour in the fridge. Meanwhile, whisk the remaining 1 tbsp. kosher salt, staying 1/2 tsp black pepper, 2 cups all-purpose flour, 1 tbsp. garlic powder, 2 tbsp. paprika, 1 teaspoon cayenne pepper, 1 tbsp. onion powder, plus one tbsp. ground mustard together into a huge bowl.
- ❑ Preheat an air fryer into 390°F. Coat the fryer racks together with cooking spray. Remove the chicken in the buttermilk, allowing any excess to drip off. Dredge in the flour mixture, shaking off any excess. Put one layer of chicken in the basket, with distance between the bits. Air fry, turning the chicken hallway through, until an instant-read thermometer registers 165°F from the thickest part
- ❑ Cook for 18 to 20 minutes, then complete.

30. Keto Chocolate Chip Muffins

Ingredients:

- ¼ tsp salt
- 1 Tbsp. powdered stevia
- ¼ cup whole milk
- 1 egg
- 1 cup almond flour

- 1 ½ tsp baking powder
- ½ cup mini dark chocolate chips (sugar free)

Method:

- Preheat your air fryer to 350 degrees F.
- In a large bowl, stir together the almond milk, stevia, salt, cinnamon, and baking powder.
- Add the milk and eggs and then stir well.
- Split the muffin batter involving each muffin cup, filling around 3/4 of this way complete.
- Set the muffins to the air fryer basket and cook for 14 minutes or till a toothpick comes out when put to the middle.
- Eliminate from the fryer and let cool.

31. Crispy Chickpeas

What, I've got in here are some chickpeas.

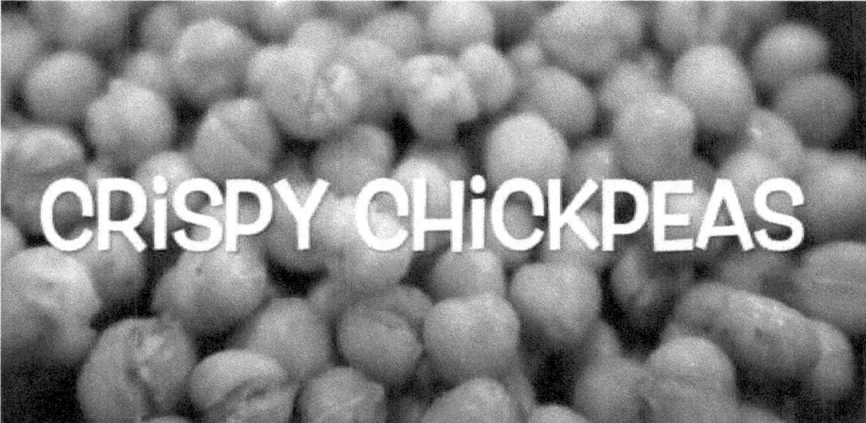

Ingredients:

- Chickpeas
- Olive oil

- Per-peril salt

Method:

I've drained and washed chickpeas and then what I'm going to do is add on some olive oil and then also the periphery salt. The reason I put some olive oil on is because it just helps the pair of results stick to the chickpeas.

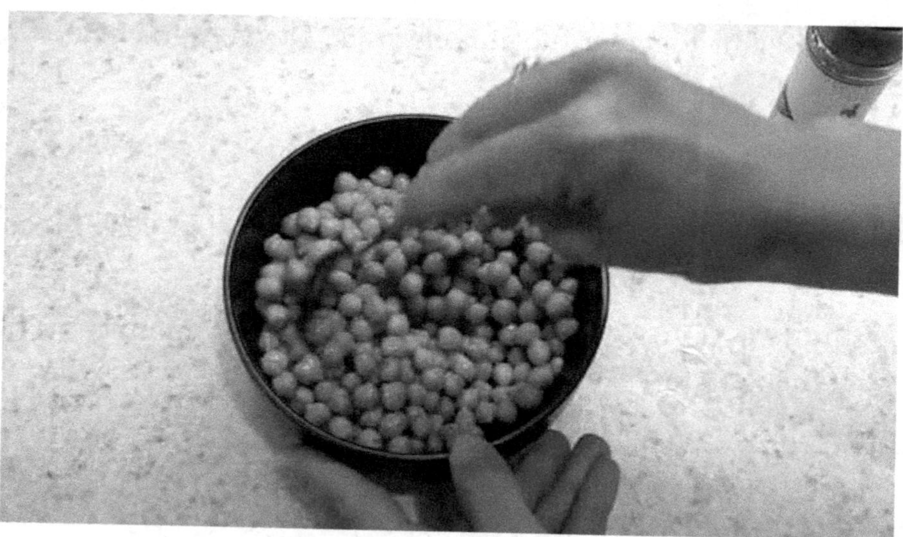

Then I'm just going to mix everything in together and pop them into the air fryer for about 15 minutes. On the chip setting these are great little snacks to make like pre dinner snacks. Instead of having crisps or if you're watching a movie, instead of having popcorn these are good little things. Also, if you are having a salad they're really nice to go in your salad as well.

32. Keto Blueberry Muffins

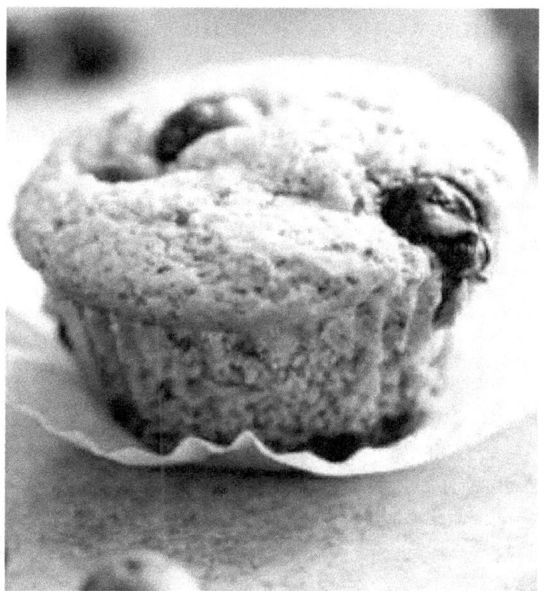

Ingredients:

- 1 egg
- ¼ tsp salt
- 1 cup almond flour
- 1 Tbsp. powdered stevia
- 1 ½ tsp baking powder
- ¼ cup whole milk
- ¼ tsp ground cinnamon
- ½ cup frozen or fresh blueberries

Steps:

1) Preheat your air fryer to 350 degrees F.
2) In a large bowl, stir together the almond milk, stevia, salt, cinnamon, and baking powder.
3) Add the milk and eggs and then stir well.

4) Split the muffin batter involving each muffin cup, filling roughly 3/4 of this way complete.

5) Set the muffins to the air fryer basket and cook for 14 minutes or till a toothpick comes out when put to the middle.

6) Eliminate from the fryer and let cool.

33. Air Fryer Donuts

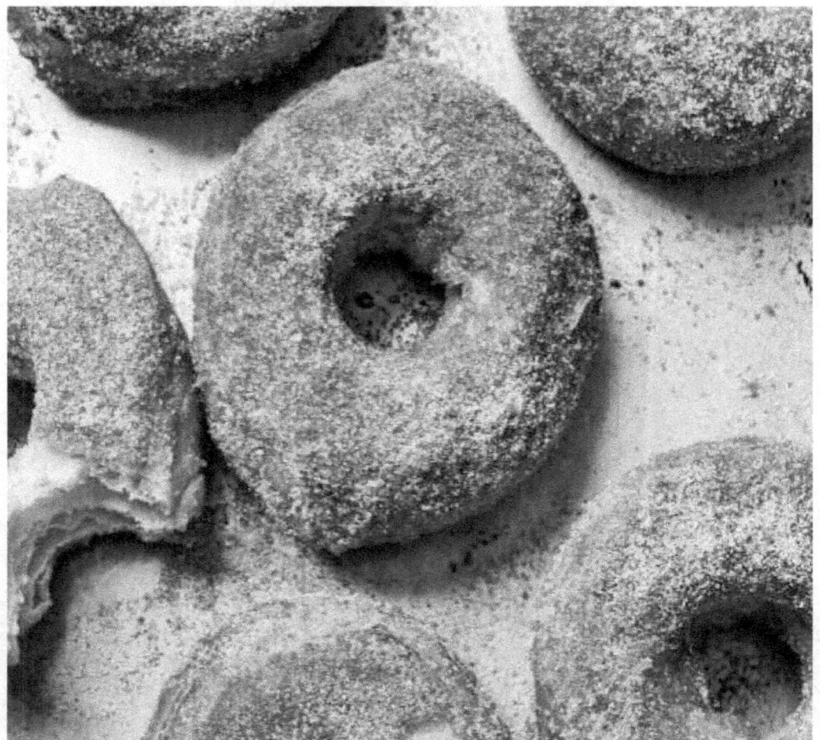

Ingredients

- ground cinnamon
- granulated sugar
- Flaky large snacks,
- Jojoba oil spray or coconut oil spray

Instructions

★ Combine sugar and cinnamon in a shallow bowl; place aside.

★ Remove the cookies from the tin, separate them and set them onto the baking sheet.

★ Utilize a 1-inch round biscuit cutter (or similarly-sized jar cap) to cut holes from the middle of each biscuit.

★ Lightly coat an air fryer basket using coconut or olive oil spray (don't use nonstick cooking spray like Pam, which may damage the coating onto the basket)

★ Put 3 to 4 donuts in one layer in the air fryer (that they shouldn't be touching). Close to the air fryer and place to 350°F. Transfer donuts into the baking sheet.

★ Repeat with the rest of the biscuits. You can also cook the donut holes they will take approximately 3 minutes total

★ Brush both sides of this hot donut with melted butter, put in the cinnamon sugar, and then turn to coat both sides.

34. Sausage and Spinach Omelet

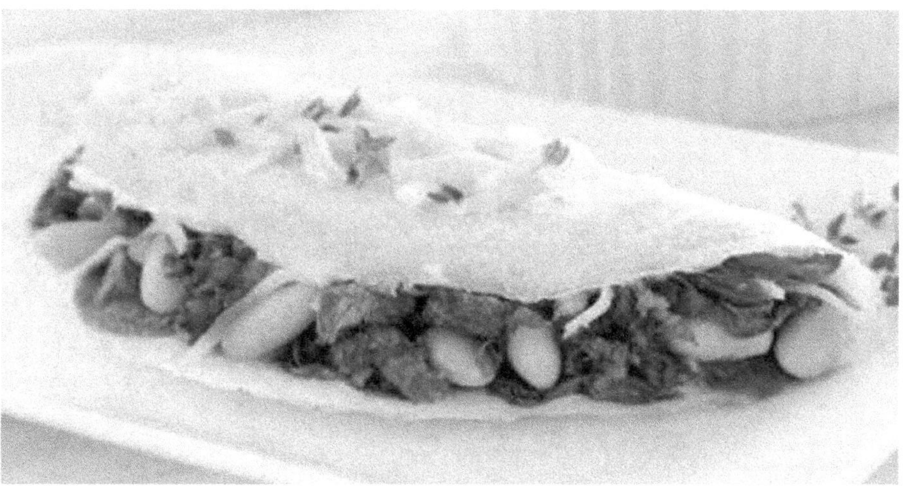

Ingredients:

½ cup baby spinach

4 eggs

¼ cup cheddar cheese, grated

½ cup cooked, crumbled sausage

3 Tbsp. heavy whipping cream

½ tsp salt

¼ tsp ground black pepper

Directions

I. Preheat the air fryer at around 330 F.

II. In a small bowl, whisk together the eggs, cream, pepper and salt.

III. Fold in the cooked sausage and sausage.

IV. Pour the mixture into the prepared baking pan then place the pan on your

V. Cook for approximately ten minutes or till the eggs are completely set.

VI. Sprinkle the cheeses round the boiled eggs and then return the pan into the fryer

VII. Fryer for another two minutes to melt the cheese.

35. Air Fryer Potato Wedges

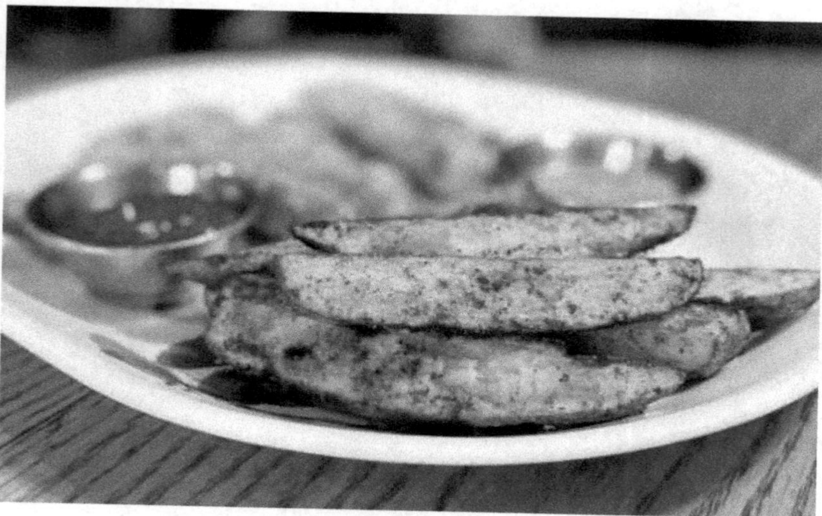

Perfectly crisp and seasoned potato wedges directly from your air fryer. It will not get any simpler than this!

Ingredients

- ➔ 2 medium Russet potatoes, cut into wedges
- ➔ 1/2 tsp sea salt
- ➔ 1 1/2 tsp olive oil
- ➔ 1/2 tsp chili powder
- ➔ ⅛ teaspoon ground black pepper
- ➔ 1/2 tsp paprika
- ➔ 1/2 tsp parsley flakes

Instructions

- ❖ Place potato wedges in a large bowl.
- ❖ Put 8 wedges at the jar of the air fryer and cook for 10 minutes.
- ❖ Flip wedges with tongs and cook for another five minutes.

36. Chocolate Chip Cookies in Air fryer

They are my day pick-me-up, my after-dinner treat, also, sometimes, a part of my breakfast. I keep either frozen cookies or baked biscuits in my freezer -- true my friends know and have come to appreciate when they come around for dinner or even a glass of wine.

The kind of chocolate chip cookie I enjoy all, depends upon my mood. Sometimes I need them super doughy, and sometimes challenging and crisp. If you're searching for one someplace in between -- gooey on the inside and crunchy on the outside -- I have discovered the foolproof way of you. It entails cooking them on your air fryer.

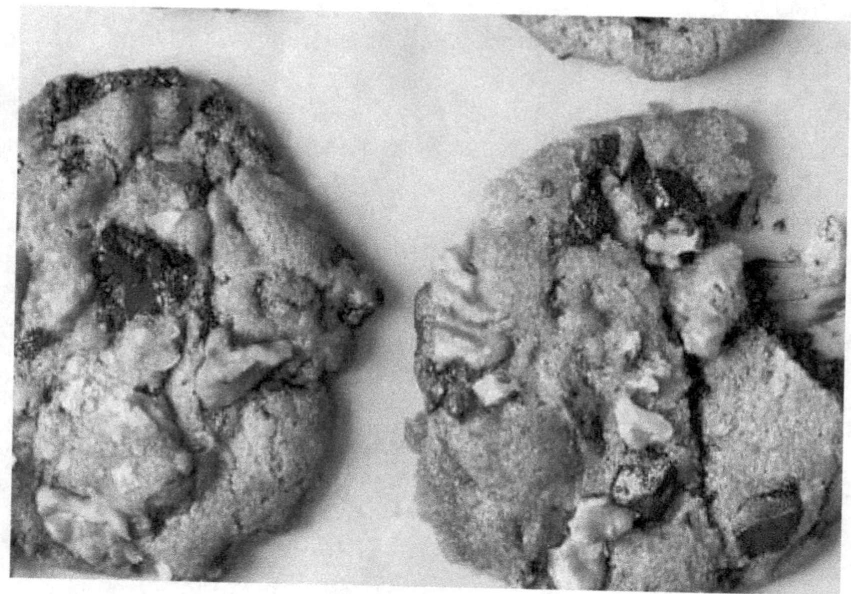

When using your fryer to create biscuits, be certain that you always line its base with foil to aid with simple cleanup. You will also need to line the basket or racks using parchment paper. Buy paper which has holes in it, cut some slits to the newspaper, or make sure you leave space around it which will allow for even cooking and flow of the air. With these suggestions, you're on your way to cookie victory!

Ingredients:

- Granulated sugar
- vanilla extract
- dark brown sugar
- 1 tsp kosher salt
- 2 large eggs
- 3/4 cup chopped walnuts
- 1 tsp baking soda
- Flaky sea salt, for garnish (optional)
- all-purpose flour
- Cooking spray

INSTRUCTIONS

- ❖ Put 2 sticks unsalted butter in the bowl of a stand mixer, fitted with the paddle attachment and also let it sit till softened. Insert 3/4 cup granulated sugar and 3/4 cup packed dark brown sugar and beat it on medium speed till blended and fluffy within 3 to 4 minutes. Add 1 tablespoon lemon extract, 2 big eggs, and 1 tsp kosher salt, and beat until just blended. After that, add 1 tea-spoon baking soda plus 2 1/3 cups all-purpose flour in increments, mixing until just blended.
- ❖ Add 2 cups chocolate balls and 3/4 cup chopped peppers and stir with a rubber spatula until just blended.
- ❖ Preheat in an air fryer, at 350°F and set to 5 minutes. Line the fryer racks with parchment paper, make sure you leave space on all sides for air to leak.
- ❖ Reduce 2-tablespoon scoops of this dough on the racks, setting them 1-inch apart. Gently flatten each spade marginally to earn a cookie form.
- ❖ Sprinkle with flaky sea salt, if using. Bake until golden brown, about 5 minutes. Remove the racks out of the fryer and let it cool for 3 to 5 minutes to place. Repeat with the remaining dough.

37. Crispy Coated Veggies

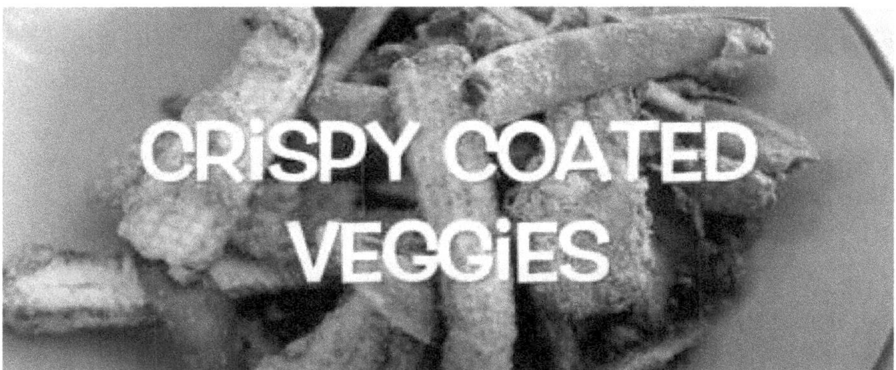

Ingredients:

- Vegetables
- Egg
- Paprika

- Salt & Pepper

Method:

I'm making some crispy coating of vegetables in this bowl. I have got one egg beaten up. This is actually almond flour but you can use normal flour and then I popped in some paprika. I've also put in some salt and pepper here too. Then I'm going to dip my veggies into my egg and then I'll put them into the flour mixture, then into the air fryer for probably about eight minutes.

38. Ranch Pork Chops in Air fryer

Ingredients

- 4 boneless, center-cut pork chops, 1-inch thick
- aluminum foil
- cooking spray
- 2 Tsp dry ranch salad dressing mix

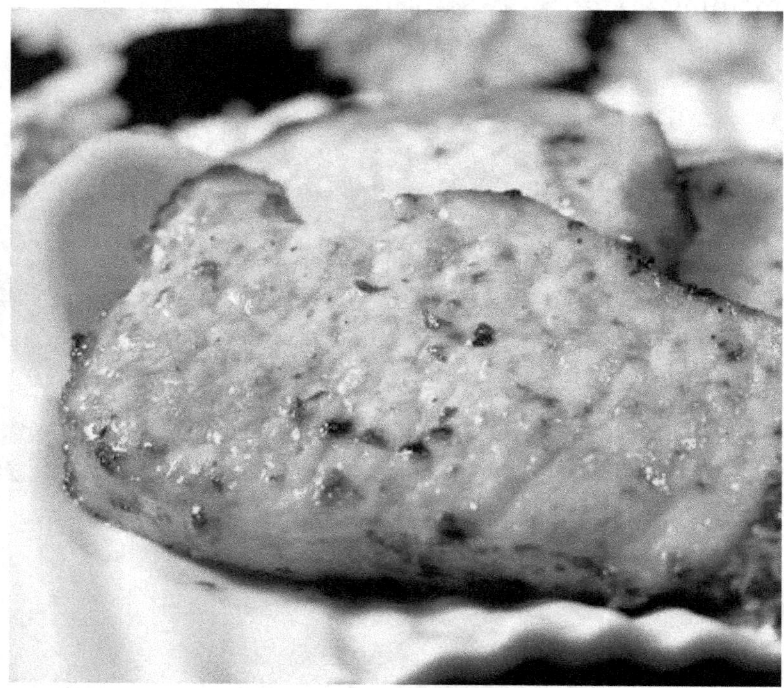

Directions

- ★ Put pork chops on a plate and then gently spray both sides with cooking spray. Sprinkle both sides with ranch seasoning mixture and let them sit at room temperature for 10 minutes.
- ★ Spray the basket of an air fryer with cooking spray and preheat at 390 degrees F (200 degrees C).
- ★ Place chops in the preheated air fryer, working in batches if needed, to guarantee the fryer isn't overcrowded.
- ★ Flip chops and cook for 5 minutes longer. Let rest on a foil-covered plate for 5 minutes prior to serving.

39. Quesadillas

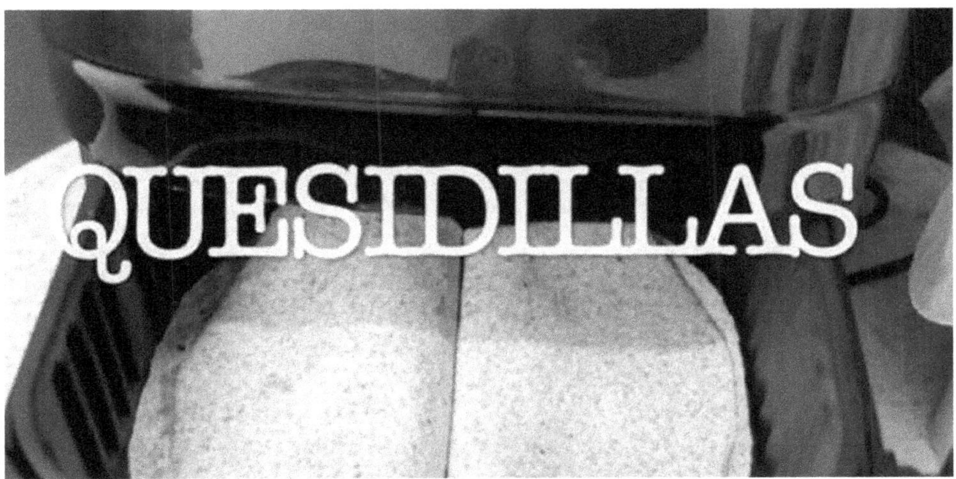

Ingredients:

- Refried Beans
- Cheese
- Peppers
- Chicken

Method:

I'm going to be using the El Paso refried beans in the tin. I will spread that onto the wrap and then I'm just going to sprinkle some cheese on top.

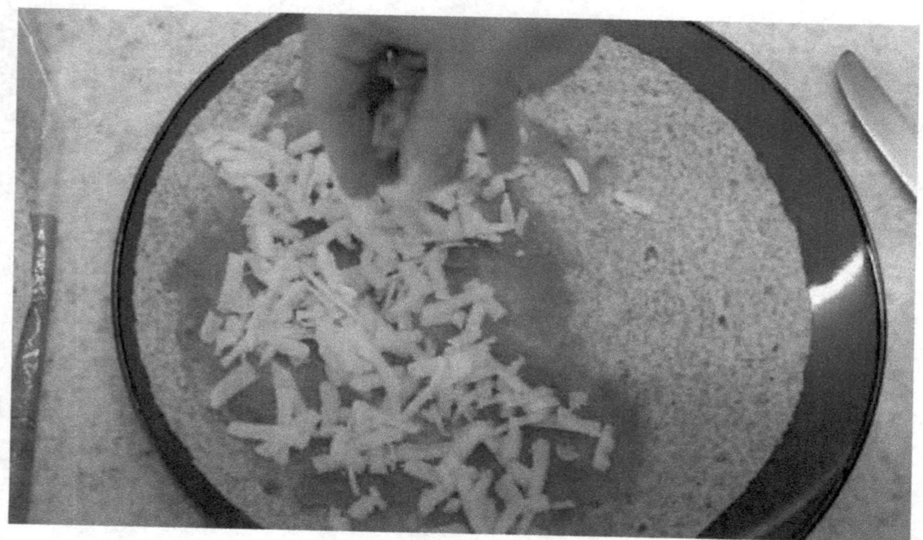

This is a really basic wrap so usually when we have routes we'll add some like peppers in here as well and loads of other bits like chicken. I just wanted to show you how well they cook in the air fryer. You pop them in on the pizza setting and in 8 to10 minutes they are done. Really crispy and ready to eat.

40. Pecan Crusted Pork Chops at the Air Fryer

The air-fryer makes simple work of those yummy pork chops. The chops make good leftovers too, since the pecan crust does not get soggy!

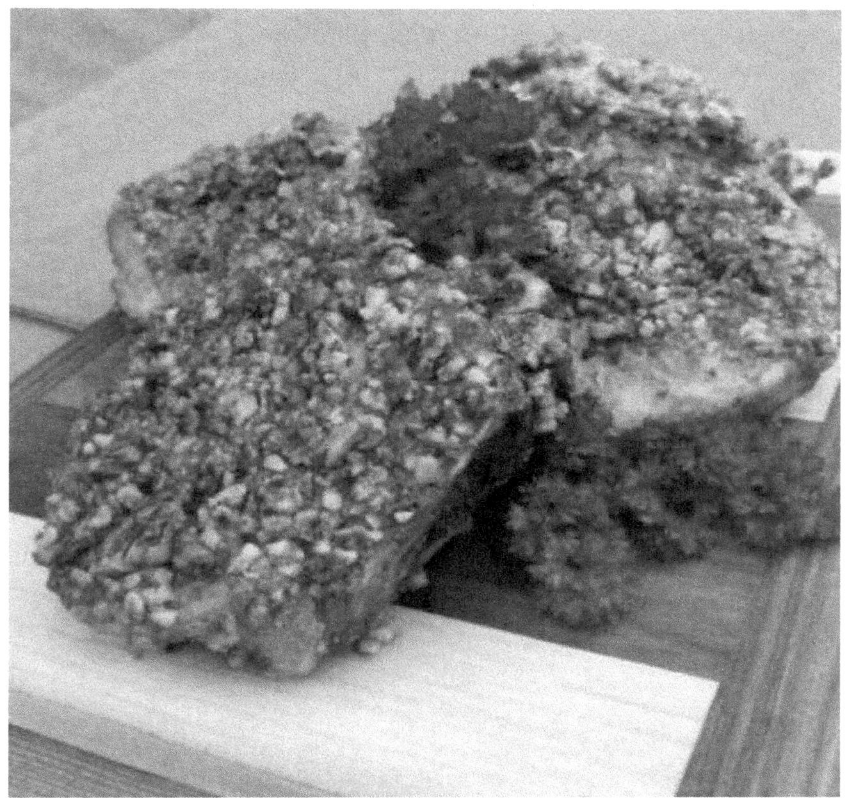

Ingredients:

- Egg
- Pork
- Pecans
- Simmer

Instructions

➢ Add egg and simmer until all ingredients are well blended. Place pecans onto a plate.

➢ Dip each pork dip in the egg mix, then put onto the plate together with the pecans

➢ Press pecans firmly onto either side until coated. Spray the chops on both sides with cooking spray and set from the fryer basket.

➢ Cook at the fryer for 6 minutes. Turn chops closely with tongs, and fry until pork is no longer pink in the middle, about 6 minutes more.

41. Crispy Chicken Thighs

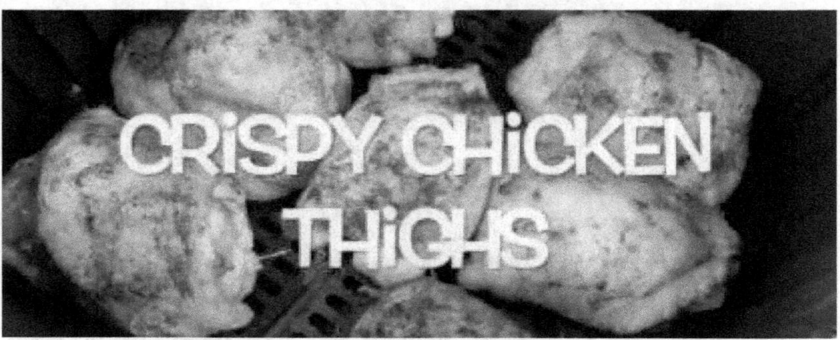

Ingredients

- Chicken thighs
- Pepper
- Olive oil
- Paprika
- Salt

Method:

I've got some chicken thighs. These have got bone-in and skinned on so what I've done is just put some olive oil on top of them with some paprika and some salt and pepper. Then I just rubbed everything into the chicken skin so I'm going to pop these into my air fryer. Press the chicken button and let the air fryer just do its thing.

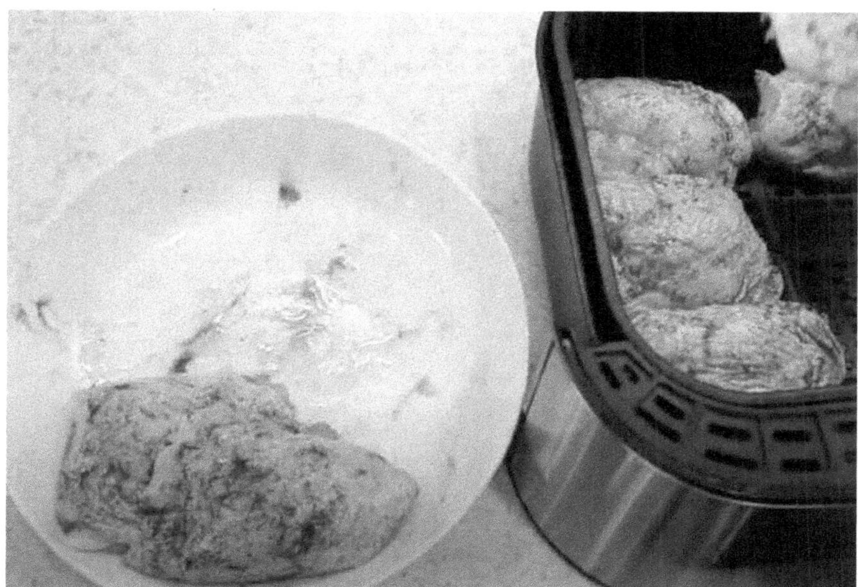

This skin is super crispy that is perfectly done and it's been in there for 20 minutes. I just wanted to show you all the fat that came out of that chicken so here are all the oils that came off.

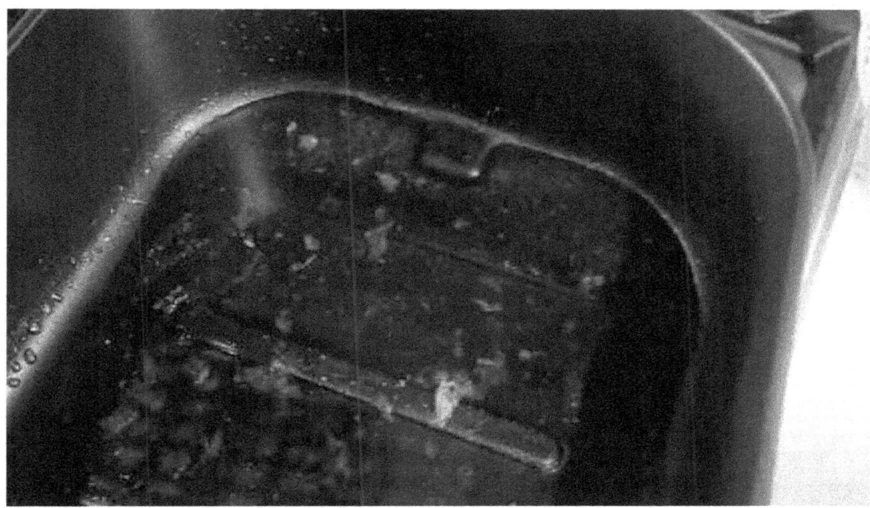

So those are what your chicken would be sitting in but instead it's all just tripped underneath the air fryer.

42. Bacon-Wrapped Scallops with Sirach Mayo

This yummy appetizer is ready quickly and easily in the air fryer and served with a hot Sirach mayo skillet. I use the smaller bay scallops because of this. If you're using jumbo scallops, it'll require a longer cooking time and more bits of bacon.

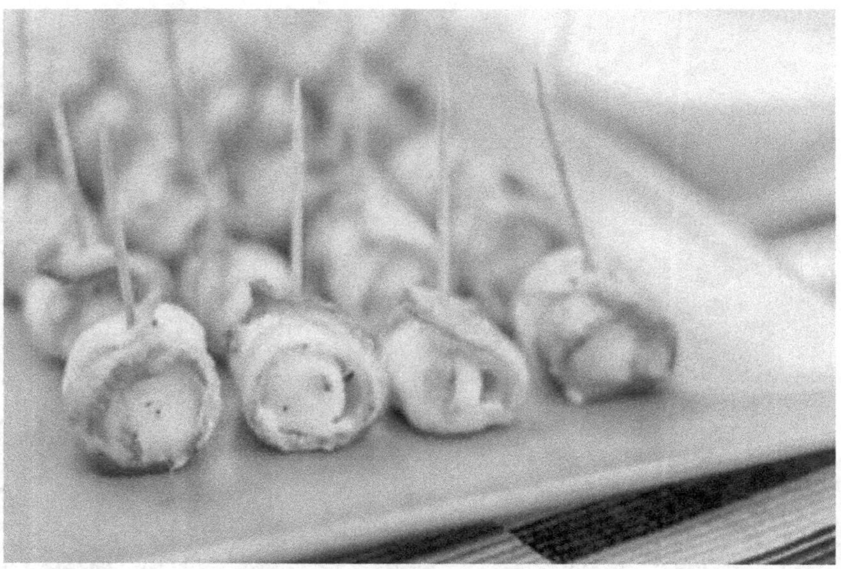

Ingredients

- 1/2 cup mayonnaise
- 1 pinch coarse salt
- 2 tbsp.Sirach sauce
- 1 pound bay scallops (about 36 small scallops)
- 1 pinch freshly cracked black pepper
- 12 slices bacon, cut into thirds
- 1 serving olive oil cooking spray

Instructions

★ Mix mayonnaise and Sirach sauce together in a little bowl.

★ Preheat the air fryer to 390 degrees F (200 degrees C).

★ Season with pepper and salt. Wrap each scallop with 1/3 piece of bacon and fasten with a toothpick.

★ Spray the air fryer basket with cooking spray. Put bacon-wrapped scallops from the basket in one layer; divide into two batches if needed.

★ Cook at the air fryer for 7 minutes. Check for doneness; scallops should be wheat and opaque ought to be crispy. Cook 1 to 2 minutes more, if needed, checking every moment. Remove scallops carefully with tongs and put on a newspaper towel-lined plate to absorb extra oil out of the bacon.

43. Homemade Chips

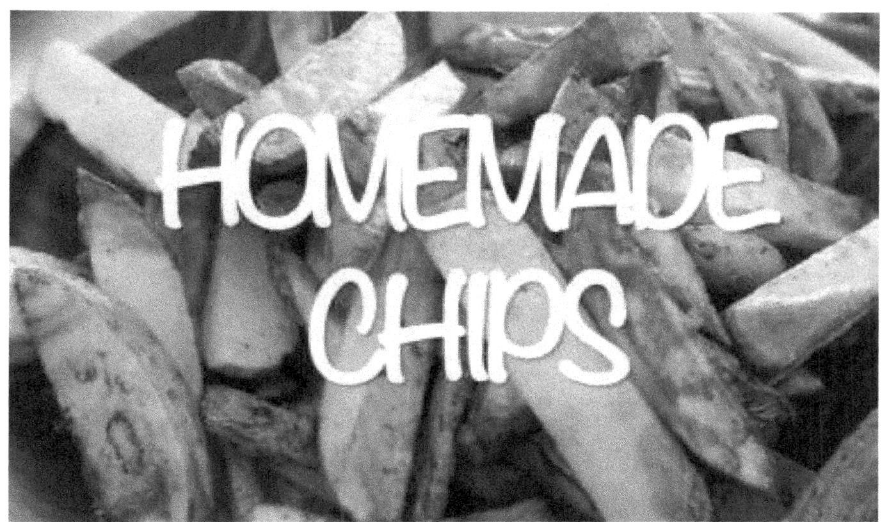

Ingredients

- Chip
- Olive oil
- Paprika
- Salt

Method:

Now I'm going to do some chips. I've just cut up some potatoes into chip shapes and then I am going to put some olive oil on top. Some paprika and some salt and the main reason I'm putting olive oil on top is basically for the paprika and the salt to stick to the surface of the chips. I'll just pop these in and then I'll put them onto the chip setting and let them cook away for about 18 minutes. I will be staring these halfway through because I'm doing quite a few chips as well. I will probably have to put these on for another 10 minutes after the 18 minutes is done.

44. Easy Air Fryer Pork Chops

Boneless pork chops cooked to perfection with the help of an air fryer. This recipe is super easy and you could not ask for a more tender and succulent chop.

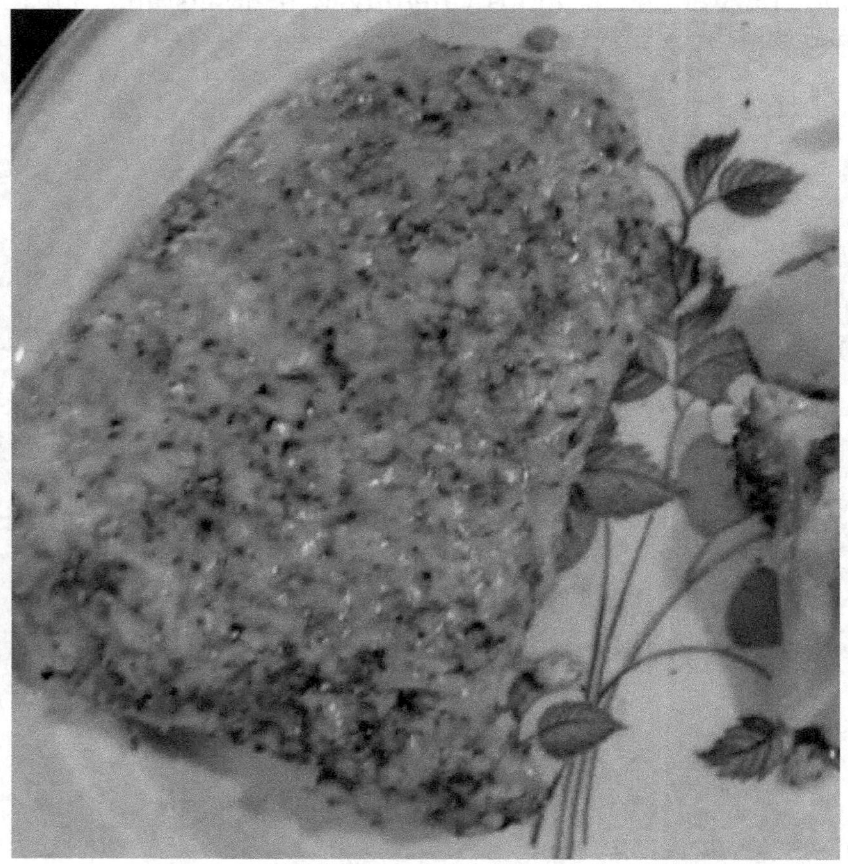

Ingredients

- 1/2 cup grated Parmesan cheese
- 1 tsp kosher salt
- 4 (5 oz.) center-cut pork chops
- 2 tbsp. extra virgin olive oil
- 1 tsp dried parsley
- 1 tsp paprika
- 1 tsp garlic powder

- 1/2 teaspoon ground black pepper

Instructions

- ❑ Preheat the fryer to 390 degrees F.
- ❑ Combine Parmesan cheese, paprika, garlic powder, salt, parsley, and pepper in a level shallow dish; combine well.
- ❑ Stir every pork chop with olive oil. Dredge both sides of each dip from the Parmesan mixture and put on a plate.
- ❑ Put 2 chops from the basket of the fryer and cook for 10 minutes; turning halfway through cook time.

45. Corn on the Cob

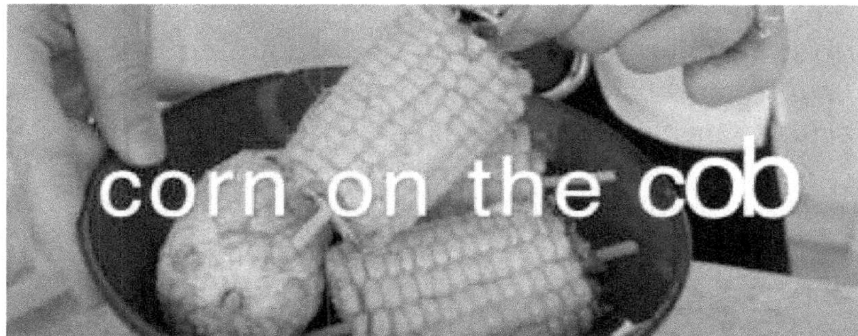

Ingredients:

- Corn
- Butter
- Salt

Method:

We're going to do some corn on the cob. What I'm going to do is just pop them into my air fryer but not put anything on top of them. I'm going to put them in on the prawn settings.

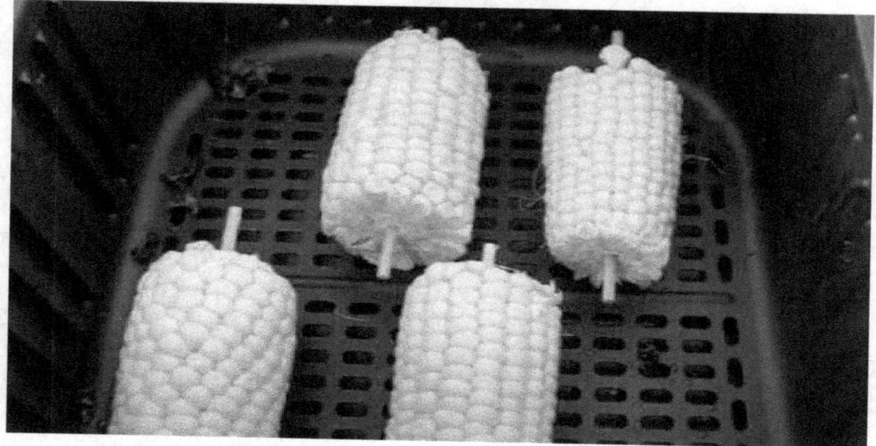

It's just eight minutes, after ten minutes like I said, I will then add some butter on top and a little bit of salt. They're ready to eat.

46. Air Fryer Broiled Grapefruit

This hot and warm grapefruit with a buttery candy topping is the best accompaniment for your Sunday brunch and makes a lovely snack or dessert. I love to add a pinch of sea salt in the end to actually bring out the tastes.

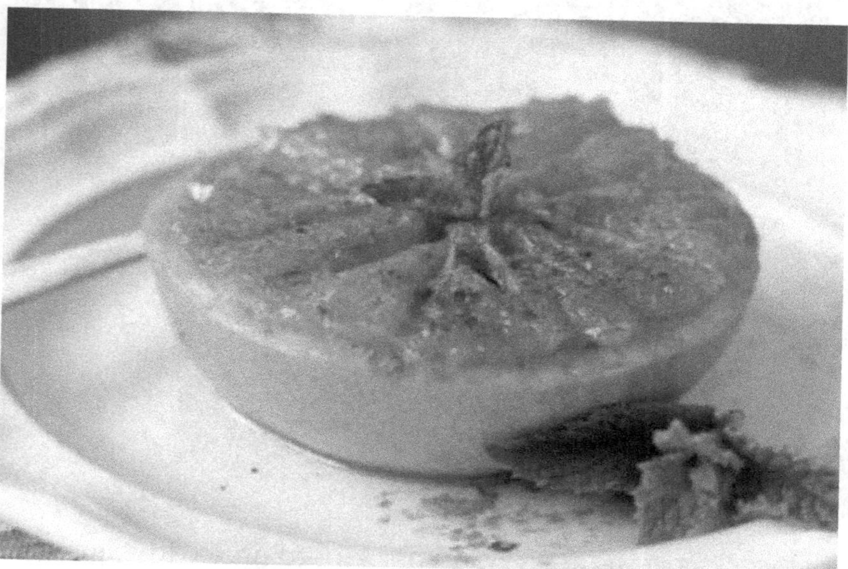

Ingredients

- 1 red grapefruit, refrigerated
- aluminum foil

- 1 tbsp. brown sugar
- 1/2 teaspoon ground cinnamon
- 1 tbsp. softened butter
- 2 tsp sugar

Instructions

- ➢ Cut grapefruit in half crosswise and slice off a thin sliver away from the base of every half, when the fruit is not sitting at level. Use a sharp paring knife to cut around the outer edge of this grapefruit and involve every section to generate the fruit easier to consume after cooking.
- ➢ Combine softened butter 1 tbsp. brown sugar in a small bowl. Spread mix over each grapefruit in half. Sprinkle with remaining brown sugar levels.
- ➢ Cut aluminum foil into two 5-inch squares and put each grapefruit half one square; fold the edges up to catch any juices. Place in the air fryer basket.
- ➢ Broil in the fryer until the sugar mixture is bubbling, 6 to 7 minutes.

47. Kale Crisps

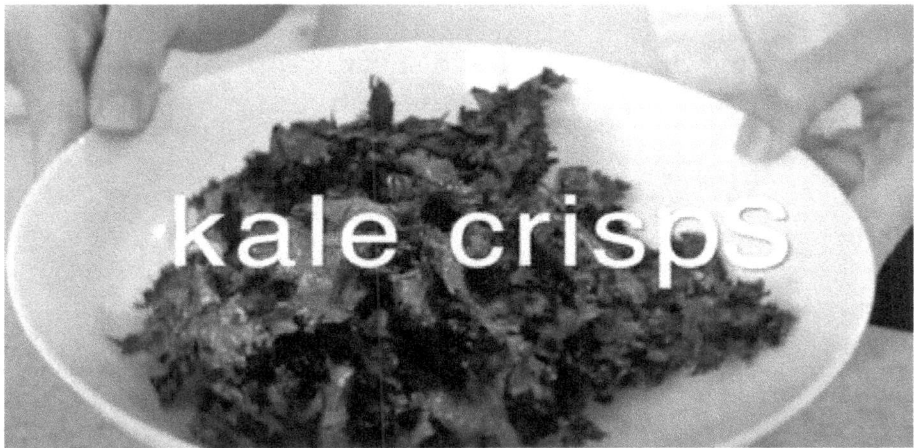

Ingredients:

- Kale
- Olive oil

- Salt

Method:

I'm going to make some kale crisps now. So, the first thing we're going to do list, get my kale and chop off the thick stocky bits. Once I've chopped that out, I will then just dice my kale up into kind of chunks and then I'll pop them into a bowl. Put some olive oil on top and some salts give everything a mix around.

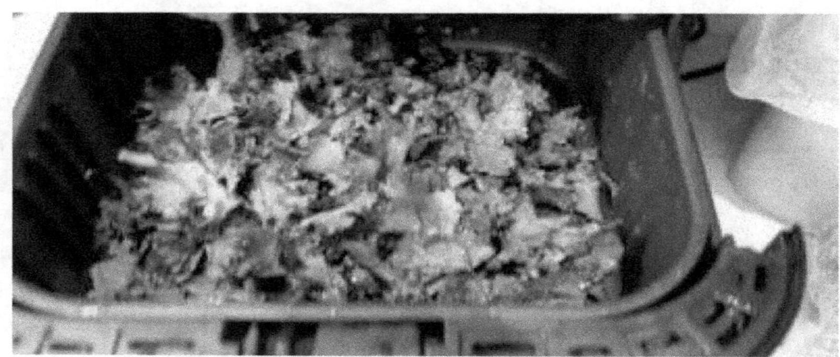

I'll pop them into my air fryer and on the prong setting. The reason I put them on the prong setting is because that's just a quick eight minute setting and that's the perfect amount of time that these kale crisps take to cook. When they come out, they are super nice and crunchy and they taste delicious.

48. Air Fryer Brown Sugar and Pecan Roasted Apples

A sweet and nutty topping made with brown sugar and pecans adds amazing flavor to apples since they cook to tender perfection at the air fryer.

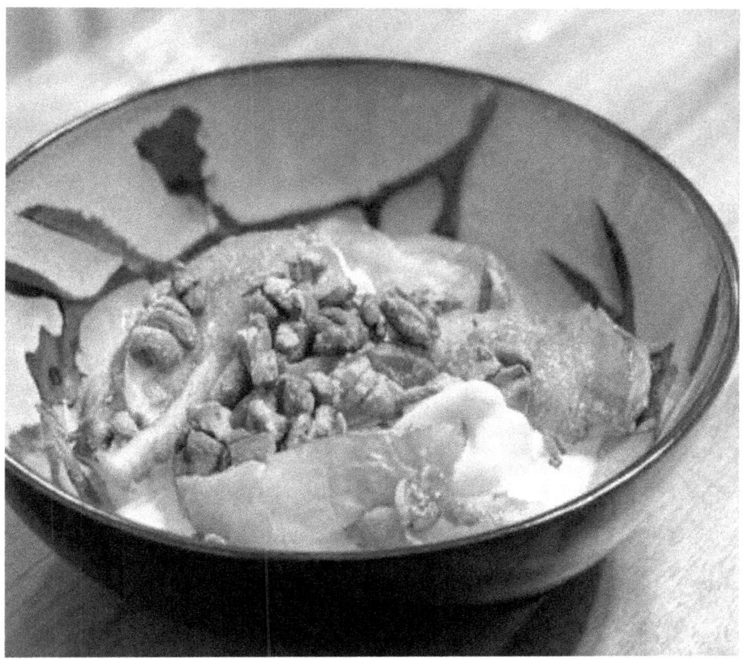

Ingredients

- 1/4 tsp apple pie spice
- 2 tbsp. coarsely chopped pecans
- 1 tbsp. brown sugar
- 1 tbsp. butter, melted
- 1 tsp all-purpose flour
- 2 medium apples, cored and cut into wedges

Instructions

➔ Preheat the air fryer to 350 degrees F

➔ Put apple wedges in a skillet drizzle with butter and toss to coat. Arrange apples in one layer in the air fryer basket and then sprinkle with pecan mixture.

➔ Cook in the preheated air fryer until apples are tender, 10 to 15 minutes.

49. Sausage Rolls

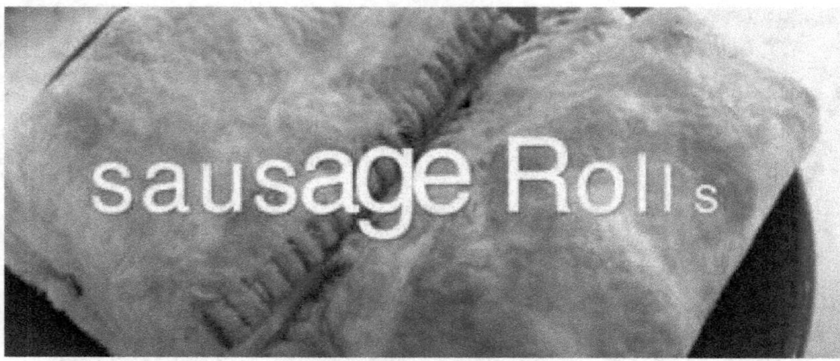

Ingredients:

- Sausage
- Puff pastry
- Cheese
- Chutney
- Milk

Methods:

Today we're going to make some really easy sausage rolls. So, I've just got some puff pastry and some sausages. What I'll do is I'll cut the puff pastry into four pieces. I'll then lay a sausage into each one of the pieces along with some grated cheese.

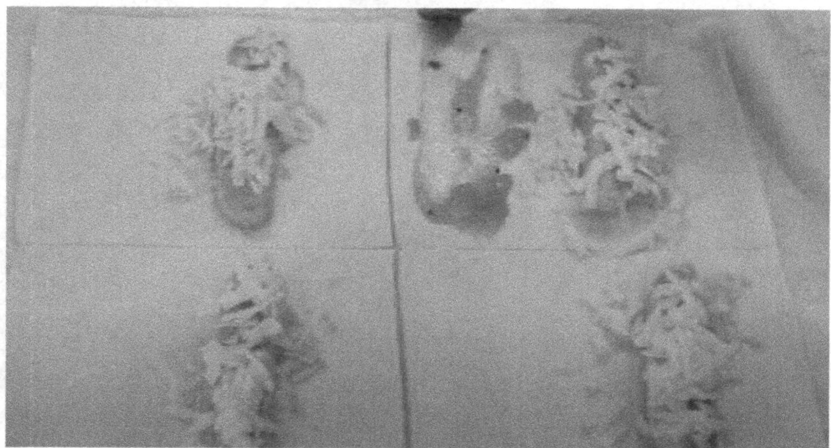

I like to have some chutney in the house as well. I'll just fold over the pastry and then secure it with a fork at the edges. So, it doesn't open up. I then just also get a bit of milk as well or you can use a beaten egg and just brush it over the top so it goes nice and golden brown. I'll pop it into my air fryer on the chip setting because they do need a good18 minutes in there to make sure the sausages are nice and cooked.

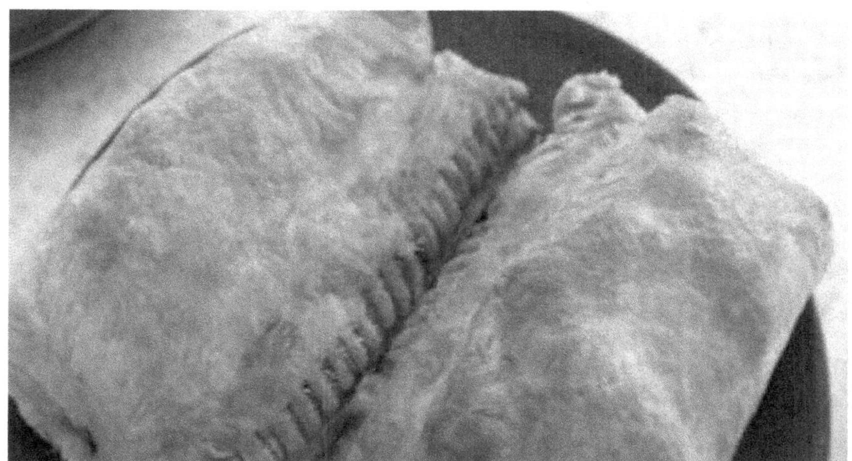

After the 18 minutes they're ready to eat.

50. Air Fryer French Fries

It will not get more classic than French fries; the normally accepted technique is fairly, dare I say, air tight, but I really do have one additional trick in shop! Last, dip them in honey mustard, hot ketchup, garlic aioli, or all 3 blended together, such as I did

Ingredients

- 1 lb. russet potatoes, peeled
- 1/2 tsp kosher salt
- 2 tsp vegetable oil
- 1 pinch cayenne pepper

Instructions

- ❖ Slice segments into sticks too around 3/8 inch-wide.
- ❖ Cover potatoes with water and let boil for 5 minutes to discharge excess starches.
- ❖ Drain and cover with boiling water with several inches (or put in a bowl of boiling water). Let sit for 10 minutes.

- ❖ Drain potatoes and move onto several paper towels. Transfer to a mixing bowl drizzle with oil, season with cayenne, and toss to coat.
- ❖ Stack potatoes in a dual layer in the fryer basket. Slide out basket and throw fries; keep frying until golden brown, about 10 minutes longer. Toss chips with salt in a mixing bowl.

51. Cheese on Toast

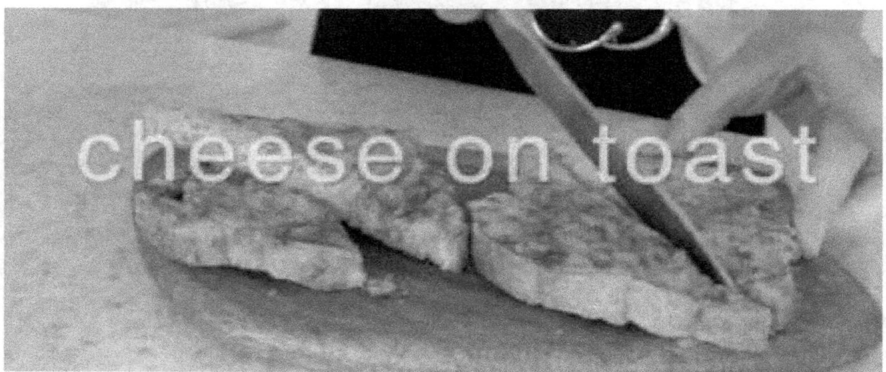

Ingredients:

- Bread
- Garlic butter
- cayenne pepper

Method:

I'm going to show you how to make a really quick and easy cheese on toast. How I make my cheese on toast is I get the bread and I put garlic butter on each side of the bread.

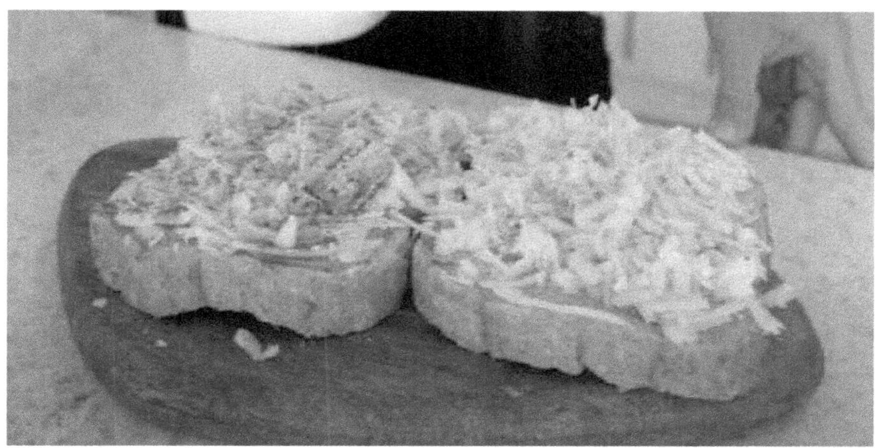

For me this is a very important step. I then grate quite a generous amount of cheese and then sprinkle it over the top. I will also add a little dash of cayenne pepper on top. Pop into my air fryer on the pizza button so that is for eight minutes at 160 degrees. Once the time is up, it comes out perfect every single time with a real nice crunchy piece of toast.

52. Tomato Pork Chops

It is a rather quick and easy recipe.

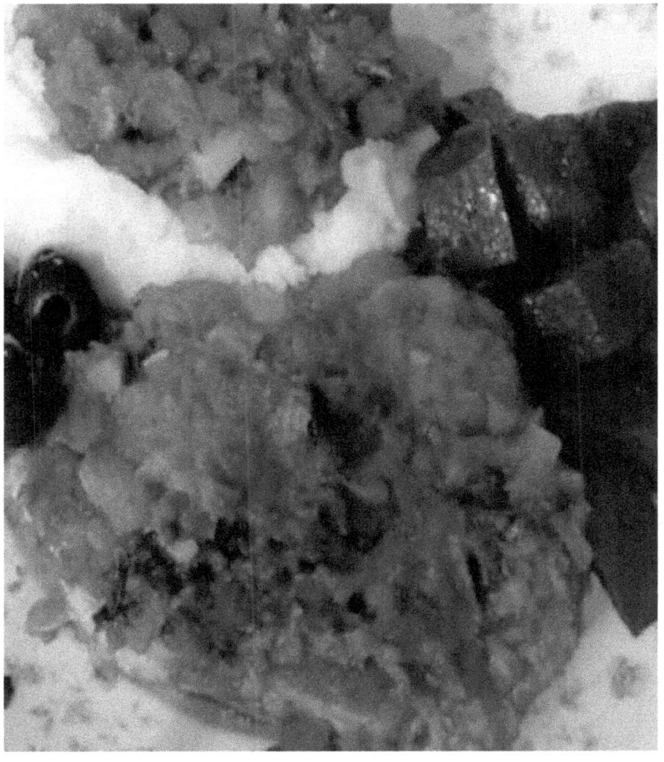

Ingredients

- 1 bell pepper - sliced, your color option
- 1 (15 oz.) can tomato sauce
- garlic powder to flavor
- 4 pork chops
- 1 tsp, sliced
- pepper and salt to taste

Directions

- Dredge the pork chops in flour, add to the pan and brown well on both sides.
- Add the onion and bell pepper, stir and cook for 5 minutes in the air fryer, or until nearly tender. Return pork chops to skillet and pour into the sauce. Permit the sauce to begin bubbling and reduce heat.
- Simmer for half an hour and season with garlic powder, pepper and salt to taste.

53. Veggie Egg Bread

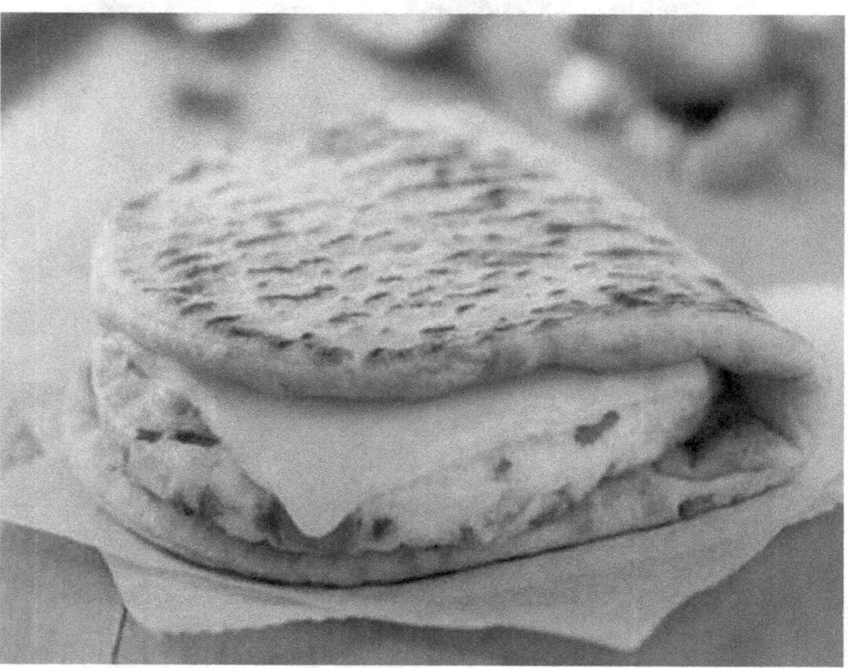

Ingredients:

- 1 tsp salt
- ½ pound cream cheese
- 10 eggs
- 4 cups grated zucchini
- 1 cup grated cheddar cheese
- ½ cup chopped tomatoes
- ½ tsp ground black pepper
- ½ cup sliced mushrooms, cooked
- ½ cup almond flour
- 2 tsp baking powder

Directions

- ❖ Be sure the pan will fit on your air fryer- normally a seven inch round pan will do the job flawlessly.
- ❖ Stir together the almond milk, pepper, salt and baking powder.
- ❖ In another bowl, beat the cream cheese until its smooth and nice afterward insert the eggs. Beat until well blended.
- ❖ Add the zucchini into the cream cheese mixture and stir until incorporated.
- ❖ Add the dry mix to the cream cheese jar and then stir well.
- ❖ Pour into the prepared pan and then cook at the fryer for 45 minutes

54. Easy Muffins

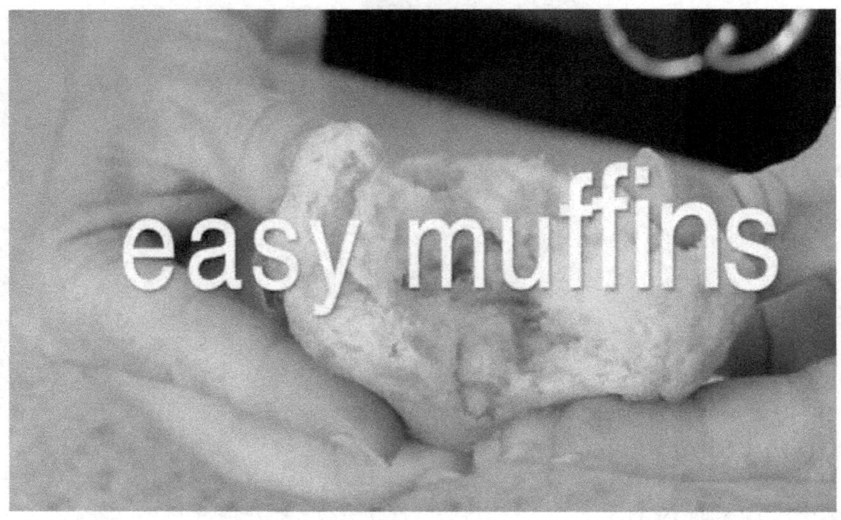

Ingredients:

- Sugar
- Butter
- Flour
- Eggs
- Milk
- Salt

Method:

We're going to make cupcakes. I have got a hundred grams of sugar, 250 grams of butter, 250 grams of flour, 4 eggs, a splash of milk and a dash of salt. We're just going to whisk this all up. I have got some of these cupcake holders. They're silicon ones. I'm going to add it to those and then we'll put them into the air fryer on the cupcake setting and let them cook away.

55. **Almond Flour Pancake**

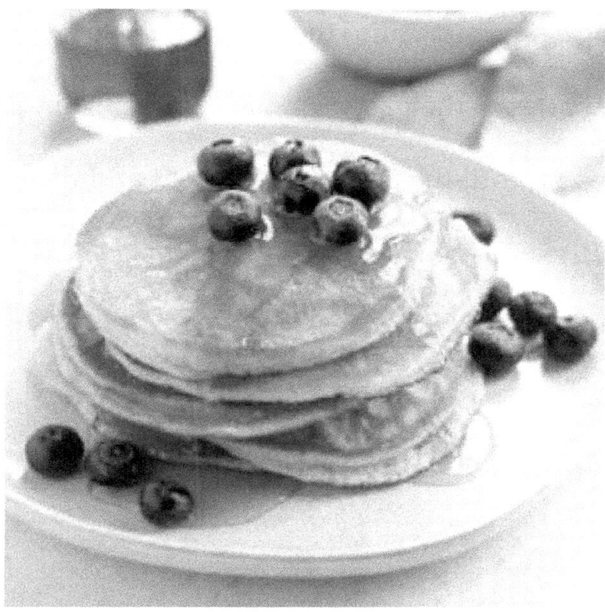

Ingredients:

- 1 teaspoon vanilla extract
- 1 1/4 cup almond milk
- two Tbsp. granulated erythritol
- 1 teaspoon baking powder
- 2 eggs
- 1/2 cup whole milk
- 2 Tbsp. butter, melted
- 1/8 tsp salt

Directions

- ❖ Be sure the pan will fit on your air fryer- normally a seven inch round pan will do the job flawlessly.
- ❖ Put the eggs, butter, milk and vanilla extract in a blender and puree for around thirty minutes.

- ❖ Add the remaining ingredients into the blender and puree until smooth.
- ❖ Pour the pancake batter to the prepared pan and set from the fryer.
- ❖ Cook for 2 minutes or until the pancake is puffed and the top is gold brown.
- ❖ Slice and serve with keto sugar free!

56. Zucchini and Bacon Egg Bread

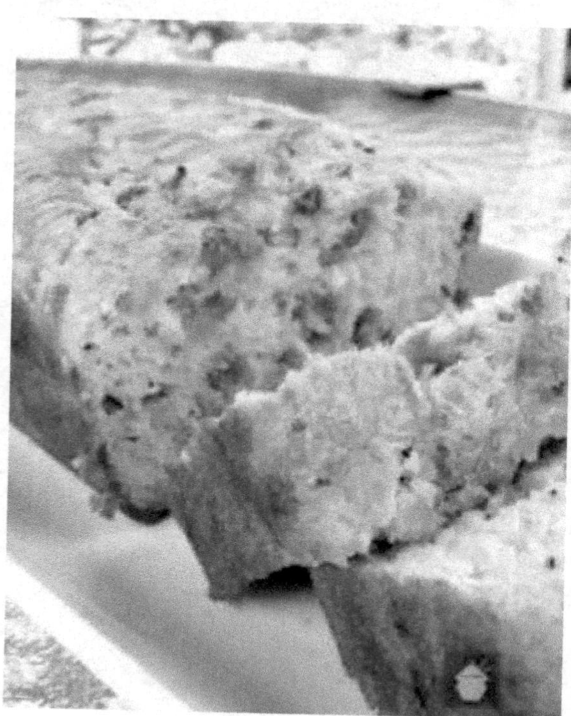

Ingredients:

- ½ cup almond flour
- 1 tsp salt
- ½ pound cream cheese
- 10 eggs
- 2 tsp baking powder
- ½ tsp ground black pepper

- 1 pound bacon cooked and crumbled
- 4 cups grated zucchini
- 1 cup grated cheddar cheese

Directions

- Be sure the pan will fit on your air fryer- normally a seven inch round pan will do the job flawlessly.
- Stir together the almond milk, pepper, salt and baking powder.
- In another bowl, beat the cream cheese until its smooth and nice afterward insert the eggs. Beat until well blended.
- Add the zucchini into the cream cheese mixture and stir until incorporated.
- Add the dry mix to the cream cheese jar and then stir well.
- Pour into the prepared pan and then cook at the fryer for 45 minutes

57. Raspberry Almond Pancake

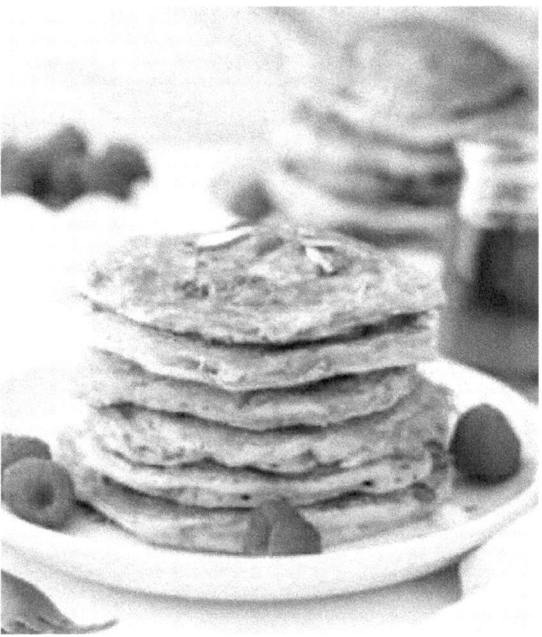

Ingredients:

- 1/2 cup whole milk
- 2 Tbsp. butter, melted
- 1 teaspoon almond extract
- 2 eggs
- two Tbsp. granulated erythritol
- 1 teaspoon baking powder
- 1/8 tsp salt
- 1 1/4 cup almond milk
- 1/4 cup frozen or fresh desserts

Directions

I. Preheat your air fryer to 420 degrees F and line a baking pan using parchment paper. Be sure the pan will fit on your air fryer- normally a seven inch round pan will do the job flawlessly.

II. Put the eggs, butter, milk and almond extract in a blender and puree for around thirty minutes.

III. Add the remaining ingredients into the blender and puree until smooth.

IV. Pour the pancake batter to the pan and stir in the raspberries

V. Lightly.

VI. Put in the fryer.

VII. Slice and serve with keto sugar free!

58. Maple Brussel Sprout Chips

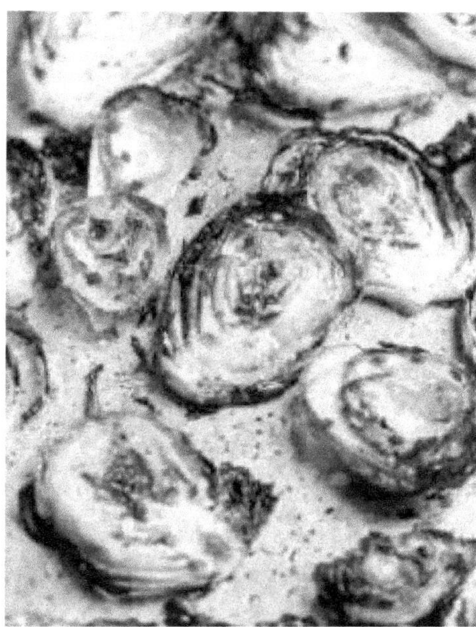

Ingredients:

- 2 Tbsp. olive oil
- 1 tsp sea salt
- 1 Pound Brussel Sprouts, ends removed
- 1 tsp maple extract

Method:

- ➢ Preheat your air fryer to 2400 degrees F and line the fryer tray with parchment paper.
- ➢ Peel the Brussels sprouts leaf at a time, putting the leaves in a massive bowl as you pare them.
- ➢ Toss the leaves using the olive oil, maple extract and salt then disperse onto the prepared tray.
- ➢ Bake for 15 minutes at the fryer, tossing halfway through to cook evenly.
- ➢ Serve warm or wrap in an airtight container after chilled.

59. Sweet and Tangy Apple Pork Chops

That is a recipe that I made using the thought that apples and pork go beautifully together! The seasonings provide the pork a pleasant and slightly spicy flavor. The apple cider increases the sweetness, while still bringing an exceptional tartness, since it's absorbed into the meat. Serve with applesauce, if wanted. Hope you like it!

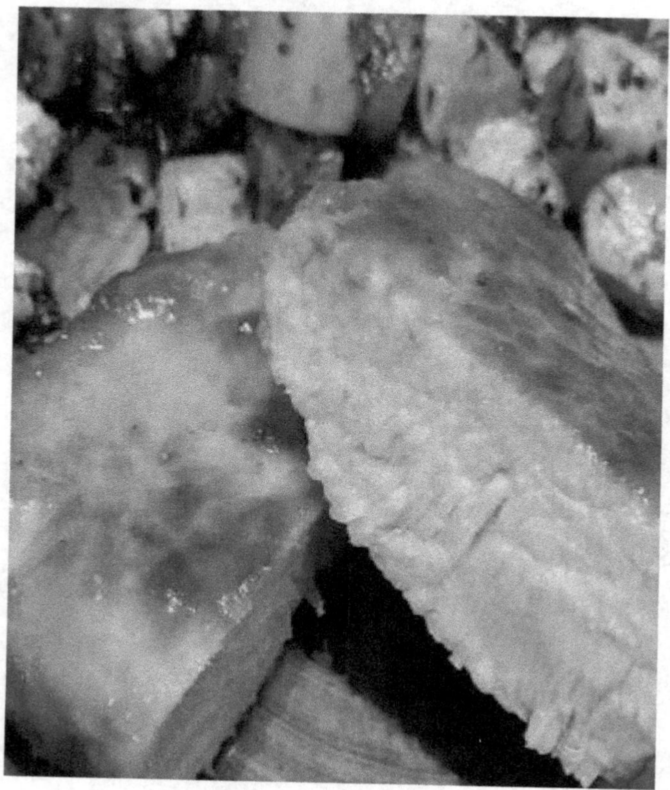

Ingredients:

- 3 tbsp. brown sugar
- 1/2 tsp garlic powder
- 2 tbsp. honey mustard
- 1 tsp mustard powder
- 1/2 teaspoon ground cumin
- 1 lb. pork chops
- 2 tbsp. butter

- 1/2 tsp cayenne pepper (Optional)
- 3/4 cup apple cider

Instructions

- ❑ Mix brown sugar, honey mustard, mustard powder, cumin, cayenne pepper, and garlic powder together in a small bowl. Rub pork chops and let sit on a plate for flavors to split into pork chops, about 10 minutes.
- ❑ Melt butter in a large skillet over moderate heat; include apple cider. Organize coated pork chops from the skillet;
- ❑ Cook until pork chops are browned, 5 to 7 minutes each side.

60. Maple Brussel Sprout Chips

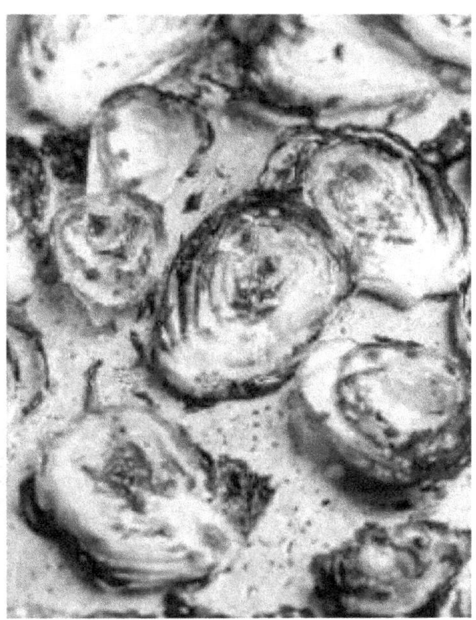

Ingredients:

- 2 Tbsp. olive oil
- 1 tsp sea salt
- 1 Pound Brussel Sprouts, ends removed
- 1 tsp maple extract

Method:

- ➢ Preheat your air fryer to 2400 degrees F and line the fryer tray with parchment paper.
- ➢ Peel the Brussels sprouts leaf at a time, putting the leaves in a massive bowl as you pare them.
- ➢ Toss the leaves using the olive oil, maple extract and salt then disperse onto the prepared tray.
- ➢ Bake for 15 minutes at the fryer, tossing halfway through to cook evenly.
- ➢ Serve warm or wrap in an airtight container after chilled.

61. Blueberry Pancake

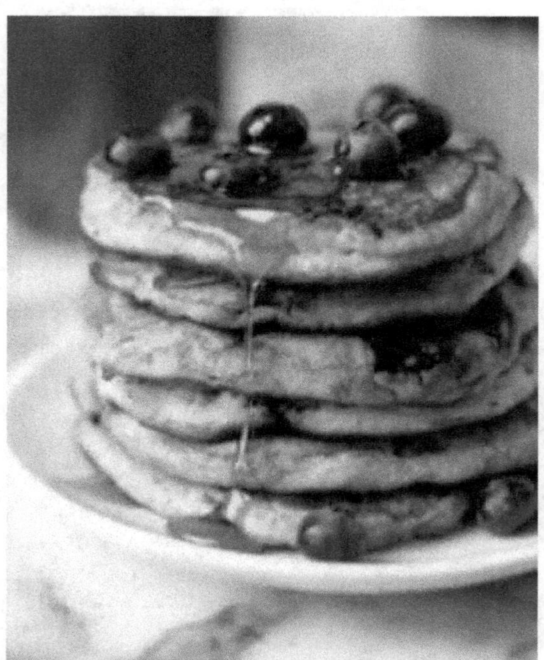

Ingredients:

- 2 Tbsp. butter, melted
- 1 teaspoon vanilla extract
- 1 1/4 cup almond milk

- 2 eggs
- 1 teaspoon baking powder
- 1/8 tsp salt
- 1/4 cup frozen or fresh blueberries
- 1/2 cup whole milk
- Two Tbsp. granulated erythritol

Directions

1. Preheat your air fryer to 400 degrees F and line a baking pan using parchment paper. Be sure the pan will fit on your fryer- normally a seven inch round pan will do the job flawlessly.
2. Put the eggs, butter, milk and vanilla extract in a blender and puree for around thirty minutes.
3. Add the remaining ingredients into the blender and puree until smooth.
4. Pour the pancake batter to the pan and stir in the blueberries
5. Put in the fryer.
6. Slice and serve with keto sugar free!

62. Chocolate Croissants

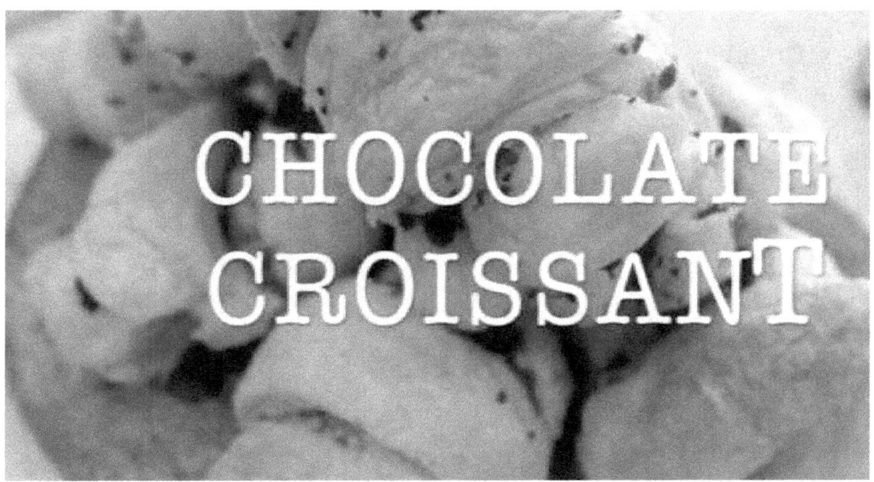

Ingredients

- Puff pastry
- Flake chocolate

Method:

I wanted to show you how to make some chocolate croissants in your air fryer as well. So, what I have got here is one roll of puff pastry and then to go on top to make it chocolatey, I have got some flake chocolate. What I'm going to do is roll out my puff pastry and then I'm going to crumble some flake chocolates all over the pastry.

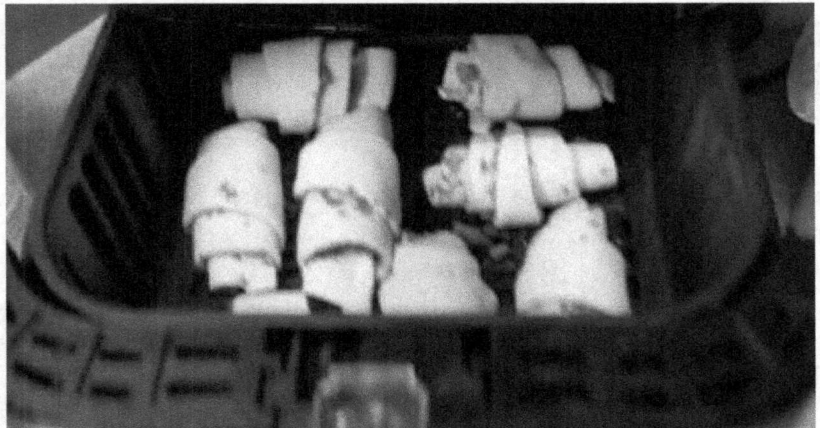

I'm then going to cut my pastry into eight. I'm going to cut them into fours and then I'll cut each four diagonally and then I'll roll them up into a croissant shape. Pop them into my air fryer, cook them on the muffin button which is a twelve minutes setting and then when they come out they are really really nice, chocolatey and delicious.

63. Strawberry Pancake

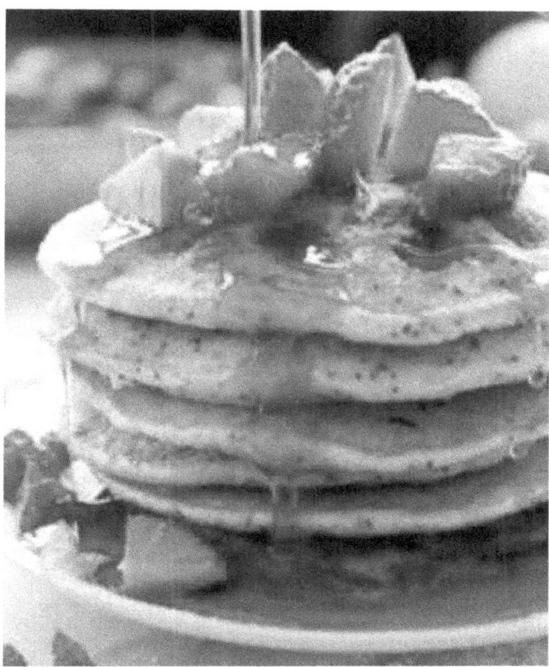

Ingredients:

- 1 teaspoon baking powder
- 1/8 tsp salt
- 1/4 cup fresh chopped tomatoes
- 2 eggs
- 1 teaspoon vanilla extract
- 1 1/4 cup almond milk

Directions

I. Pre-heat the air fryer for around 15 minutes.

II. Put the eggs, butter, milk and vanilla extract in a blender and simmer for about half an hour.

III. Add the remaining ingredients into the blender and puree until smooth.

IV. Pour the pancake batter to the pan and stir in the berries gently.

V. Put in the fryer.

VI. Slice and serve with keto sugar free!

64. Cheesy Zucchini Bake

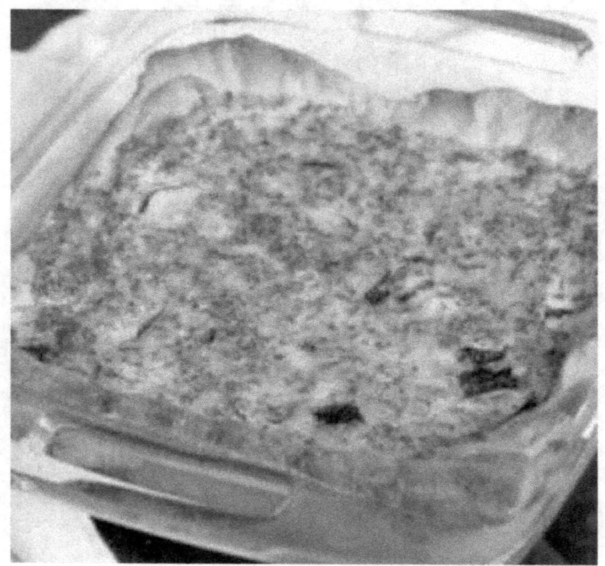

Ingredients:

- 2 tsp baking powder
- ½ tsp ground black pepper
- 1 tsp salt
- ½ cup almond flour
- 4 cups grated zucchini
- ½ pound cream cheese
- 10 eggs
- 1 cup grated cheddar cheese

Method:

1. Be sure the pan will fit on your air fryer- normally a seven inch round pan will do the job flawlessly. If it's possible to fit a bigger pan, then do so!

2. Stir together the almond milk, pepper, salt and baking powder.

3. In another bowl beat the cream cheese until its smooth and nice afterward insert the eggs. Beat until well blended.

4. Add the zucchini into the cream cheese mixture and stir until incorporated.

5. Add the dry mix to the cream cheese jar and then stir well.

6. Pour into the prepared pan and then cook at the fryer for 45 minutes.

65. Basil-Garlic Grilled Pork Chops

I had been tired of the exact same old agendas, and opted to try out something new... WOW! These chops are excellent!! They're fantastic for casual entertaining or family dinner. Together with the fresh basil and grated garlic, the taste is quite refreshing! Everybody will adore these!

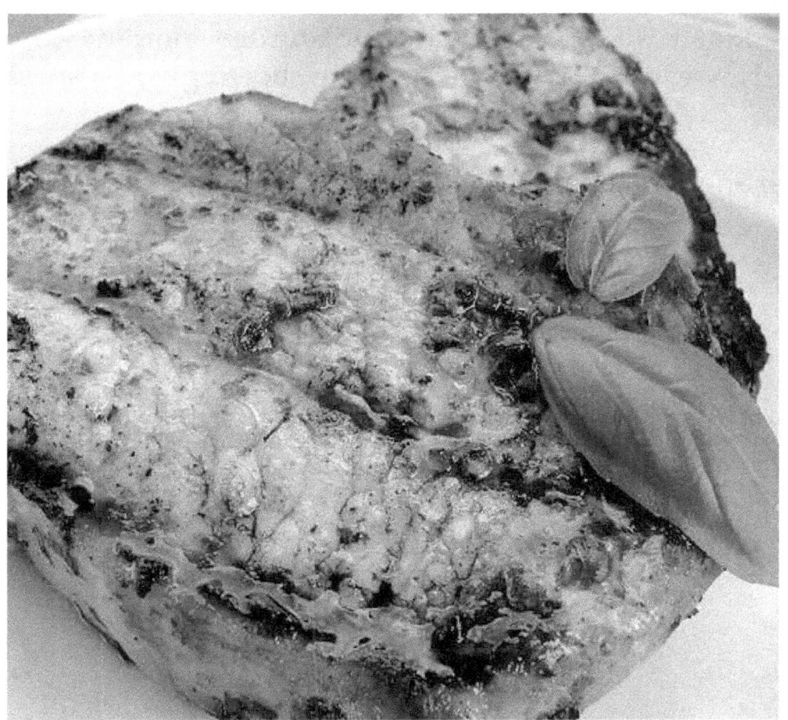

Ingredients

- 4 (8 ounce) pork chops
- 4 cloves garlic, minced

- ¼ cup chopped fresh basil
- 1 lime, juiced
- salt and black pepper to taste

Instructions

❖ Toss the pork chops with all the carrot juice in a bowl until evenly coated. Toss with ginger and garlic. Season the chops to taste with pepper and salt. Set aside to marinate for half an hour.

❖ Cook the pork chops on the fryer till no longer pink at the middle, 5 to 10 minutes each side.

66. Full English breakfast

Full English breakfast is one that my family really really likes. We have lived in England for a while so my kids really look forward to Saturday morning so that we make full English breakfast. However today I'm going to be showing you a special way to make it stress free.

I'm going to be starting off with the hash browns.

Ingredients:

- Potatoes
- Cheese
- Egg
- Salt
- Pepper
- Chili Flakes
- Sausage

Method:

So, the hash brownies are going to be composed of potatoes. I'm going to be using two, then I'm also going to be using cheese. This is shredded cheese and this is like the equivalent of one and a half cups of cheese. We are also going to be using one egg, this is one raw egg and some all-purpose flour, and this is the equivalent of two huge teaspoons of flour. We will be using some pepper along with chili flakes and finally of course some salt to taste. Right, so these are the ingredients that I'm going to be using for the hash browns.

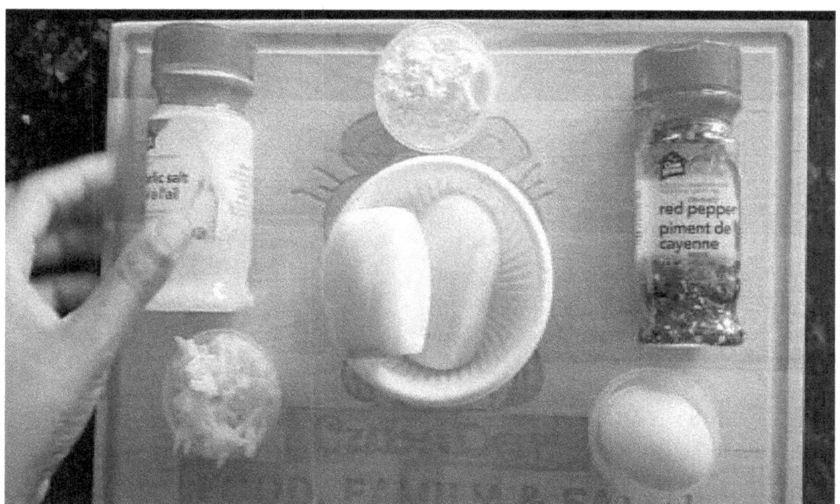

Before we start off with hash browns let's move on to all the other ingredients or condiments that are going to make up the English breakfast so part of the traditional ones we also use would be the eggs so this will make up we're going to make sunny side up eggs I'mgoing to be using some tomatoes some sausage, so this is not this is not the same way you have a traditional English breakfast.

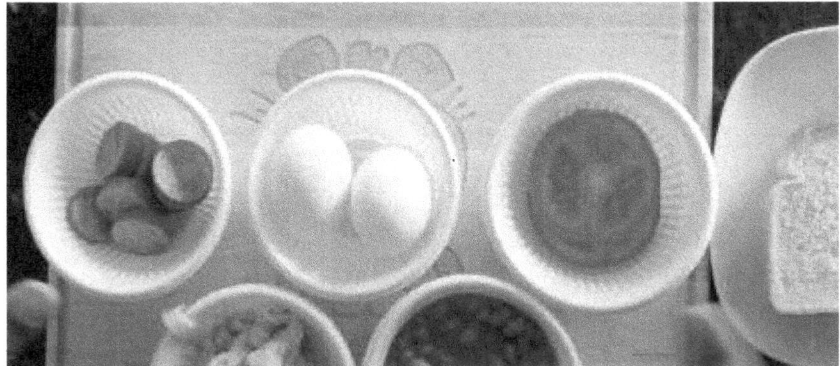

This isn't the same kind of way the sausage is or the way to slice but this is fine. Then we're going to be including baked beans right. So, this is a shop bought and actually there's still one more ingredient I'm going to be using: bacon. This is raw thinly sliced bacon and we have two slices of bread right. So, that's all the components or the condiments are going to go into the full English breakfast.

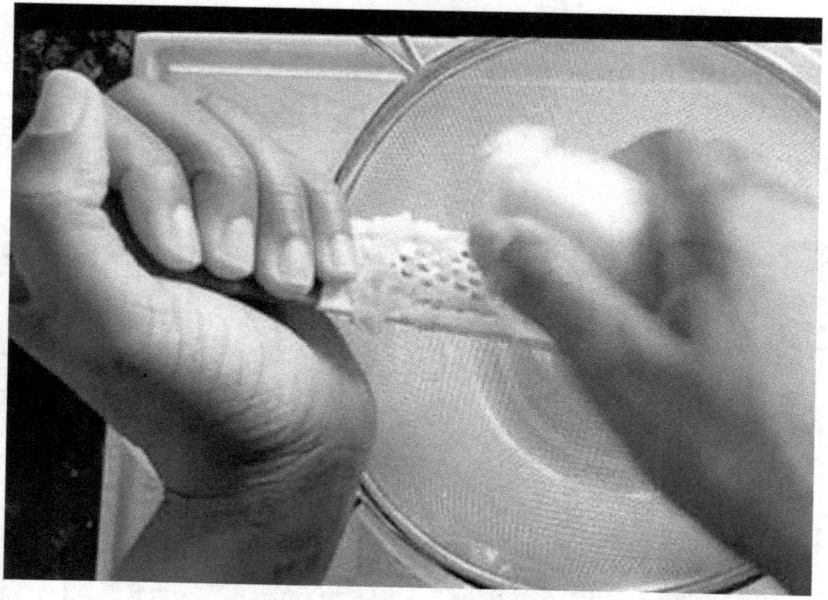

Let's start off straight away with the hash browns because all these other things are pretty much ready to go. Let's start with the preparation of the hash browns. So the first thing I'm going to be doing to grate the potatoes. With grated you can use any size. I want to use the really thin size because I want it more or less almost if it's already mashed or boiled. Because I'm going to be putting it in an array, I want it to take as little time as possible in order to get the potatoes done. If you've had English breakfast before let me know what you include or what you remove. I know people have different types of English breakfast at different times. Yeah, I know there's the black pudding, if you're a traditional English person you probably like black pudding instead.

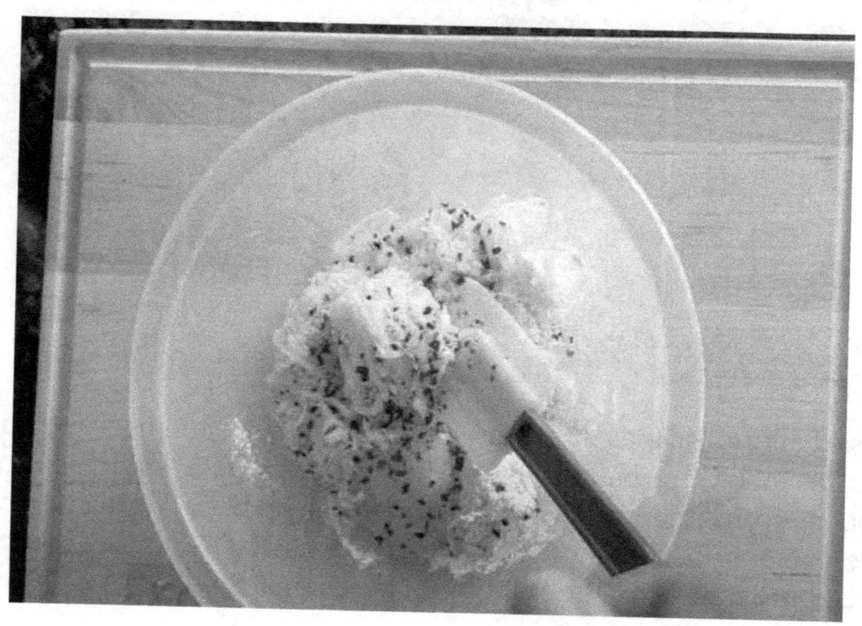

We're done with the grating of the potatoes and I've rinsed it out in sense that I've put some water in. I'm giving it a good squeeze to make sure all the water is gone. This helps to remove the majority of the starch in the potatoes. So it's completely up to you, if you want to skip this process in the sense that you want to rinse out some of the water from the potatoes. Okay so that done, the next thing we're going to move on to the mixing. I'm going to put in my flour. This is two teaspoons but it seems like I'm going to use only one. Then I remember eggs, had a full raw egg for my potato to make the hash browns. I also have some cheese, add some salt to taste and some chili flakes. I like something hot and spicy and yeah that's why I add that. So, I give this a really good mix for hash browns, people usually sometimes add butter so it's completely up to you what you want to include in your own hash browns. I'm just keeping my own soft shots sweet and simple. You can add or subtract as much as you want.

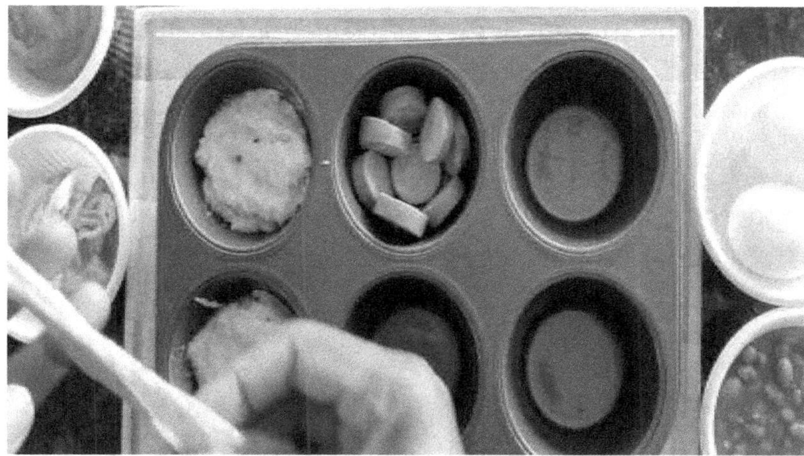

I'm going to give my tray a spray just to oil it, because what I'm going to do guys, this is something different. I'm going to start off with the hash browns. I'm putting everything and it's going to come out like a cup sort of like a cupcake, because my cans are a bit deep. I'm going to spread it into two sections right because I want it to cook all the way through so the potatoes are going to come out, sort of like a cupcake or potato cups. I'm also going to give this another spray right now, this is different.

I'm going to put in oops my sausages right, to line them all in here. As I'm using the air fryer for everything stress less so hopefully this should work for a bachelor or spencer or a small family or just making breakfast for somebody for just one person in the family. This works pretty good. I'm going to put them in first so the next thing that is going to be included in the air fryer all three of them are going in now is the bacon. I'm going to put the bacon this way, alternatively, I could have chopped up the bacon and put them in one of these sections. Maybe I would actually just do that so that you have a look-see at its rest of the bacon. I'm just going to cut this one in here.

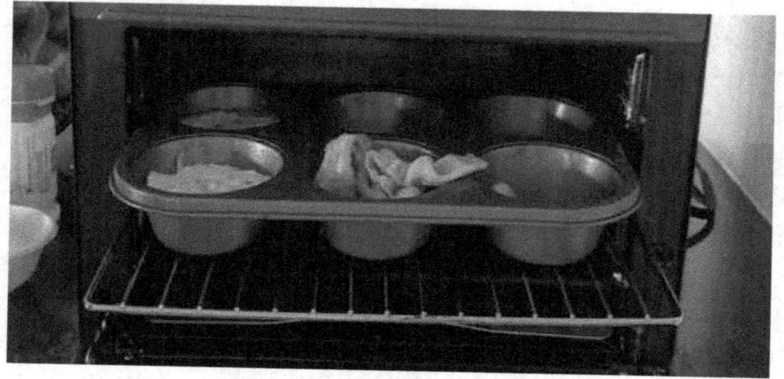

Throw it into the extra bit there again, I'm not going to be bothered about these bacon, because you know they're going to come up with their own oil. It's going to go into the air fryer oven. Put it in the air fryer oven and let it fry just turning the timer to one hour. It's an air fryer oven and the specific degree setting should be up on your screen and yeah so once this is ready again, like I said it's halfway into the cooking of the sausages of the hash browns and the bacon.

I'm now going to include the baked beans and the eggs because those ones will actually take less time compared to what you've got in the oven. I've had these in the air fryer and I can see that my bacon is coming out nicely.

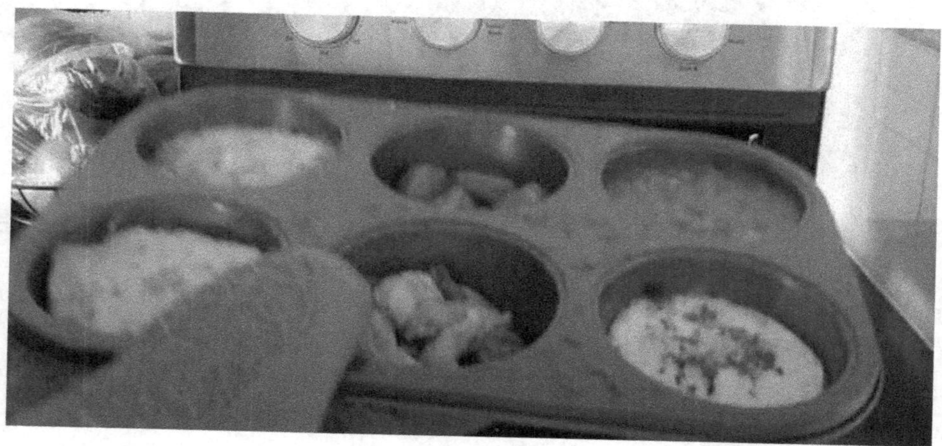

You see that so it depends on you if this is how you like your bacons this is the point in which you take them out. So, I'm just going to chuck the monotone section of the cupcake bits. What I'm going to do is to put the ones that are under done on the top and the ones that are already getting as crisp, I'm going to put them at the bottom. Now I'm just trying to get my stuff together. I'm scooping out all the sausages tone section so that I have two sections free for me to put my eggs and my baked beans. I'm going to have the egg sunny side up, I'm not going to spray the container again because all the bacon oil is in the egg, is in the cupcake holder. I'm just going to break two eggs and putting two into one section and then add some salt and some chili flakes. Our egg begins to cool, then I'm also going to put in the baked beans right in the final section. We are all good to go so I just want to show you guys what it looks like.

We've got the eggs we've got the baked beans we've got everything in the section in the containers. I'm going to have the the tomatoes, I'm just going to line them on top here and yeah voila. I know for some people it's a lot of work but this is really stress less. The only bit where you have lots of work to do is with the grating of the potatoes and that's pretty much it. We're going to allow these now to cook all the way through by the time the egg is done and the baked paint is ready, the entire dish should be ready. We're about 30 minutes into the entire thing and it's looking really really good. I just want to bring this and mix up the sausages a bit, yeah and put this back because you need a couple of minutes to go. You can see the egg, you can see the bacon everything is looking wonderful. I'm going to move this all the way back because I want to put my tomatoes just to give it a little bit of somehow grilled max and then my bread right just to heat it up.

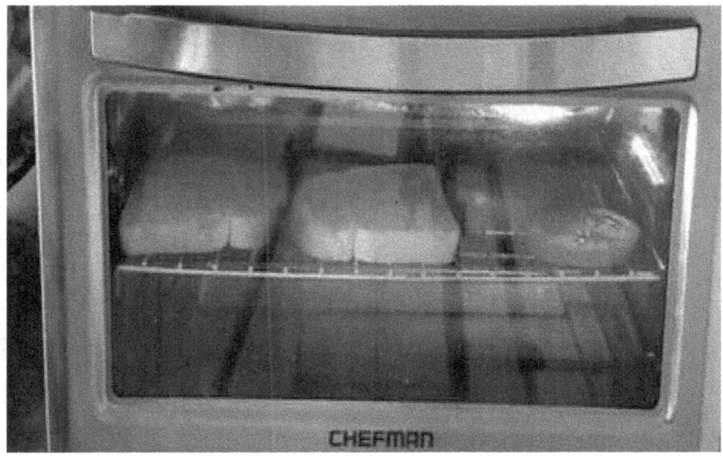

Let it give me somewhat like a mini toast. I'm going to shut this down now its done 30 minutes and it's done right. I'm not looking to get toasted bread but I just want this really warm. It's not toasted but it's warm and really crispy. I'm going to get the bread out of the way and the same thing with the tomatoes. So they're just warm so that when the breakfast is being eaten it's really nice and warm and fuzzy. Let's get onto plating it okay we are all ready, can you see that looks really good so and this is every single thing in one place right. So, our potatoes looks properly cooked a bit hot, our hash browns potatoes looks good and you can see our sausages. It did really really well cooked properly right and the same thing with the bacon so you can see all crispy or crunchy. I was able to achieve breakfast.

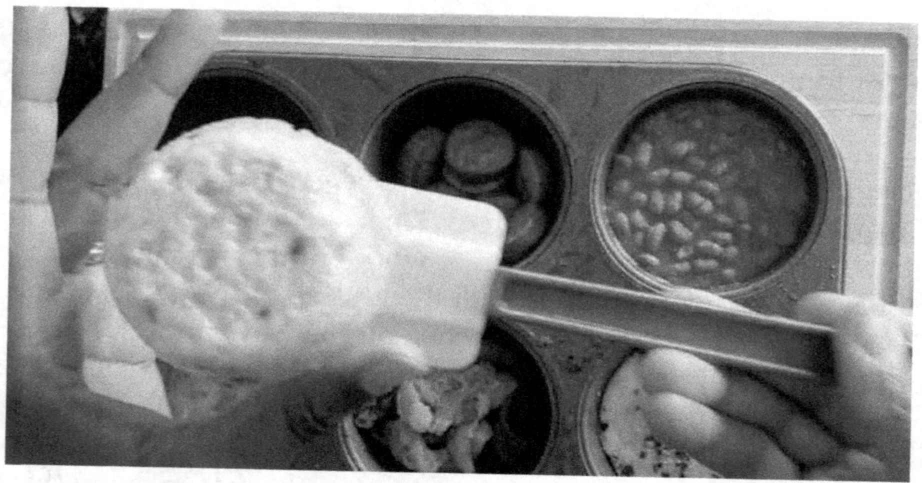

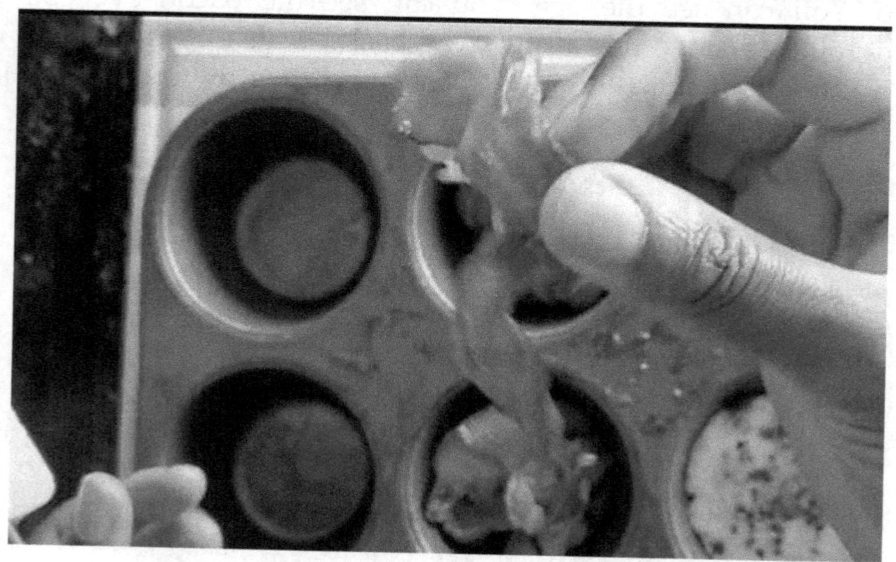

It took me about 30 minutes to make the entire dish so you can see my eggs yummy yummy yummy. I'm just going to dish this out and yeah so you can see the entire dish all presented for you. This is our English breakfast right you have the bread, we've got the bacon, I'm going to put in the sausages. This is a wonderful breakfast. All I really did was just to check it up at various times and baked beans is ready. This could actually is pretty decent meal and I think can it's perfect for more than one person. We have got egg there's not mushroom, there is no black pudding but this is completely fine the way it is right. So, this is what our full English breakfast looks like on some days and I've got the eggs, I've got the bacon, I still have some bacon there in the tray because I did make a lot so, still have some eggs.

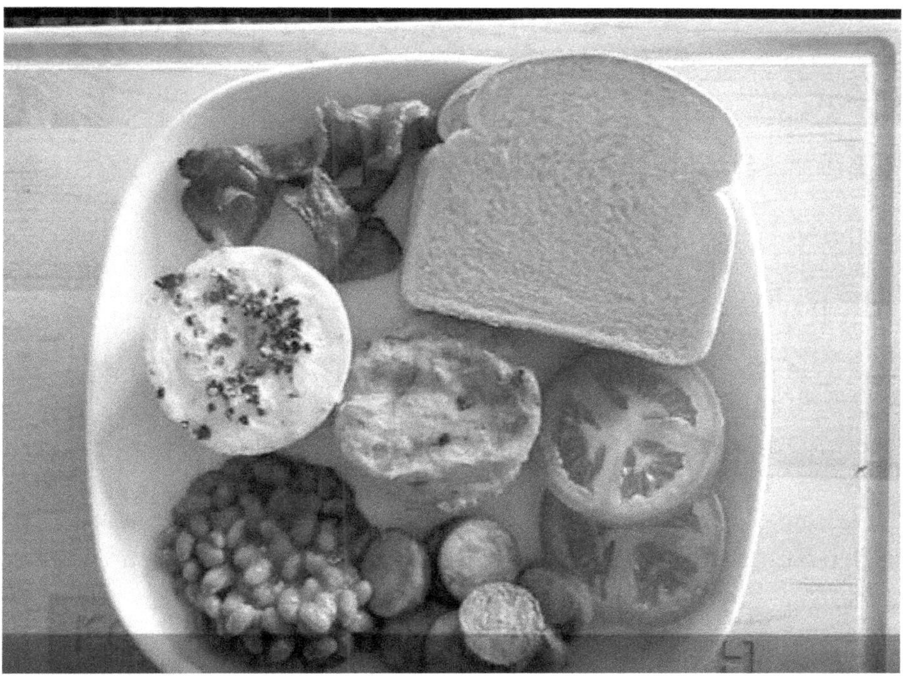

I have got some bacon some bread, yeah with a glass of milk or a cup of coffee you're good to go.

67. Garlic Brussel Sprout Chips

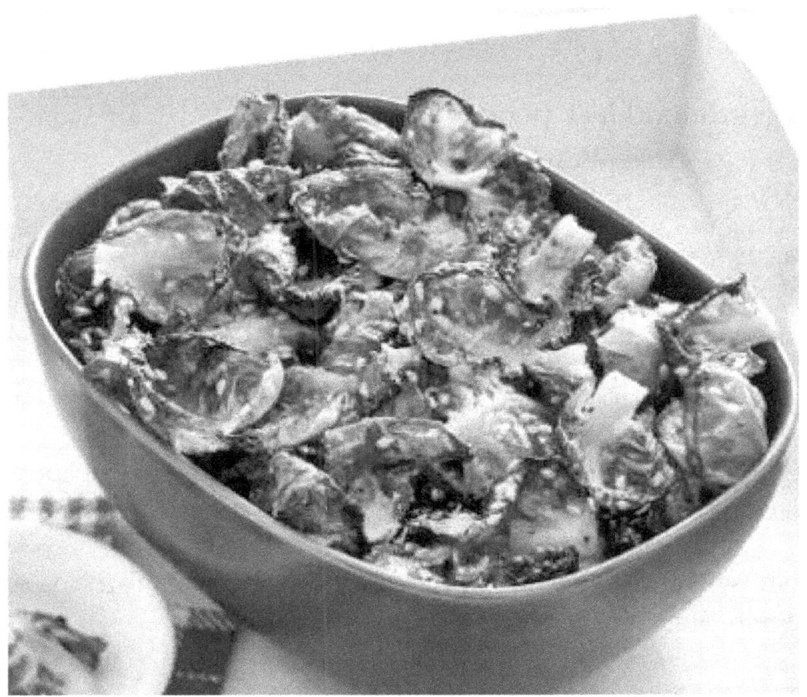

Ingredients:

- 1 tsp sea salt
- 1 Pound Brussel Sprouts, ends removed
- 2 Tbsp. olive oil
- 1 tsp garlic powder

Method:

- ❖ Preheat your air fryer to 2400 degrees F and line the fryer tray with parchment paper.
- ❖ Peel the Brussels sprouts leaf at a time, putting the leaves in a massive bowl as you pare them.
- ❖ Toss the leaves together with olive oil, garlic powder and salt then disperse onto the prepared tray.
- ❖ Bake for 15 minutes at the fryer, tossing halfway through to cook evenly.

68. Home and Asparagus

Ingredients:

- 1/4 teaspoon ground black pepper
- 1/4 tsp salt
- 1 lb. asparagus spears

Directions

- ❑ Preheat your air fryer to 400 degrees F and line your fryer tray using a
- ❑ Set the cod filets onto the parchment and sprinkle with the pepper and salt and rub the spices to the fish.
- ❑ Top the fish with the remaining components then wrap the parchment paper around the fish filets, surrounding them entirely.
- ❑ Put the tray in the fryer and bake for 20 minutes.

69. Herbed Parmesan Crackers

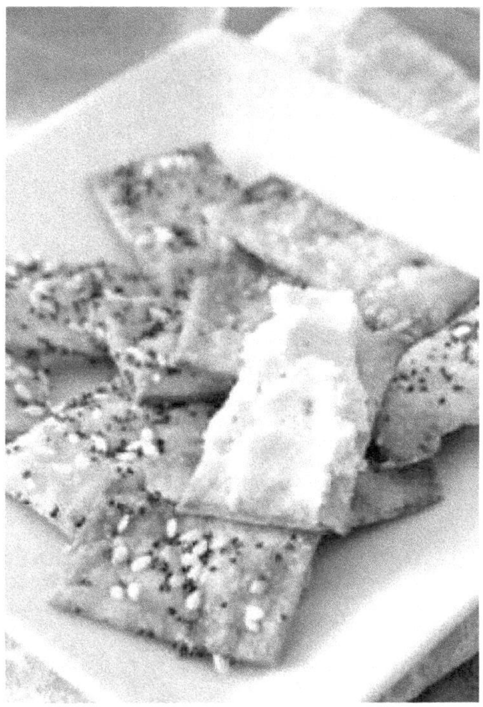

Ingredients:

- 2 Tbsp. Italian seasoning
- ½ cup chia seeds
- 1 ½ cups sunflower seeds
- 1 egg
- 2 Tbsp. butter, melted
- Salt
- ½ tsp garlic powder
- ½ tsp baking powder
- ¾ cup parmesan cheese, grated

Method:

- ❑ Set the sunflower seeds and chia seeds in a food processor until finely mixed to a powder. Put into a large bowl.
- ❑ Add the cheese, Italian seasoning, garlic powder and baking powder to the bowl and combine well.
- ❑ Add the melted butter and egg and stir till a wonderful dough forms.
- ❑ Put the dough onto a sheet of parchment and then put the following slice of parchment on top.
- ❑ Roll the dough into a thin sheet around 1/8 inch thick.
- ❑ Remove the top piece of parchment and lift the dough with the underside parchment and set onto a sheet tray which can fit in the air fryer.
- ❑ Score the cracker dough to your desired shape and bake for 40-45cminutes.
- ❑ Break the crackers aside and enjoy!

70. Salmon and Asparagus

Ingredients:

- ¼ tsp ground black pepper
- 1 ¾ pound salmon fillets
- ¼ tsp salt
- 1 pound asparagus spears
- 1 Tbsp. lemon juice
- 1 Tbsp. fresh chopped parsley
- 3 Tbsp. olive oil

Method

- ➔ Preheat your air fryer to 400 degrees F and line your fryer tray using a long piece of parchment paper.

- ➔ Set the salmon filets onto the parchment and sprinkle with the salt and pepper and rub the spices to the fish.
- ➔ Top the fish with the rest of the ingredients then wrap the parchment paper around the fish filets, surrounding them completely.
- ➔ Put the tray in the fryer and bake for 20 minutes.

71. Super Seed Parmesan Crackers

Ingredients:

- ½ tsp baking powder
- 1 egg
- 2 Tbsp. butter, melted
- 1 cups sunflower seeds
- ¾ cup parmesan cheese, grated
- 2 Tbsp. Italian seasoning
- ½ cup chia seeds
- ½ cup hulled hemp seeds
- ½ tsp garlic powder
- Salt

Method:

- ★ Preheat your air fryer to 300 degrees F.
- ★ Put into a large bowl.
- ★ Add the cheese, Italian seasoning, garlic powder and baking powder to the bowl and combine well.
- ★ Add the melted butter and egg and stir till a wonderful dough forms.

- ★ Put the dough onto a sheet of parchment and then put the following slice of parchment on top.
- ★ Roll the dough into a thin sheet around 1/8 inch thick.
- ★ Remove the top piece of parchment and lift the dough with the underside parchment and set onto a sheet tray which will fit from the air fryer.
- ★ Score the cracker dough to your desired shape and bake for 40-45 minutes.
- ★ Break the crackers aside and enjoy!

Conclusion

We have included 70 best recipes for you in this book. So, just try it out and then give us feedback with images of cooking.

Bariatric Air Fryer Cookbook

70+ Healthy, Tasty Recipes for After-Surgery Recovery and Lifelong Weight Management

Haile Banister

Table of Contents

Introduction

Weight loss surgery has proved to be an invaluable tool in the process of losing weight and becoming healthier. However, this tool must be used correctly in order to achieve positive results. The most important step is to follow your doctor's Directions and accordingly try to ease back into eating and taking care of your healing body. In the long-term, you must be careful of not only your portion sizes and also of what foods are good for you and which ones you should avoid.

Bariatric surgery, on its own, is not enough to enable you to lose weight and keep it off. After the bariatric surgery, your diet will have to change drastically. You will need to follow a healthy diet of bariatric recipes to ensure your long-term weight loss.

Eat healthy

The most important step in following a bariatric diet is to eat healthily.

. In general, your bariatric diet should consist only of 'FOG' foods, which are as follows:

Farm- The food that is raised on farms i.e. chicken, eggs, dairy products.

Ocean- The food that comes from the ocean i.e. fish.

Ground- The food that is grown in the ground i.e. fruits, vegetables, nuts, whole grains.

Proteins-the essential part of diet

Proteins are one of the most important nutrients required by your body. You need up to 80 grams/day of proteins, in order to stay healthy. However, now that your stomach is down to the size of a golf ball, 80 grams is a big percentage of the available space.

If you are not eating enough proteins, your body will begin to break down muscle, in order to get the number of proteins required by the body.

This can cause nausea, irritability, weakness, and tiredness.

Proteins can be found in a number of foods including, meat, fish, dairy products, legumes, and nuts.

Stages of a bariatric diet

The stages of a bariatric diet in the first few months may vary, depending on the type of weight loss surgery you had. This is a general, four-stage plan for successful healing and weight loss process. However, it is important to follow your surgeon and dietitian's Directions, before you follow any diet.

Stage 1: clear liquids

Basically, clear liquids, as the name implies, are liquids you can see through. Apart from water, there are several other liquids, which are included in this category as well:

- Pulp-free juices that have been diluted 50/50 with water (however, orange juice and tomato juice are not considered clear liquids)
- Clear beef, chicken, or vegetable broth (high-protein broths)
- Clear, sugar-free gelatin
- Sugar-free ice pops
- Decaf coffee
- tea
- Sugar-free, noncarbonated fruit drinks
- Flavored sugar-free, noncarbonated water
- Clear liquid supplements

Stage 2: full liquids

Full liquids are liquids or semi-liquids, which are pourable at room temperature. You also cannot see through them. You can start to have these liquids as early as the second day after surgery, provided you can tolerate clear liquids.

Full liquids include all those liquids which are in their clear liquid phase as well as the following foods:

- Low-fat soups that have been strained or puréed.
- Cooked wheat or rice cereals that have been thinned and are of a soupy consistency
- All juices (diluted fruit juice, 50/50 with water)
- Skimmed or 1 percent milk; plain, low-fat soy milk; or buttermilk (or lactose-free milk if you're lactose intolerant)
- Sugar-free custards or puddings
- Sugar-free hot chocolate
- Protein shakes with at least 10 grams of protein per 100 calories
- No-sugar-added or light yogurt

Stage 3: smooth foods

Smooth foods, also known as puréed foods, are those foods which have been put through the food processor in order to turn them into a puree with a smooth texture. You may follow the stage three for up to four weeks, depending on your surgeon's recommendations.

Smooth foods include the following:

- Blended low-fat cottage cheese
- Blended scrambled eggs
- Mashed potatoes made with skim milk
- Sugar-free applesauce
- Blended meats
- Part-skim ricotta cheese

Stage 4: soft foods

The stage 4 diet is the easiest to follow, as you can easily fulfill your protein requirements without using supplements. Your diet can include the following soft foods:

- Finely ground tuna
- Soft, tender, moist proteins like chicken salad (no onions or celery), turkey, veal, pork, beef, shrimp, scallops, and white fish that have been minced or ground in the food processor
- Soft, cooked vegetables
- Canned fruit packed in its own juice or water
- Eggs
- Low-fat soft cheese
- Low-fat cottage cheese
- Beans
- Crackers

Bariatric recipes

A good bariatric recipe is one which is high in protein and low in fat. Fish and lean meat are the excellent sources of proteins. Fried foods and recipes with lots of oil and butter must be avoided at all costs. Therefore, baking and grilling is a better option than frying. Spices and lemon juice can also be used, as they provide healthier flavors as compared to the oil and butter.
You should also try to avoid foods that are heavy in carbohydrates like pasta or white bread. Whole wheat bread and brown rice are better alternatives.

Best ways to prepare bariatric recipes

The preparation of bariatric food is the most important step in determining whether the food is healthy and meets all the requirements of a bariatric diet. Therefore, the following things must be kept in mind, when preparing your food:

- The food must be baked, grilled, poached or broiled. Frying is not an option.
- Use skimmed milk instead of whole milk.
- Use chicken or vegetable broth instead of oil.
- Oil must be replaced with applesauce or yogurt.
- Add spices or lemon juice to add flavors instead of olive oil or butter.

Chapter 1: Tips for Weight Loss

This is by no means an exhaustive list but just something to let you kick start the weight loss journey if you haven't already. The tips are all quickly actionable and easy to follow, though some may require a little more effort than the other, these are all ideas which have been known to work for people in pursuit of weight loss.

Record what you eat - Get a notebook if you are of the more pen and paper variety, or simply just use the note function on your smartphone to record down the food that you are consuming throughout the day. This gives you a sense of accountability when you sit down at the end of the day and review what you have eaten. You might be surprised at the amount of food you have taken in, and this will serve as a timely reminder to do better the next day. Get an accountability partner - Many people do better in tasks that require discipline when they are required to report to somebody else.

Getting an accountability partner will give that added sense of responsibility as well as the desire not to disappoint the partner when you report on your weight loss daily activities. Having someone to cajole and encourage you during this period can also be immensely gratifying, and that could be the added push to keep you on track for the weight loss journey.

Get enough sleep - It is by no means a measure of surprise to know that lack of sleep hampers your weight loss efforts by the simple increase of the hormone cortisol in our body system. Cortisol increases our appetite and hunger sensations, which is why getting sufficient sleep can do simple wonders in letting you shed the excess pounds. You will feel less cranky and more energized too!

Be mindful when eating - We get the feeling of fullness and satiation when we concentrate on the food that we are chewing and not get distracted by the ever-present mobile devices or the other assorted distractions available in this modern world while we have our meals. When eating, just eat! I know, it is easier said than done, but you can try counting the number of chews for that mouthful of food, get to seven or ten chews before swallowing. It helps to focus your mind back onto the food that you consume, and as a bonus, you are helping your stomach with better digestion as well!

Avoid processed foods - Yeap, that means the ice-creams, donuts and creamy cakes have got to take a backseat when it comes to your food selection. Pile on the whole and natural foods because those are nutrient dense items that will ensure you do not take in empty calories. Most of the processed food found today contain quite a bit of sugar and are pretty much deficient in the nutrients department, hence the term empty calories! The sugar eats into your daily calorie limit while not providing you with the essential nutrients your body needs. Go for chicken meat instead of chicken nuggets, whole potatoes instead of fries. You get the idea. Putting whole foods on your platter gives you more bang for the buck regarding your daily calorie limit, where you ensure that the calories you take in supplies your body with the nutrients that it needs to function well.

How can Hypnosis change the way you think?

Human information on the genuine substance of daze and entrancing is gotten from the Assumption Satisfaction Hypothesis of Dreams by Joe Griffin. For, obviously, dreaming is the most profound daze of all. At the point when the baby initially starts to show REM (quick eye development) rest, it is the most crucial type of daze that creates in the belly. Dreams deactivate the enthusiastic excitement, permitting the mind to react newly to each new day,thus safeguarding our senses' uprightness.

Because of the reasonable physiological similitudes with the territory of REM rest, we allude to daze as the REM state in the human giving methodology.

Profound daze reflects numerous parts of REM rest when instigated by spellbinding, for example, impenetrability to outside tangible data, less agony affectability, muscle loss of motion, and so forth Moreover, parts of how the REM state functions when we dream equal techniques utilized for daze enlistment. To help create daze, numerous hypnotists may utilize cadenced movement (for instance, making dull hand developments or getting people to gaze at turning optical figments), which connections back to the crude cerebrum of fish that we have advanced from. Obviously, on account of their consistent need to move, steer and equilibrium themselves in water, which they do by 'turning' their balances, fish respond incredibly capably to cadence. Centering consideration mirrors retention in a fantasy. Another closeness is in the focal point of consideration:

creating a noisy clamor or unexpected development can place an individual in a daze, as that quickly catches their consideration and includes electrical cerebrum action known as the direction reaction, a similar PGO waves as found in REM rest. The direction reaction fires angrily when we initially begin to dream.

The fantasy hypothesis of assumption satisfaction clarifies that this is the instrument for making the mind aware of the presence of unexpressed passionate feelings of excitement that should be released in a fantasy. Considerably more likenesses exist. As we nod off, the profound unwinding that psychotherapists use as enlistment into daze matches what occurs. Also, whenever clients are loose, the guided symbolism we use to permit them to see and beat their issues from an alternate point of view equal dream material emerging, the distinction being that the advisor manages the interaction in a misleadingly incited daze, while the 'fantasy script symbolism' in our rest gives the 'unused enthusiastic feelings of excitement from the earlier day.' As we probably are aware, allegory, when given to an individual in a daze, is profoundly incredible in treatment; and dreams are illustrations. Clear daze encounters may include mental trips. For instance, clients may report the glow of the sun they envisioned on their appearances, and dreams are additionally illusory. Exploration has shown that in the two conditions, a similar cerebrum pathways are dynamic. Likewise, visionaries additionally immediately experience wonders that can be actuated in a daze, like an amnesia (for the fantasy), sedation and absense of pain, body hallucinations, catalepsy, separation, and twisting of time.

Be that as it may, similarly as spellbinding isn't a daze, so the REM state isn't a fantasy. In actuality, it is the venue wherein the fantasy happens. The fantasy script isn't like the REM theater, our inward 'reality generator' as Joe Griffin appeared, and inside, it is carried on or made genuine.

In a wide range of daze, the REM state at that point is dynamic. It's not simply a condition of 'loose' or 'latent.' It's dynamic. All types of learning, scholarly or something else (counting molding, treatment, and teaching), are engaged with programming inborn and learned information, and furthermore when we wander off in fantasy land and take care of issues. At the point when we are damaged, the REM state is the medium through which the mind catches the horrible mishap and turns into a learned part of the models of endurance. Along these lines, the REM state, especially on the off chance that we are associated with conveying treatment, is fundamentally critical to comprehend.

Chapter 2: Breakfast

Italian Poached Eggs

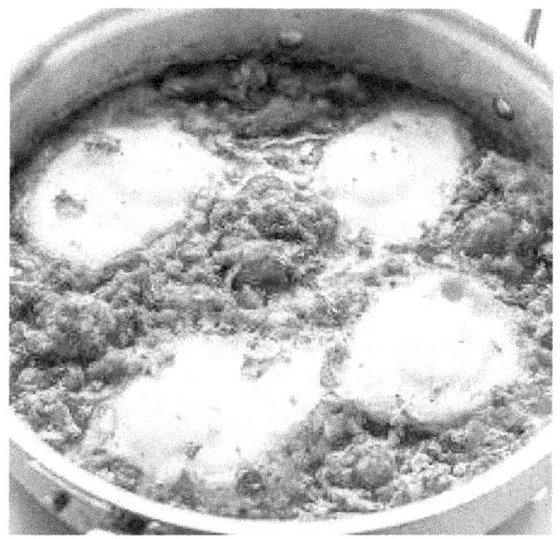

Serves: 6

Time: 30 minutes

Ingredients

16 oz. marinara sauce

4 shredded basil leaves

3-4 roasted red pepper, sliced

Pepper

4 eggs

Salt

Directions

Grab a skillet and let it heat up. Add the marinara sauce and the peppers then mix them together and allow them to heat up.

Once they are hot, use a spoon to make four wells into the marinara sauce. Now, crack one egg into each of the wells you have made.

Sprinkle pepper and salt over each of the eggs.

Allow this to cook for about 12 minutes. You can cook the eggs as long as you want until it reaches your desired doneness. You can also place a lid on your skillet so that the eggs cook a bit faster.

Remove the skillet from the stove and sprinkle the torn basil over the top. Scoop the eggs out along with a bit of sauce and enjoy.

Egg Burrito

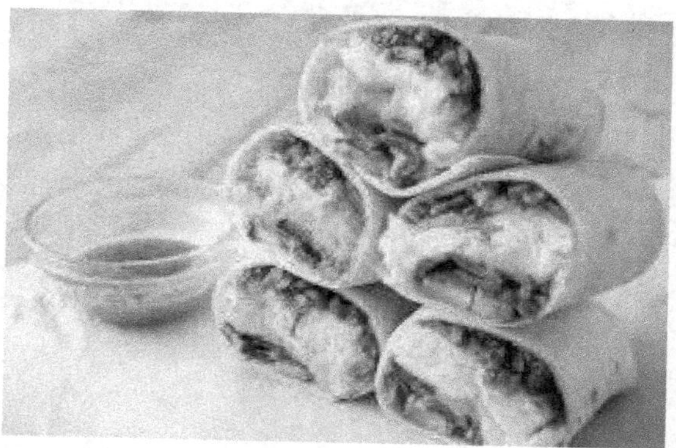

Serves: 4

Time: 30 minutes

Ingredients

Pepper

1 tbsp. shredded Mexican cheese blend

Salt

2 tbsp. salsa

1 egg + 1 egg white

1 oz. protein of choices such as ground beef, chicken, or tofu

2 tbsp. plain fat-free Greek yogurt

Directions

Place the egg white and egg into a small bowl. Whisk until well combined. Spray cooking spray on a skillet. When warmed, pour eggs into the hot pan. Tilt pan to spread the eggs evenly on the bottom. Let it sit until edges are set. Sprinkle with pepper and salt then gently flip over.

Allow the other side to cook until the eggs are done. Place on a plate. Put your protein of choice and cheese onto the center of the egg. Roll up the egg in the form of a burrito. Add salsa and Greek yogurt, if desired.

Bunless Breakfast Sandwich

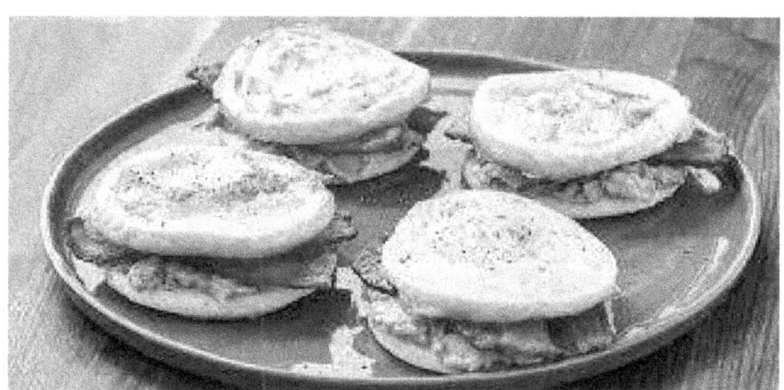

Serves: 4

Time: 35 minutes

Ingredients

¼ c shredded cheddar cheese

2 eggs

2 tbsp. water

½ avocado, mashed

2 sliced cooked bacon

Directions

Place two canning jar lids into a skillet and spray with cooking spray. Let everything warm up. Crack one egg in each lid and whisk the egg gently with a fork to break the yolks.

Pour a small amount of water into the pan and put the lid on the skillet. Allow to cook and steam the eggs. Cook for three minutes. Take off the lid and put cheese on just one of the eggs. Allow cheese to melt for about one minute.

Put the egg without the cheese on a plate. Add avocado and then the bacon on top. Put the other egg on top with the cheesy side down. Enjoy.

Chocolate Porridge

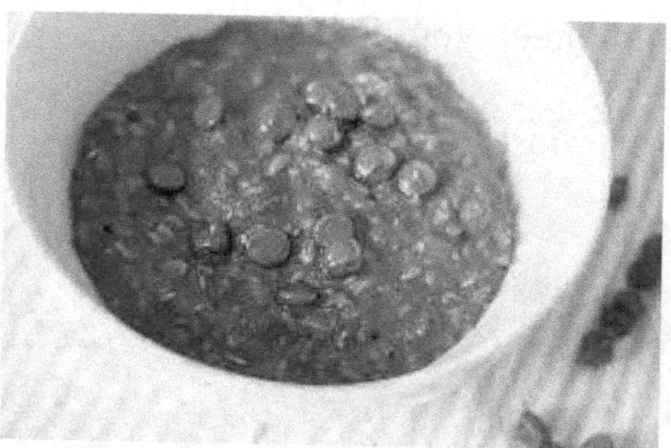

Serves: 4

Time: 5 minutes

Ingredients

Chopped nuts, fruits, or seeds of choice

4 tbsp. porridge oats

1 c skim milk

Sugar-free syrup

1 square dark unsweetened chocolate

1 tbsp. cocoa powder

Directions

Place the chocolate, cocoa powder, oats, and milk in a microwavable bowl.

Cook for two minutes. Give everything a good stir and cook for an additional 15 to 20 seconds.

Put in a serving bowl and add desired toppings. Enjoy.

Cheesy Spiced Pancakes

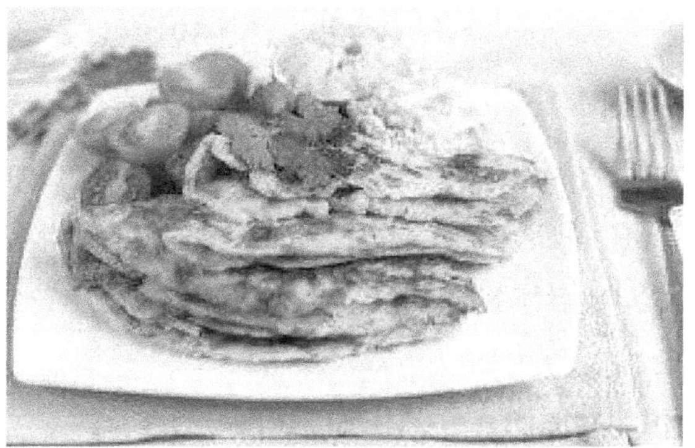

Serves: 4

Time: 55 minutes

Ingredients

Pancakes:

1 tbsp. artificial sweetener

1 tsp. mixed spice, ground

Low-fat cooking spray

8 oz. spreadable goat cheese

Pinch salt

3 eggs, separated

½ c all-purpose flour

Optional Adult Toppings:

Sweetener

1 measure Brandy

4 tangerines, peeled

2 oz. cranberries

Directions

To make the pancakes: Combine the egg yolks, cheese, and mixed spice. Add the salt and flour and mix well.

Beat the egg whites until they are stiff peaks and whisk in sweetener. Fold this into the cheese mixture.

If using the optional topping, place sweetener and tangerines into a pot. Stir occasionally until tangerines begin to release some juices and begin to look a bit syrupy. Add the Brandy and cranberries. Let this cook for few minutes. Keep warm until ready to use.

Spray the skillet with cooking spray. Allow to warm up. Add three large spoonful of batter into the pan. Cook for about two minutes until bubbles form on top. Flip and cook until the other side is browned. Remove from the pan and keep warm. Continue until all batter has been used. You should get 12 pancakes from this batter.

Divide among four plates and spoon the topping. Enjoy.

Pumpkin Pie Oatmeal

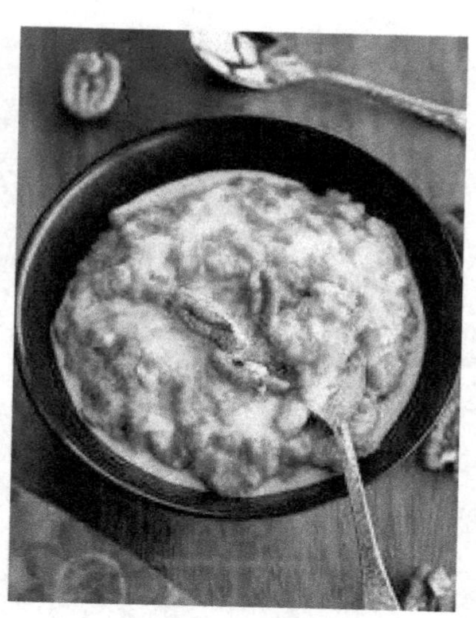

Serves: 6

Time: 10 minutes

Ingredients

½ c canned pumpkin

1 tsp. Truvia

Dash ground cloves

1/3 c old fashioned oats

Dash ground ginger

½ c no salt 1% cottage cheese

1/8 tsp. cinnamon

Directions

Place the sweetener, spices, pumpkin, and oats into a microwavable bowl. Mix to combine. Microwave on high for 90 seconds. Add the cottage cheese and stir well. Microwave for another 60 seconds. Wait for few minutes before eating then enjoy.

Egg Muffin

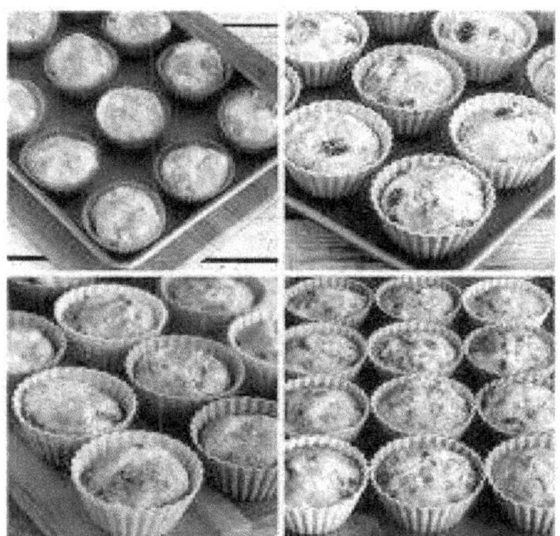

Serves: 4

Time: 45 minutes

Ingredients

¼ tsp. salt

12 slices turkey bacon

¼ tsp. Italian seasoning

6 large eggs

¼ tsp. pepper

¾ c shredded low-fat shredded cheese of choice

½ c 1% milk

Directions

Spray cooking spray into muffin pan. Your oven needs to be warmed to 350.

Place three slices of bacon on the bottom of each muffin cup.

Mix all remaining ingredients together until well combined. Reserve ¼ cup of shredded cheese. Put a fourth cup of this mixture into every muffin cup. Add a bit more cheese on top.

Bake for about 25 minutes. The eggs should be set.

Flour-Less Pancakes

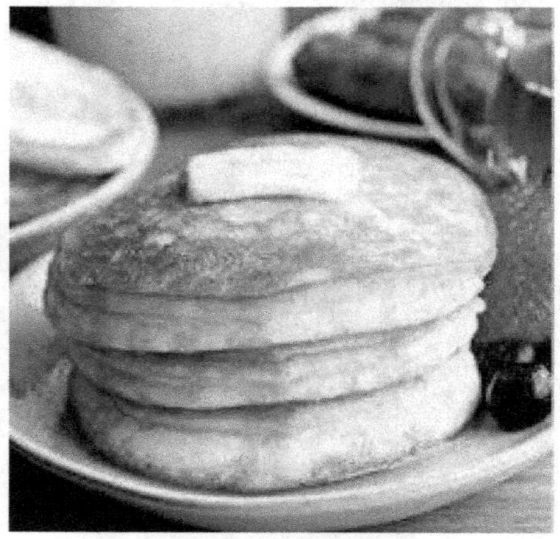

Serves: 8

Time: 70 minutes

Ingredients

Milk to mix

1 egg

Low-fat cooking spray

1 c rolled oats

1 banana

Directions

Place the banana, egg, and oats into a food processor. Process until smooth. Add a small amount of milk and blend again. Add the milk until the mixture has reached a runny consistency. Three tablespoons should be the maximum amount you use.

Allow to sit for about 15 minutes. This lets the mixture thicken slightly.

Spray a small amount of cooking spray into a skillet. Allow to get warm. Add a spoonful of the batter to form a small pancake. Put as many as your pan will allow. Just make sure you have room to flip each. Allow the first side to cook for about a minute until bubbles begin to form on the surface. Flip and cook until browned. Remove from the skillet onto a plate and keep warm while you continue to cook the remaining batter.

Serve warm with fruit, yogurt, sugar-free syrup, a dusting of powdered sugar, or a drizzle of lemon. You might prefer them plain. Either way, enjoy.

Broccoli Quiche

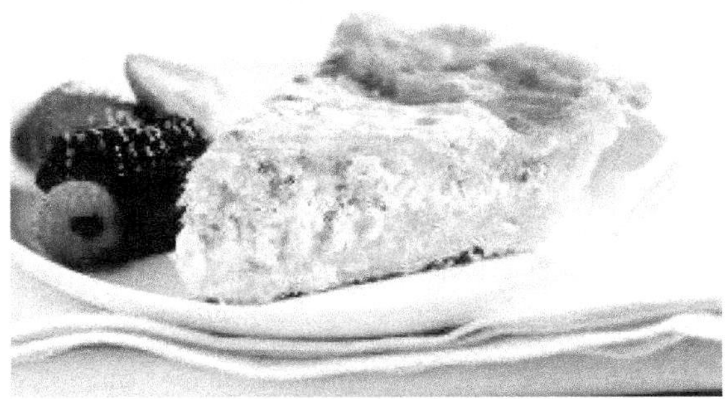

Serves: 4

Time: 60 minutes

Ingredients

½ c fat-free half and half

3 oz. low-fat Swiss cheese

¼ c skim milk

½ c canned mushrooms

1 c egg substitute

1 large head broccoli

Directions

Your oven should be set to 400. Coat a pie plate with nonstick spray.

Put the broccoli in a steamer basket. In a pot that the basket will fit into, add about an inch of water. Place a steamer basket into the pot then steam for about five minutes. Allow to cool slightly then give the broccoli a rough chop.

Put the mushrooms and broccoli into the pie plate.

Whisk together the half and half, skim milk, and egg substitute. Whisk until well combined.

Pour the egg mixture over the mushrooms and broccoli. Add some cheese on top.

Cook for about 40 minutes until the eggs are set.

Cut into four equal servings and enjoy.

Oatmeal Cookie Shake

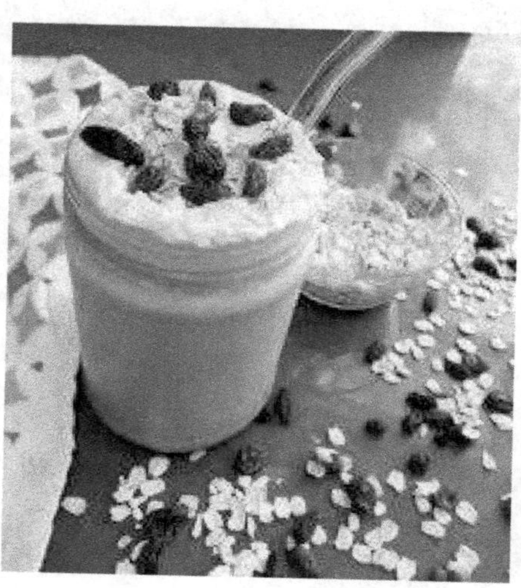

Serves: 8

Time: 20 minutes

Ingredients

Low-fat cream, cinnamon, and nuts - garnish

1 c low-fat nut milk

Ice

½ tsp. cinnamon

¼ tsp. vanilla

1 scoop vanilla whey protein powder

1 tbsp. oatmeal

Directions

Place the protein powder, mice, milk, vanilla, cinnamon, and oatmeal into a strong blender, and pulse couple of times until all of the ingredients come together.

Pour the shake into a glass and top with some cinnamon, cream, and nuts.

Soft Eggs with Chives and Ricotta

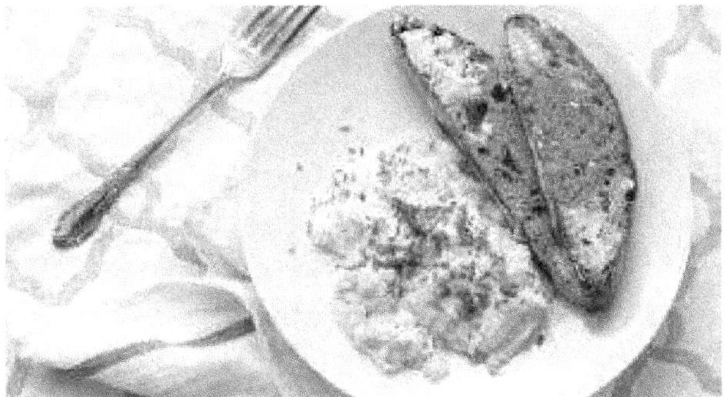

Serves: 4

Time: 40 minutes

Ingredients

2 eggs

Olive oil

½ c milk

1 tbsp. chopped chives

½ c ricotta

Directions

Add the eggs and milk to a jar. Place the lid on tightly and shake it until everything is mixed together well.

Grab yourself a skillet and place it on the stove. Once it is warm, pour the eggs into the skillet and scramble them. Allow them to cook until they are soft-set. Once soft-set, let it cook and gently stir them once in a while.

After the eggs are done, stir the ricotta and the chives. Add the eggs to a plate and drizzle some oil over the top if you would like.

Ham and Egg Roll-Ups

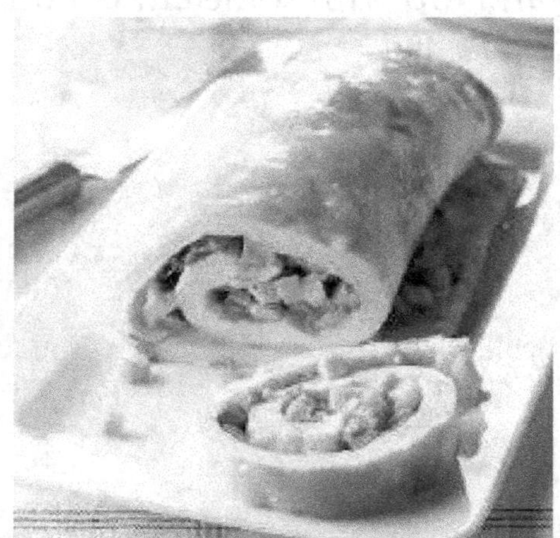

Serves: 6

Time: 35 minutes

Ingredients

2 tsp. garlic powder

1 c baby spinach

1 c chopped tomatoes

10 eggs

Pepper

2 tbsp. butter

Salt

1 ½ c shredded cheddar cheese

20 ham slices

Directions

Turn oven to broil. Crack all the eggs into a bowl and beat together. Add the garlic powder, pepper, and salt. Mix well.

Warm a skillet on stove top. Add the butter and allow it to melt. Add the eggs and scramble until they are done. Mix the cheese, stirring until it melts. Fold in the spinach and tomatoes.

Put two pieces of ham on a cutting board. Add a spoonful of eggs then roll up. Repeat this process until all ham and eggs are used.

Place the roll-ups on a baking sheet and broil about five minutes.

Cottage Cheese Pancakes

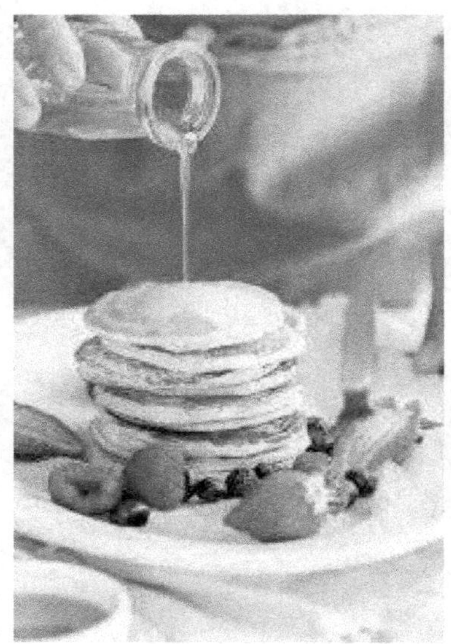

Serves: 7

Time: 45 minutes

Ingredients

1/3 c all-purpose flour

½ tbsp. canola oil

½ tsp. baking soda

3 eggs, lightly beaten

1 c low-fat cottage cheese

Directions

Sift the baking soda and flour in a small bowl.

Mix the remaining ingredients together.

Mix the flour into the wet ingredients and stir to incorporate.

Spray cooking spray into a skillet and warm. When warmed, place one-third cup of the batter into the pan and cook until you see bubbles. Flip and cook until the other side is browned.

Serve warm with sugar-free syrup. Enjoy.

Mocha Frappuccino

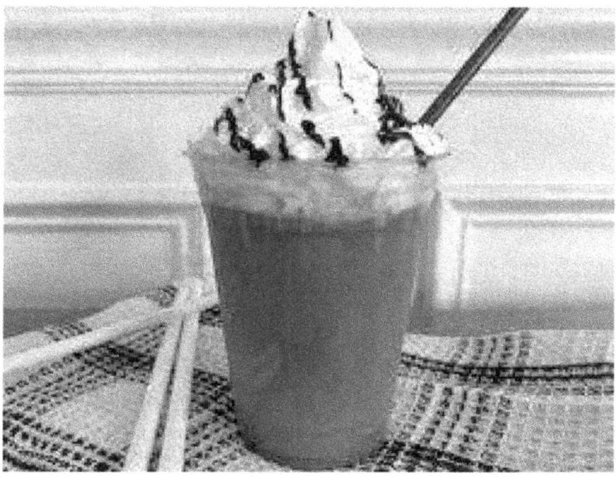

Serves: 4

Time: 15 minutes

Ingredients

¼ c brewed coffee

Low-sugar chocolate syrup

¼ c unsweetened almond milk

Low-fat whipped cream

½ c 0% fat Greek yogurt

1 c ice

3-4 drops liquid sweetener

1 tbsp. cocoa powder

Directions

Place the coffee, ice, milk, cocoa, yogurt, and sweetener in a blender and pulse until all of the ingredients come together and it's all smooth.

Pour the Frappuccino into a glass and swirl some whipped cream and chocolate syrup over the top.

PB&J Pancakes

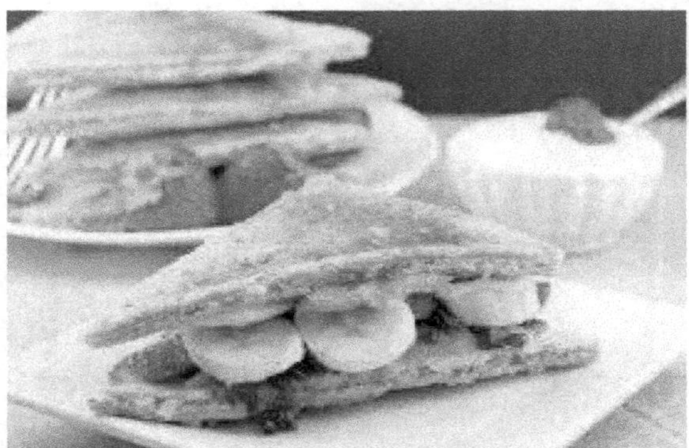

Serves: 8

Time: 50 minutes

Ingredients

½ c instant oatmeal

1 c frozen mixed berries

½ c low-fat cottage cheese

4 large egg whites

2 tbsp. powdered peanuts

Directions

The ingredients have to be put in the blender in a specific order. You will add the cottage cheese first. Next, will be the oatmeal. Followed by the powdered peanuts. Last, will be the egg whites. Blend until smooth and the consistency is of a pancake batter. Pour into a bowl and add the mixed fruit. Spray a skillet with cooking spray. Put ¼ cup batter into the heated skillet and cook until the top forms bubbles. Flip and cook until browned on the other side. Should make between four and seven pancakes. Serve warm with sugar-free syrup.

Breakfast Popsicles

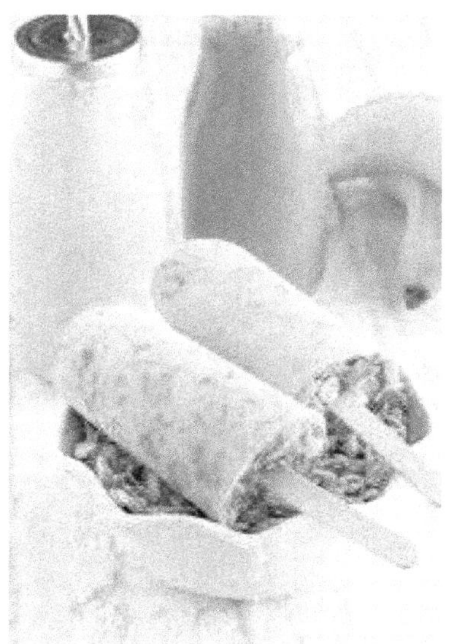

Serves: 4

Time: 50 minutes

Ingredients

½ c oats

1 c Greek yogurt

1 c mixed berries

½ c 1% milk

Directions

Mix together the yogurt and milk. Divide the mixture equally into popsicle molds. Place some berries into each one. Divide the oatmeal mixture equally into each popsicle mold. Place a popsicle stick into each and place in the freezer. Freeze at least four hours. If popsicles are reluctant to come out of their molds, dip into warm water for a few seconds. Enjoy.

Chapter 3: Protein Shakes & Smoothies

Blueberry Cacao Blast V 20

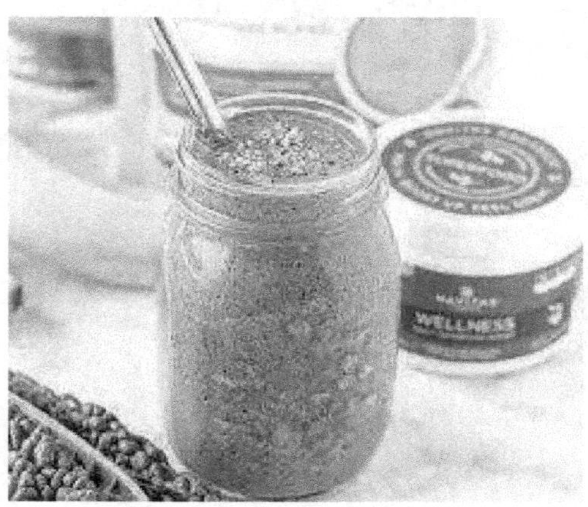

Serves: 1

Time: 5 minutes

Ingredients:

1 cup blueberries

1 tablespoon raw cacao nibs

1 tablespoon Chia seeds

1 dash cinnamon

½ Spinach (chopped)

½ Cup Bananas (chopped)

1½ Cup Almond milk

2 scoops Whey protein powder

Directions:

Place raspberries, cacao nibs, Chia seeds and cinnamon in a blender.

Add enough almond milk to reach the max line.

Process for 30 seconds or until you get a smooth mixture.

Serve immediately in the chilled tall glass.

Cucumber and Avocado Dill Smoothie V 20

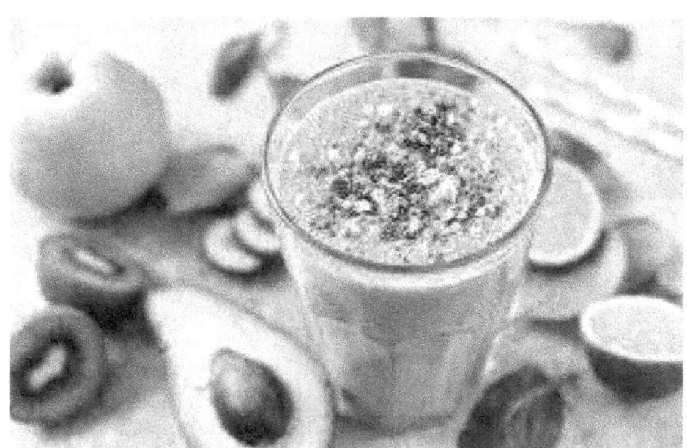

Serves: 2

Time: 5 minutes

Ingredients:

1 cucumber, peeled, sliced

2 tablespoons dill, chopped

2 tablespoons lemon juice

1 avocado, pitted

1 cup coconut milk

1 teaspoon coconut, shredded

2 kiwis, peeled, sliced

Directions

In a blender add all ingredients and blend well.

Drain the extract and discard residue.

Serve and enjoy.

Coco - Banana Milkshake V 20

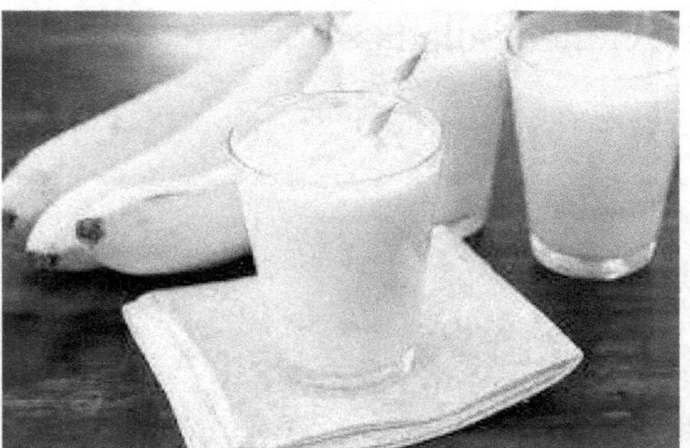

Serves: 1

Time: 5 minutes

Ingredients

1 cup coconut milk

2 ripe bananas

2 tablespoons cinnamon

¼ teaspoon cardamom powder

2 scoops protein powder

7 ice cubes

Directions

In a blender add coconut milk with cardamom powder, cinnamon, bananas and blend well.

Pour into glass and add ice chunks.

Serve and enjoy.

Stuffed Southwest Style Sweet Potatoes

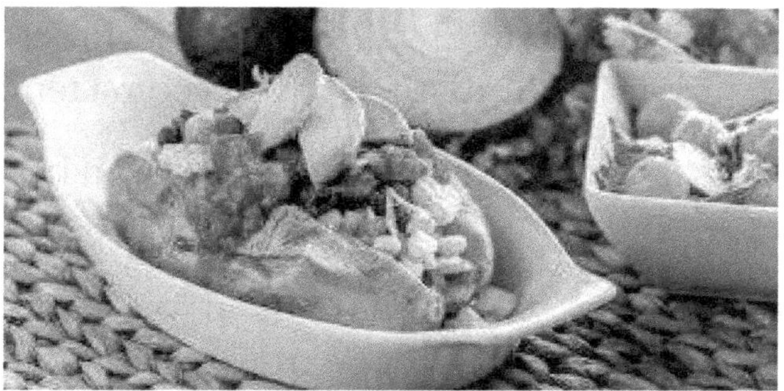

Serves: 4

Time: 60 minutes

Ingredients:

Pepper

Salt

Chopped cilantro, 2 tbs

Frozen corn kernels, ½ cup

Ground cumin, 1 tsp

Cooked black beans, ½ cup

Chopped tomatoes with juices, 1 cup

Chili powder, ½ tsp

Diced red onion, 1 small

Olive oil, 1 tsp

Small sweet potatoes, 4

Minced garlic, 1 clove

Directions:

Set your oven to 400 degrees.

Sit the sweet potatoes on a cookie sheet and allow them to bake in your heated oven for 30 minutes.

Take the potatoes out of the oven and prick them a few times and then place them back in for another 30 minutes, or until they have become tender.

As the sweet potatoes are baking, place a pan on medium heat and allow it to heat up.

Add in the olive oil and the onions and allow them to cook for two minutes. The onions should be soft, but they should not be translucent.

Add in the garlic and allow it to cook for 30 seconds or until you can start to smell the garlic.

Mix in the salt, chili powder, and cumin. Mix everything together until well combined. Mix in the cilantro and season the mixture with a bit more pepper and salt.

Taste and adjust the flavorings as you need.

To serve the potatoes:

Take the sweet potatoes out of the oven and slice them down the middle.

Fluff the meat inside of the potato up a little and season it with a bit of salt.

Divide the filling you just made between the different potatoes.

Enjoy.

Chocolate Coconut Chia Smoothie V 20

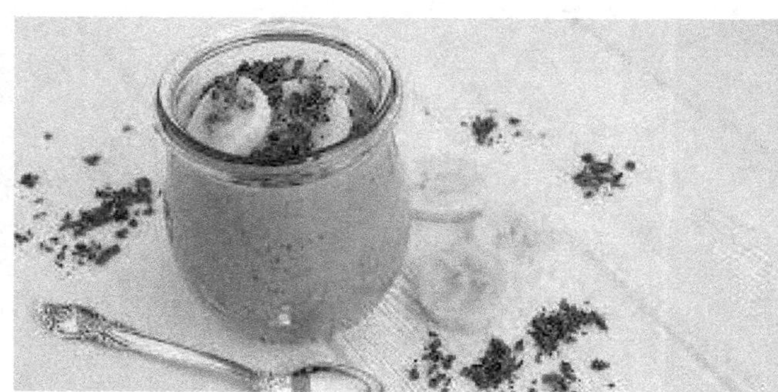

Serves: 1

Time: 5 minutes

Ingredients:

1 tablespoon raw cacao nibs

1 tablespoon Chia seeds

1 dash cinnamon

½ Spinach (chopped)

½ Cup Coconut (shredded)

1½ Cup Almond milk

Directions:

Place coconut, cacao nibs, Chia seeds and cinnamon in Vitamix.

Add enough almond milk to reach the max line.

Process for 30 seconds or until you get a smooth mixture.

Serve immediately in the tall chilled glass.

Banana-Cherry Smoothie V 20

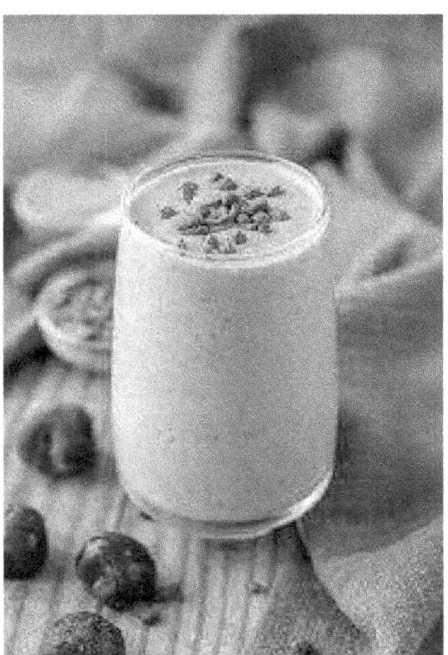

Serves: 1

Time: 5 minutes

Ingredients:

1 banana

1 cup cherries, pitted

¼ teaspoon nutmeg

1scoop protein powder

1 cup almond milk

Directions:

Place all ingredients in a blender

Process ingredients until smooth, for 20 seconds.

Serve immediately.

Avocado Smoothie V 20

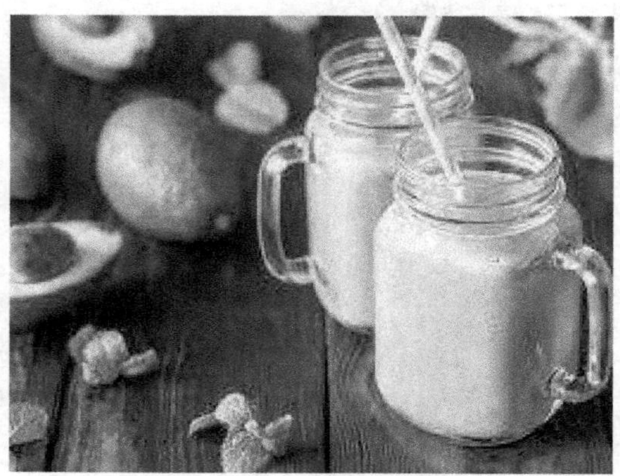

Serves: 1

Time: 5 minutes

Ingredients:

1 medium ripe avocado

¼ cup crushed peanuts

1 tablespoon flax seed

1 ½ cups vanilla Greek yogurt

1 cup Liquid (milk, water, coconut milk, etc.)

Directions:

Place all ingredients in Vitamix.

Process ingredients until smooth, for 20 seconds

Serve immediately.

Sweet Pepper Poppers

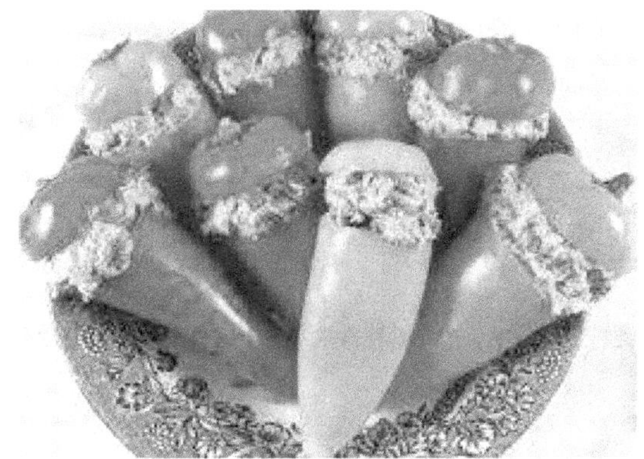

Serves: 6

Time: 20 minutes

Ingredients:

Salsa, for serving

2% shredded cheese, ½ cup

Chopped cilantro, 2 tbs

Taco seasoning packet

93% lean ground turkey, 1 pound

A bag of mini sweet bell peppers

Directions:

Start by halving the peppers and removing their seeds.

Set your oven to 350 degrees.

While the oven is heating up, brown the ground turkey.

Once the turkey is thoroughly cooked, drain off any fat that may have accumulated, and then sprinkle in the taco seasoning packet. Follow the directions on the packet for seasoning.

Place the halved bell peppers onto a baking sheet.

Ease the ground, seasoned turkey into the bell peppers.

Make sure you try to get an even amount of turkey into each bell pepper half.

Sprinkle the tops of each of the peppers with some cheese.

Place the baking tray in the oven and allow it to cook for five minutes.

Allow the peppers to cool slightly and then place over onto a serving plate.

Sprinkle them with cilantro and serve them with some salsa for dipping.

Mango Smoothie V 20

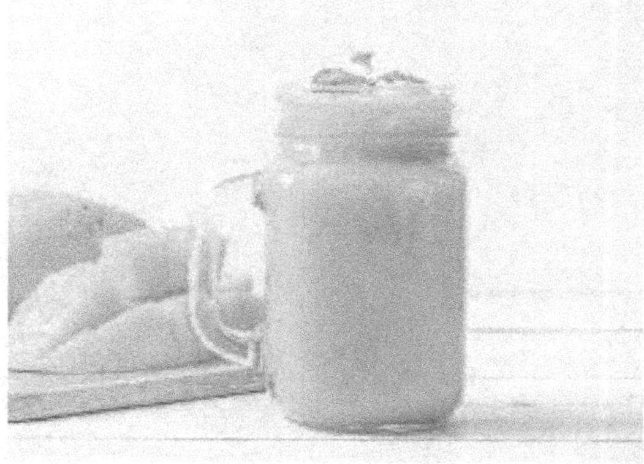

Serves: 2

Time: 5 minutes

Ingredients:

2 Mangos (seeded, diced, frozen)

Milk (1 cup)

½ cup crushed ice

1 cup plain yogurt

2 scoops protein powder

Directions:

Combine all ingredients in Vitamix.

Process for 30 seconds or until smooth

Serve immediately in a tall glass.

Pink Lady Cornmeal Cake

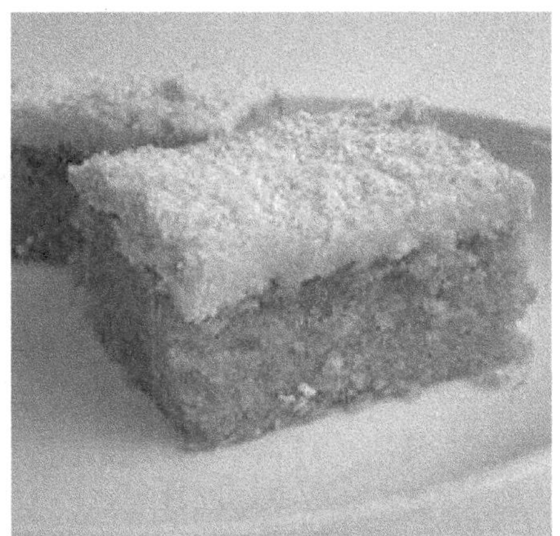

Serves: 12

Time: 1 hour 25 minutes

Ingredients:

Juice and zest of one lemon

Baking powder, 1 tsp

Ground almonds, 2 cups

Salt

Cornmeal, 1 cup

Vanilla, 1 tsp

Eggs, 3 large beaten

Splenda, ¾ cup

Butter, ⅔ cup

Pink lady apple, cored, peeled, and chopped, 1

Topping:

Pink lady apple, cored and sliced thin, 1

Confectioner's sugar, ¼ heaped cup

Zest and juice of one lemon

Crème fraîche to top

Directions:

Preheat your oven to 350 degrees. Grease and line an eight-inch round cake pan.

Place the chopped apple in a little bit of water for about six minutes until fork tender. Take off heat and drain. Let this cool.

Beat the sugar and butter together until creamy and light. Slowly mix in the eggs and beat until smooth. Mix in the baking powder, ground almonds, salt, cornmeal, and vanilla. Fold until well combined. Add in the cooled apple, lemon juice, and zest. Stir until well combined.

Carefully spoon the batter into your pan and smooth out the top. Slide into the oven for 45 minutes until golden brown and firm.

Carefully remove from oven and let it cool for around 20 minutes. Carefully turn the cake out onto a wire rack so that it can cool entirely.

While cake is cooling, make the topping. Add confectioner's sugar, four tablespoons of water, and lemon zest into a pot. Allow it to boil. Place in the sliced apples and allow it to simmer for five minutes. Spoon over the cake and let cool.

Slice into 12 even portions and serve with crème fraiche.

Bean and Spinach Burrito

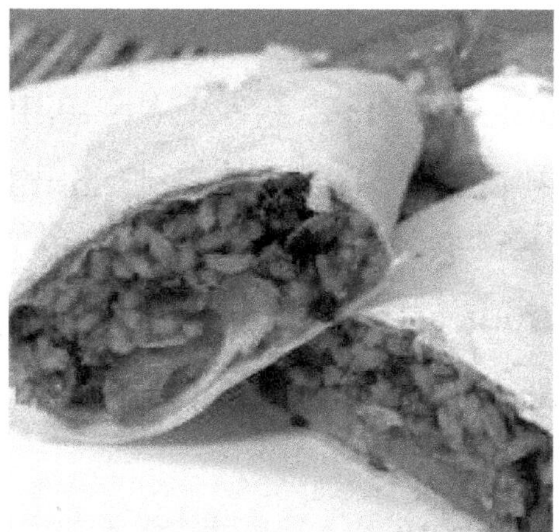

Serves: 6

Time: 30 minutes

Ingredients:

Whole grain tortillas, 6

Salt, to taste

Fat-free Greek yogurt, 6 tbs

Salsa, ½ cup

Reduced-fat grated cheddar cheese, ½ cup

Chopped romaine lettuce, ½ cup

Cooked Mexican rice, 1 ½ cups

Drained and rinsed black beans, 15 ounces

Baby spinach, 6 cups

Directions:

Set your oven to 300 degrees.

Stack all of the tortillas on top of each other and wrap them in a large piece of aluminum foil.

Sit the stack of tortillas on a baking sheet and bake them for 15 minutes until heated through.

Allow them to warm as you prepare the rest of the ingredients.

Add the spinach to the food processor and pulse it until they are finely chopped. If you don't have a food processor, you can also use a knife to slice up the leaves.

Place a large pan on medium heat and allow it to heat up.

Add in the spinach and black beans. Cook the mixture until the spinach has wilted. This should take around three minutes.

Evenly distribute this mixture between the six tortillas. Make sure that you leave about two inches on the end of the wrap to aid in folding it up.

Add about a quarter cup of the mixture to each tortilla and top with the lettuce, salsa, cheese, and the yogurt. Make sure you distribute the toppings evenly among them. Fold the tortilla over and under on the ends.

Cilantro Lime Cauliflower Rice

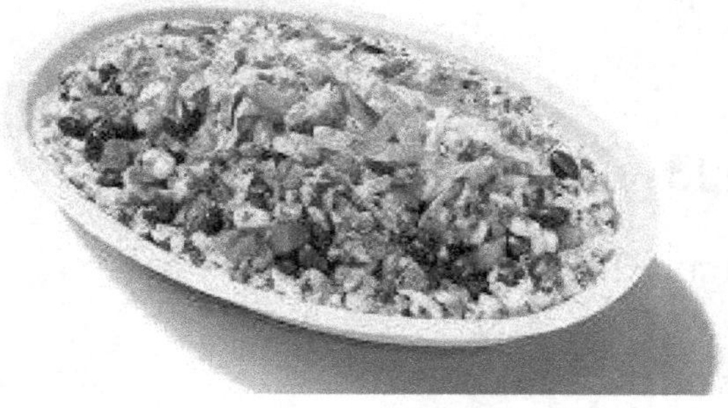

Serves: 4

Time: 6 minutes

Ingredients:

Chopped cilantro, 1 ½ tbs

Sea salt, ¼ tsp

Fresh lime juice, 1 tbs

Frozen riced cauliflower, 10 oz

Directions:

Follow the directions on the package of riced cauliflower to cook it.

As the cauliflower is cooking, chop up your cilantro.

Take the cauliflower out of the microwave and open the bag to allow all of the steam to release. Make sure that you don't get burned.

Pour the cooked cauliflower into a bowl and add in the salt, cilantro, and lime juice. Stir everything together to combine all of the flavors.

Chicken Curry

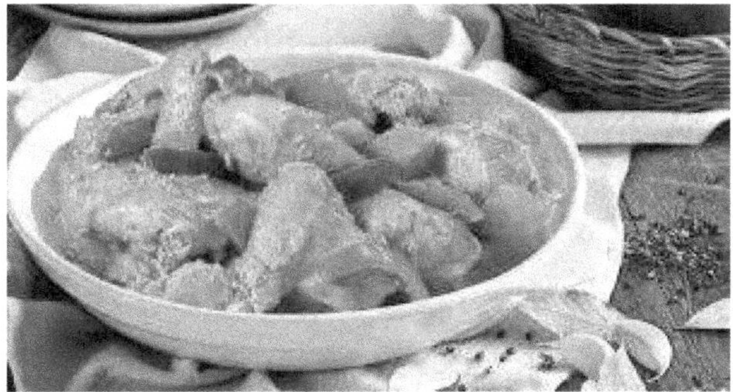

Serves: 4

Time: 60 minutes

Ingredients:

Cornmeal, 2 tbs

Cilantro, chopped, 2 tbs

Chicken stock, ¾ cup

Light coconut milk, 14 ounces

Sweet potato, 7 ounces peeled and chopped

Granny Smith apple that has been peeled, cored, and chopped, 1

Chicken breast, skinless, boneless, 1 pound, cut into cubes

Cinnamon stick

Cardamom pods, 6, crushed

Ground cumin, 1 tsp

Turmeric, 1 tsp

Red chili that has been seeded and chopped, 1

Garlic cloves, 2 crushed

One large onion that has been chopped

Low-fat cooking spray

Directions:

Coat a skillet with nonstick spray. Warm up the skillet on the burner and then add the onion and garlic, cooking until soft. This should take about five minutes. Place in the cinnamon stick, cardamom pods, cumin, turmeric, and chili and cook for an additional two minutes.

Place chicken into skillet and cook for three minutes. Stir to combine everything. Add cilantro, chicken stock, coconut milk, sweet potato, and apple. Stir well again. Partially cover the skillet and turn the heat down to a simmer. Let this cook for 35 minutes. Add water as needed.

Mix the cornmeal with a small amount of water. Mix together. Add to chicken mixture. Stir well until mixture is slightly thickened.

Serve hot over rice if desired.

Corn and Black Bean Salad

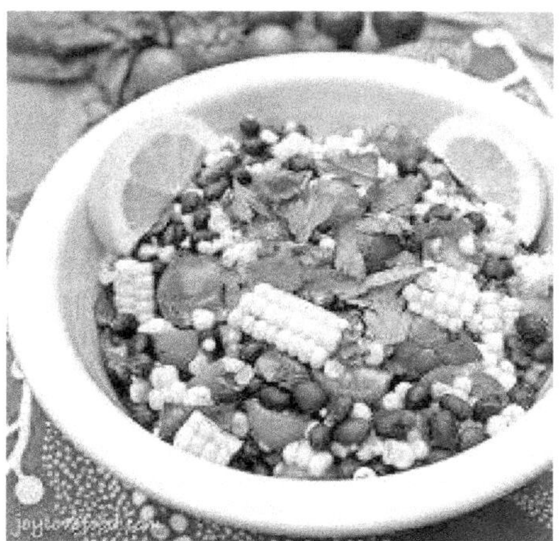

Serves: 30

Time: 6 minutes

Ingredients

Pepper, ¼ tsp

Olive oil, 2 tbs

Dash of salt

Brown sugar or honey, 1 tsp

Minced garlic, 1 tsp

Balsamic vinegar, ¼ cup

Minced red onion, 2 tbs

Chopped parsley, ¼ cup

Drained and rinsed black beans, 2, 16-ounce cans

Whole kernel corn, 1 cup

Directions:

Place the parsley, red onion, black beans, and corn in a large bowl and mix everything together.

Whisk the pepper, salt, honey, garlic, lemon juice, olive oil, and balsamic vinegar together. Make sure that all of the seasonings are mixed together well.

Pour the dressing you just made over the corn and bean mixture.

Toss everything together and allow the vegetables to marinate for at least 30 minutes before you serve them.

This will allow all of the flavors to mix together, and the flavor will be a lot more intense.

Enjoy.

Chicken Nuggets

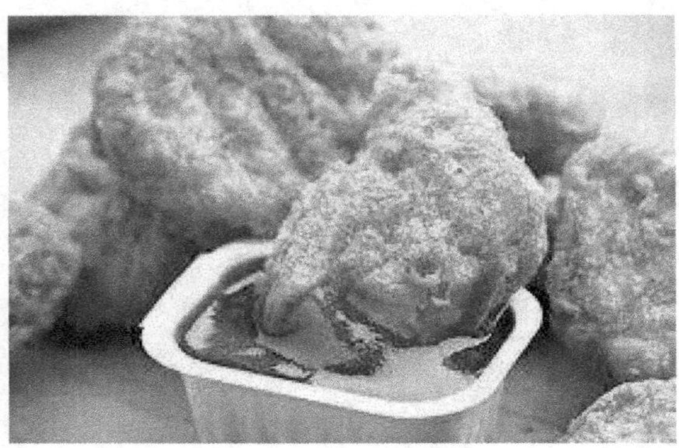

Serves: 4

Time: 50 minutes

Ingredients

2 tbsp. parmesan

3 tsp. canola oil

Nonstick spray

1 lb. chicken breasts, diced

3 tbsp. panko breadcrumbs

½ tsp. salt

¼ tsp. oregano

½ tsp. Italian herbs

¼ tsp. pepper

½ tsp. garlic salt

Directions

Heat your oven to 450.

Coat the chicken with oil. Sprinkle with pepper, garlic salt, oregano, salt, and Italian herbs. Massage into each piece of chicken.

Put the breadcrumbs and parmesan cheese into a gallon zippered bag and add the chicken. Seal the bag and shake and squeeze the chicken to coat it well.

Spray cooking spray on a cookie sheet.

Put chicken nugget in a single layer on the cookie sheet.

Spritz the chicken with some cooking spray.

Place in the oven and cook for eight minutes until no longer pink.

Chia Blueberry Banana Oatmeal Smoothie V 20

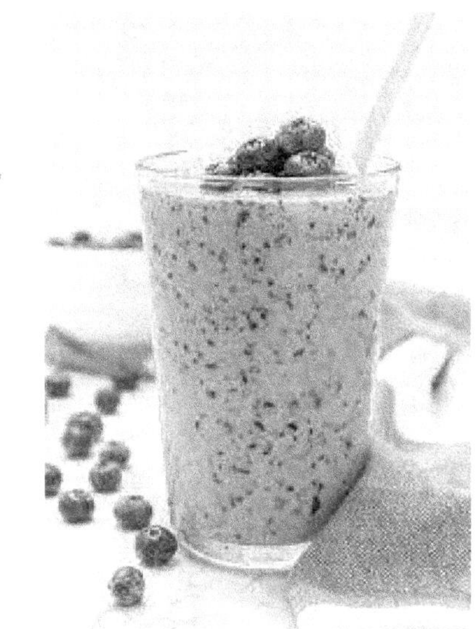

Serves: 1

Time: 10m

Ingredients:

Soy milk (1 cups)

Frozen banana (1, sliced)

Frozen blueberries (1/4 cup)

Oats (1/4 cup)

Vanilla extract (1 tsp.)

Cinnamon (1 tsp., to taste)

Chia seed (1 tbs.)

Directions:

Add all ingredients into a blender and blend until the ingredients are combined and smooth.

Serve and enjoy!

Strawberry and Cherry Shake V 20

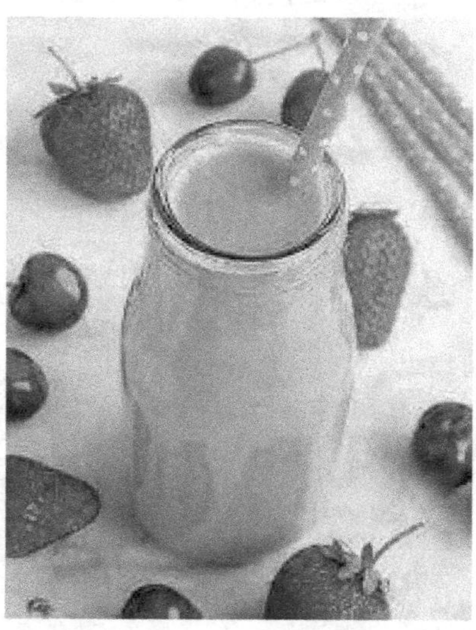

Serves: 2

Time: 5 minutes

Ingredients:

1 cup strawberries

1 cup cherries

1 cup almond milk

½ cup coconut milk

2 scoops protein powder

Few ice chunks

Directions

In a blender add all ingredients and blend well.

Serve and enjoy.

Pineapple Shake V 20

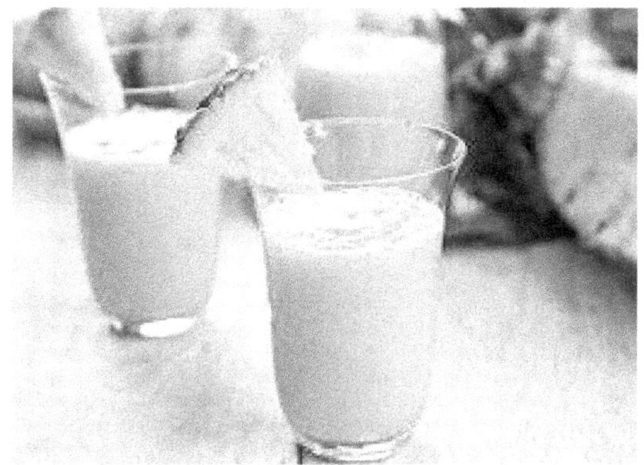

Serves: 6

Time: 20 minutes

Ingredients:

Frozen pineapple (3 cups)

Whey Protein Powder (2 scoops)

Greek yogurt (1 cup, pineapple/vanilla flavored)

Unsweetened vanilla almond milk (1 cup)

Vanilla extract (1 tbs.)

Directions:

Add the ingredients in the blender and blend until smooth.

Serve and enjoy!

Spicy Peanut Vegetarian Chili

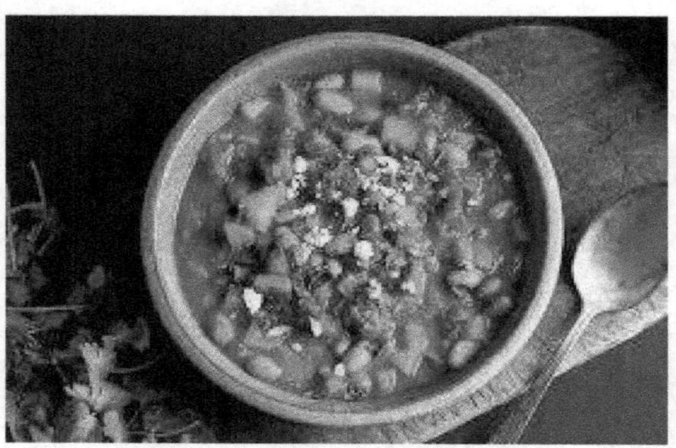

Serves: 12

Time: 50 minutes

Ingredients:

Vegetable broth, 2 cups

Tomato sauce, 15 ounces

Diced tomato, 28 ounces

Powdered peanuts, ⅔ cup

Rinsed and drained white beans, 16 ounces

Rinsed and drained, black beans, 16 ounces

Dried oregano, ¼ tsp

Chipotle chili pepper, 1 tsp (optional)

Chili powder, 2 tbs

Minced garlic, 2 cloves

Chopped onion, 1 cup

Peanut oil, 1 tbs

Directions:

In a Dutch oven, pour the oil in and let it heat up over medium-high heat.

Place in the onion and garlic and sauté them together for three to four minutes. The onions should become tender, but make sure that you don't let your garlic burn.

Mix in the salt, oregano, pepper, and chili powder. Allow this mixture to sauté for another two minutes, or until it becomes fragrant.

Mix in the broth, tomato sauce, tomatoes, powdered peanuts, corn, and cleaned beans.

Stir everything together and let it all come to a boil.

Lower the heat down to a simmer and allow the mixture to cook for 30 minutes.

If you want, this can also be fixed in a slow cooker.

Add everything to the slow cooker and mix everything together.

Cover the slow cooker and set it to high for two to three hours.

Halloumi Wraps

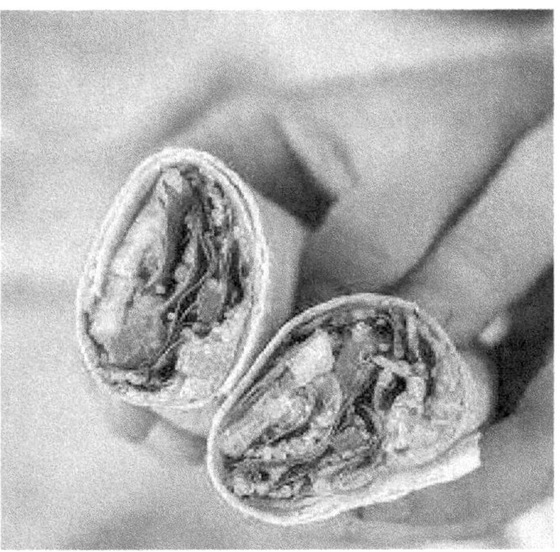

Serves: 6

Time: 30 minutes

Ingredients

Dressing:

1 olive oil

2 tbsp. sweet chili sauce

Filling and Salad:

6 radishes, sliced

9 oz. Halloumi cheese

4 spring onions, sliced

4 wraps, low-carb

1 head lettuce, leaves separated

1 lime, juiced

2 celery stalks, sliced

Directions

Combine the dressing ingredients and stir well to combine.

Slice the Halloumi into eight equal slices and coat with the dressing.

Put them on the grill or in a pan and brown on both sides about three minutes. They need to be crispy and browned on the outside.

While these are cooking, combine the radishes, lettuce, spring onions, and celery together. Add the rest of the dressing on the salad and toss.

Divide this between the wraps and place two of the grilled cheese slices on each. Serve immediately.

Enjoy.

Sichuan Roasted Eggplant

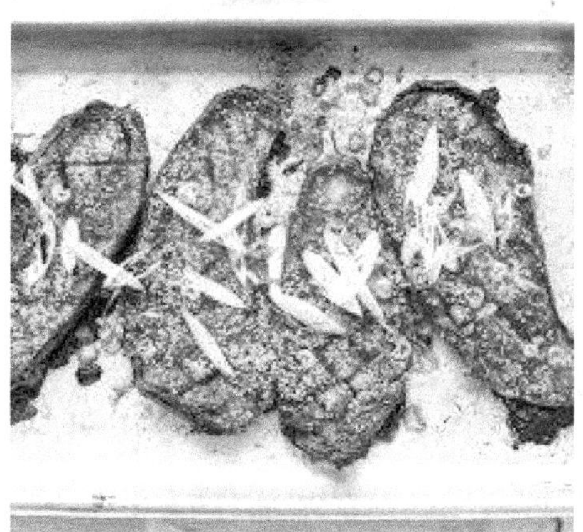

Serves: 4

Time: 80 minutes

Ingredients

1 tbsp. dark soy sauce

4 cloves crushed garlic

3 eggplants

2 tbsp. tomato paste

Pepper

3 tsp. chopped ginger

2 tbsp. olive oil

1 red chili, chopped finely

Salt

2 tbsp. sweet chili sauce

2 tsp. honey

Optional Toppings

Sesame oil

6 spring onions, chopped

Directions

Set your oven to 400. Put foil or silicone pad on a baking sheet. To make cleanup easier.

Mix pepper, ginger, honey, chili, salt, sweet chili sauce, tomato paste, oil, and soy sauce.

Slice eggplants in half lengthwise and make deep crisscross scores into the eggplants. Don't cut through the skins. Mark the flesh only. Put eggplants on the baking sheet and spoon the paste you made earlier on the flesh. Cover the eggplants loosely with foil and cook for about 30 minutes.

Remove the foil and allow to cook for another 30 minutes. They need to be brown and tender. Drizzle with some sesame oil and let stand for five minutes.

Top with chopped onions.

Enjoy.

Crustless Pizza Bites

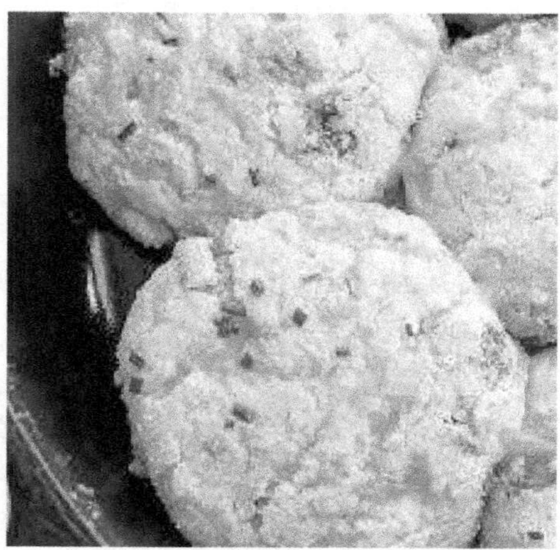

Serves: 5

Time: 45 minutes

Ingredients

Shredded mozzarella cheese

Pizza toppings of choice

Thick cut Canadian bacon

Pizza sauce

Directions

Spray cooking spray in a regular muffin tin. Put three slices of Canadian bacon in the bottom of each cup. Let the overlap to look like a three-leaf clover. Press down to form them to the cups. They don't like to stay well, but it's okay. When you put the toppings in, they will stay.

Get your cheese, sauce, and toppings together.

Put one tablespoon pizza sauce in each cup.

Add whatever toppings you would like that the cups will hold.

Sprinkle with a good amount of mozzarella cheese.

Heat your oven to 350. Put the pizzas in the oven for 27 minutes or until browned and bubbly. Watch them closely, so they don't burn.

Remove the pizzas from the pan with a fork. There will be some liquid in the bottom of the muffin cups, just throw away and enjoy your pizza bites.

Thai Sea Bass

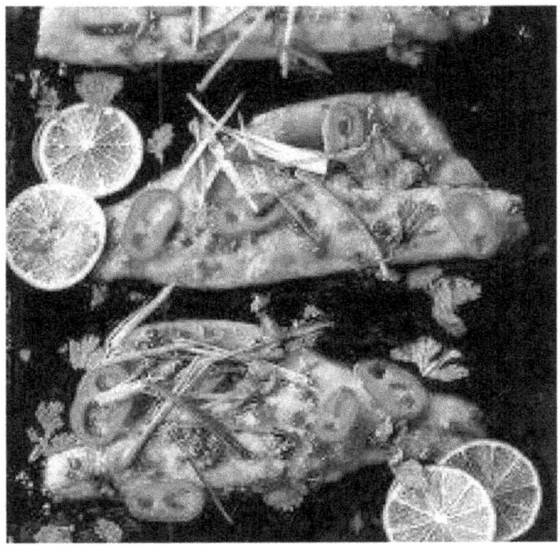

Serves: 5

Time: 20 minutes

Ingredients

2 tbsp. chopped cilantro

8 oz. bok choy, quartered

1 tbsp. soy sauce

4 oz. asparagus, trimmed

2 sea bass fillets

2 spring onions, chopped

Zest and juice of one lemon

1 mild red chili, sliced and seeded

2 cloves crushed garlic

4 tsp. grated ginger

1 tbsp. fish sauce

3 tbsp. oil

Directions

Heat your oven to 400.

Place the onions, bok choy, and asparagus in a roasting pan.

Mix lemon juice, fish sauce, garlic, lemon zest, chili, oil, soy sauce, and ginger together. Pour half over the vegetables and toss to coat. Slide this into the oven and cook for five minutes.

Take the veggies out and put the sea bass on top. Put back into the oven for another eight minutes until fish is cooked through. It should flake when you poke it with a fork.

Pour remaining dressing on top of fish, top with cilantro and enjoy.

Pacific Cod with Fajita Vegetables (Dairy-Free)

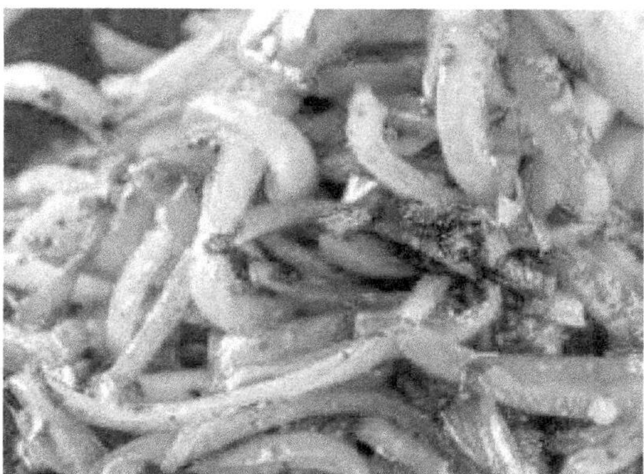

Serves: 4

Time: 20 minutes

Ingredients:

Pepper

Salt

Large julienned carrot, 1

Sliced yellow bell pepper, 2

Sliced red bell pepper, 2

Low-fat nonstick spray

Scallions, 6

Juice and zest of a lime

Wild Alaskan Pacific cod, 4, 6-ounce fillets

Directions:

Heat up your grill or broiler.

Place some aluminum foil over the grill rack and place the cod fillets on top.

Top the fillets with the lime juice, zest, and some slices of the scallions.

Allow them to grill or broil for six to eight minutes, or until it is cooked all the way through. The fish will turn opaque and will easily flake once it is cooked through.

As the fish cooks, spray a large skillet with some low-fat nonstick spray and allow it to heat up for a few moments on high.

Add in the bell peppers, the rest of the scallions, and carrot.

Allow them to cook, stirring often, for three to five minutes.

Divide your cooked veggies between four different plates and top each of them with a cod fillet.

Season the top of the fish with some pepper and salt to taste.

Mini Meatloaves

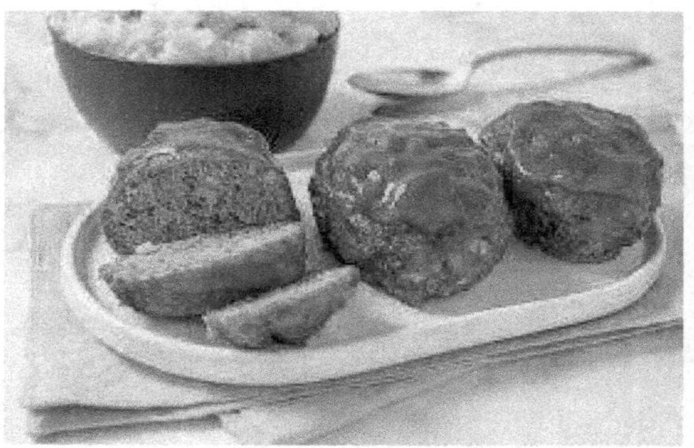

Serves: 4

Time: 50 minutes

Ingredients

¼ c whole wheat panko breadcrumbs

¾ c reduced fat shredded cheese

½ c chopped green bell pepper

¼ c egg whites

1 tsp. garlic powder

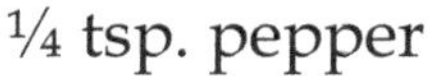

¼ tsp. pepper

3 tbsp. ketchup

½ tsp. salt

1 c chopped onion

1 tsp. onion powder

1 lb. ground beef

1 tsp. mustard

Optional Toppings:

Ketchup

Mustard

Dill pickles

Directions

Heat your oven to 375. Spray cooking spray in a regular muffin tin.

Stir together all of the ingredients, except for the cheese and toppings. Everything needs to be combined well. Divide the meat evenly among the cups and smooth out the tops.

Bake for 35 minutes until edges are browned and the meatloaf is firm.

Sprinkle with the cheese and cook for another three minutes until the cheese is melted and browned.

Take the dish from the oven and take out of the muffin pan with a knife or fork. Serve with toppings of choice and enjoy.

Salmon with Summer Salsa (Dairy-Free)

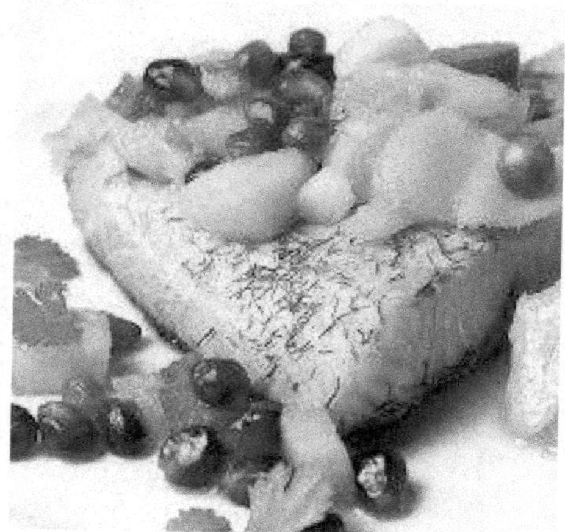

Serves: 4

Time: 55 minutes

Ingredients:

Lime wedges

Chopped cilantro, ¼ cup

Pepper

Balsamic vinegar, 1 tbs

Salt

Minced red onion, ¼ cup

Cooked corn kernels, ½ cup

Olive oil, 1 tsp

Crushed garlic clove

Chopped avocado, ½ an avocado

Chopped tomato, 1 cup

Skinless salmon, 4, 4-ounce fillets

Directions:

Set your oven to 325 degrees.

Stir all of the ingredients together, except for the lime and salmon.

Allow the mixture to refrigerate for around 30 minutes so that all of the flavors can meld together.

Place the salmon in your preheated oven and let it cook for 15 to 20 minutes, or until it has cooked all the way through. The salmon should flake easily and should be opaque when it is fully cooked.

Serve the cooked salmon topped with the salsa and lime wedge. A great summer option is to allow the salmon to cool off completely after it has cooked. Serving cool salmon with the chilled salsa is delicious.

Roasted Corn Guacamole

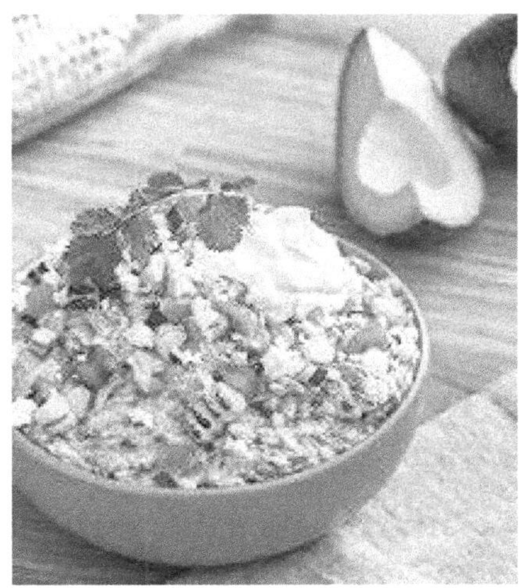

Serves: 6

Time: 15 minutes

Ingredients:

Pepper

Salt

Chili pepper, 1 tsp

Garlic powder, 1 ½ tsp

Chopped cilantro, ¼ cup

Diced onion, ¼ cup

Diced small tomato

Lime juice, 2 tsp

Large avocados, 2-3

Cumin, 2 tsp, divided

Butter, 1 tbs

An ear of corn

Directions:

Heat up a grill. Brush the corn with some butter and sprinkle it with a teaspoon of the cumin.

Lay the corn on the grill and cook it for five minutes. Make sure you turn it often during the cooking process to make sure it browns evenly.

The corn should char slightly during the cooking process.

Take it off the grill, and with a sharp knife, slice off the kernels. Set the kernels aside and discard the cob.

Pit the avocados and scoop out the meat of the avocados and place it in a bowl.

Mash up the avocados using a fork until they are creamy, but they still have a little bit of texture.

Mix in the garlic powder, chili powder, cilantro, and lime juice. Mix all of the ingredients together to make sure everything is evenly distributed.

Add in some pepper and salt to taste. Carefully stir in the corn, tomatoes, and onion.

Serve the guacamole immediately.

This is a great topper for any of the recipes in the beef and poultry sections of this book.

Spinach Green Smoothie V 20

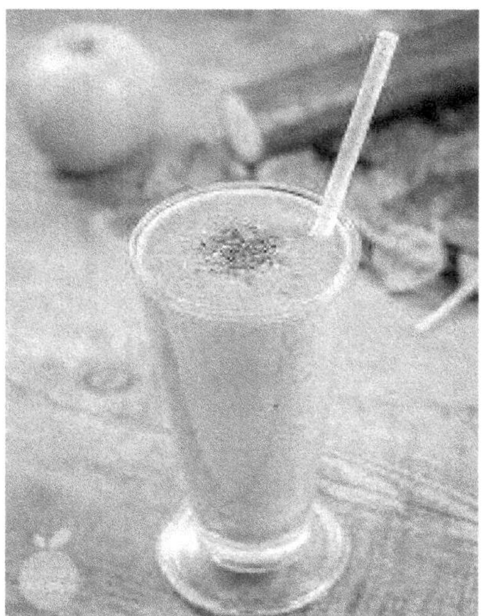

Serves: 2

Time: 5 min

Ingredients:

1 cup baby spinach leaves

2-3 mint leave

1 cup 100% grapes juice

1 cup 100% pineapple juice

2 tablespoons lime juice

2 scoops protein powder

Directions

In a blender add ingredients and blend well till puree.

Transfer to serving glasses.

Serve and enjoy.

Vegetable Chili

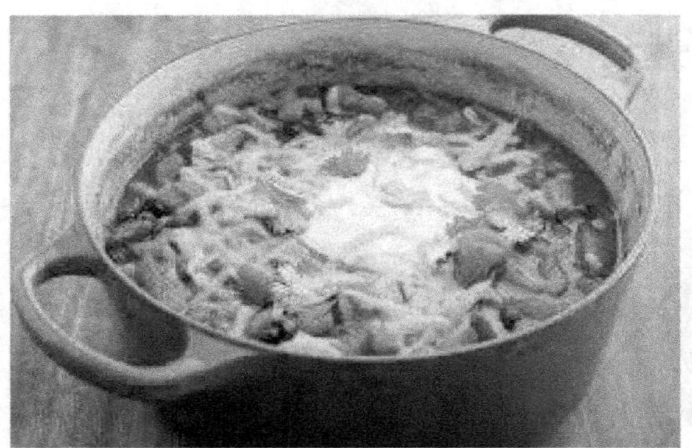

Serves: 12

Time: 8 hours 15 minutes

Ingredients:

Cilantro, ½ cup

Corn kernels, 1 cup

Vegetable broth, 2 ½ cups

Tomato paste, 6 ounces

Diced green chilis, 4 ounces

Cumin, 1 tsp

Drained black beans, 2 cans

Diced tomatoes, 2, 15-ounce cans

Salt, 1 tsp

Pepper, ½ tsp

Diced sweet potato

Diced celery, 1 cup

Diced sweet onion, 1 cup

Chili powder, 3 tbs

Sliced carrots, 2 cups

Dark red kidney beans, 1 can

Directions:

Place all of the chili ingredients, except for the cilantro, into a slow cooker.

Stir everything together and place the lid on the cooker and then set it to cook for six to eight hours on low.

Once it has finished cooking, sprinkle in the cilantro. You can also top the chili with some diced avocado, sour cream, and shredded cheese.

Black Bean, Rice, and Zucchini Skillet

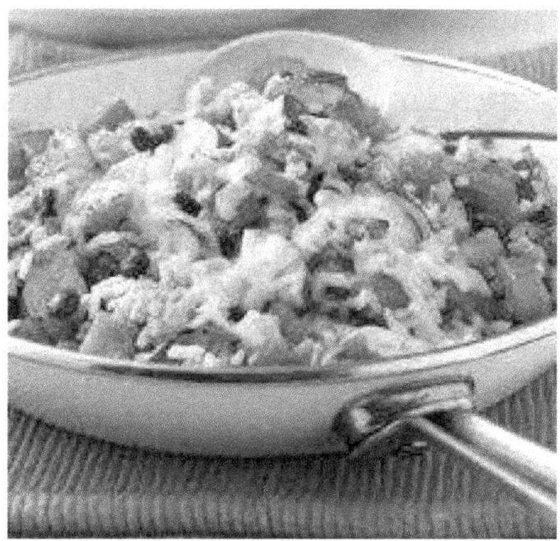

Serves: 4

Time: 25 minutes

Ingredients:

Monterey Jack and Cheddar cheese blend, shredded, ½ cup

Uncooked instant white rice, 1 cup

Dried oregano, ¼ tsp

Water, ¾ cup

Undrained fire roasted diced tomatoes with garlic, 14.5 ounces

Rinsed and drained black beans, 15 ounces

Diced green bell pepper, ½ cup

Chopped onion, ½ cup

Small sliced zucchini

Canola oil, 1 tbs

Directions:

Start out by heating the oil in a large pan over medium heat.

Once it is well heated, add in the bell pepper, zucchini, and onion. Allow the veggies to cook for five minutes, or until softened.

Make sure that you stir them occasionally.

Add in the oregano, water, undrained tomatoes, and beans.

Bring the heat up a bit and allow it to come to a boil.

Mix in the rice, stirring well to distribute all of the flavors.

Place the lid on the pan and then set it off the heat.

Allow the mixture to sit for seven minutes, or until the rice has absorbed all of the water.

Sprinkle everything with cheese and enjoy.

Mini Chicken Parmesan

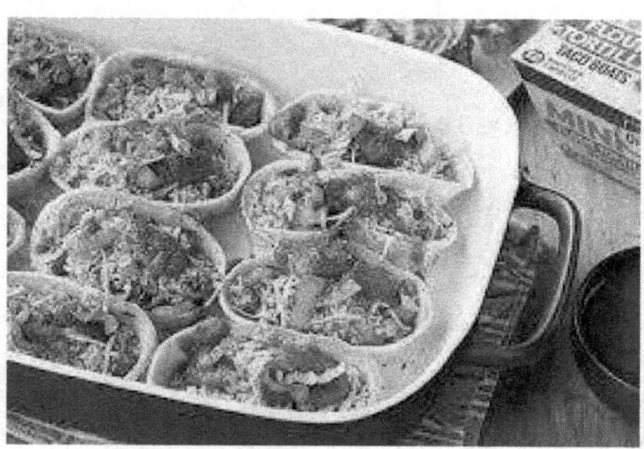

Serves: 4

Time: 35 minutes

Ingredients

1 egg

¾ c pasta sauce

1 ½ lb. ground chicken breast

¾ c mozzarella cheese, reduced fat

1 egg white

2 cloves minced garlic

6 tbsp. breadcrumbs

¾ c parmesan cheese

¾ tsp. dried basil

1/3 tsp. pepper

¾ tsp. oregano

¾ tsp. dried thyme

½ small chopped onion

¾ tsp. salt

Directions

Heat the oven to 350. Spray cooking spray into a muffin tin.

Mix the parmesan, pepper, egg, onion, salt, egg whites, garlic, oregano, breadcrumbs, thyme, basil, and chicken. Don't overmix. Make sure all the ingredients are distributed throughout the chicken.

Divide the mixture evenly into the muffin cups. Put pasta sauce over the meat mixture. Slide this in the oven for 20 minutes. Remove from the oven and add one tablespoon shredded cheese. Put back in the oven to let the cheese melt.

Take out of the muffin pan with a knife and enjoy.

Stuffed Chicken

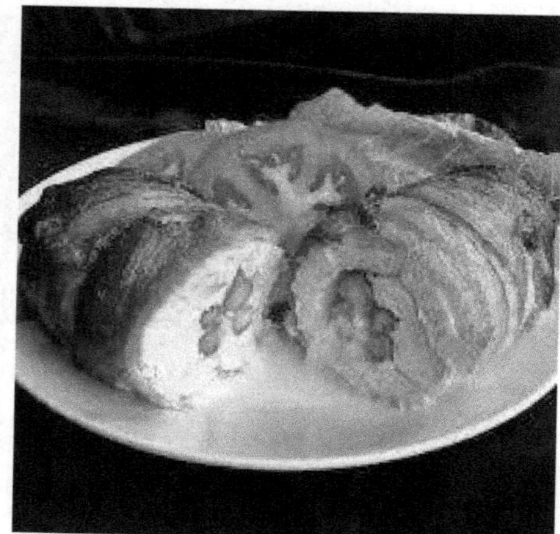

Serves: 4

Time: 40 minutes

Ingredients

Pepper

4 chicken cutlets, pounded thin

Salt

½ c breadcrumbs

Tomato sauce

¼ c parmesan, divided

Mozzarella cheese

1 egg

½ c ricotta cheese

½ pack frozen spinach, thawed and well drained

Directions

Heat your oven to 425.

Add half the breadcrumbs and parmesan cheese to a bowl, mix to combine. Set to the side.

Squeeze the spinach to get rid of all the liquid in it. Mix the rest of the parmesan with the ricotta and spinach in a bowl.

Put the cutlet on a cutting board and spread two tablespoons of the spinach on the top.

Roll up and secure with toothpicks.

In a shallow dish, whisk the eggs.

Coat each cutlet with egg and then the breadcrumbs.

Place them seam side down in a baking dish that you prepared with nonstick spray. Slide this in the oven for 25 minutes.

Take this out and top with some tomato sauce and mozzarella cheese.

Slide this back into the oven for five more minutes.

Remove from the oven and enjoy.

Fajita Chicken

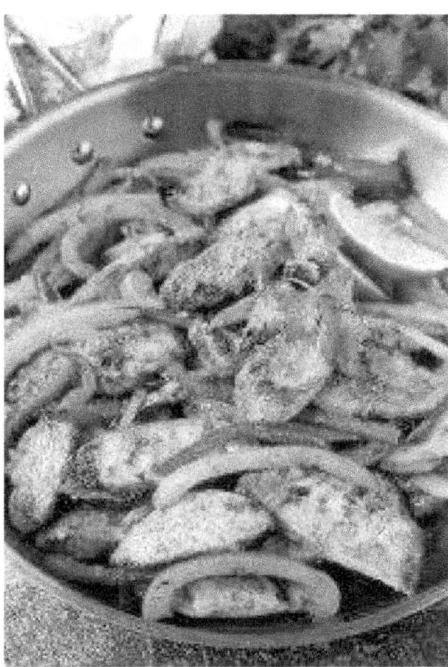

Serves: 4

Time: 8 hours 10 minutes

Ingredients

1 bag frozen pepper and onion blend

1 packet taco seasoning

Garlic powder

3 lb. frozen boneless chicken breast

3 c chunky salsa

Directions

Place the frozen chicken into a Crock-Pot. Sprinkle with taco seasoning and spoon salsa on each one. Sprinkle with garlic powder then add frozen onions and pepper on top.

Place the lid on and set on low for eight hours.

Serve as it is or shred for tacos, nachos, taco salad, fajitas, burritos or add to a baked potato. Leftovers can be stored in the refrigerator for a week or frozen.

Lamb Koftas

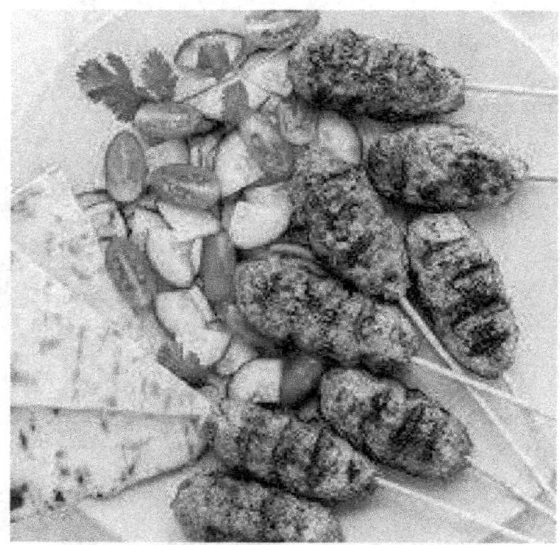

Serves: 4

Time: 40 minutes

Ingredients

2 tbsp. mint, chopped

8 oz. lean ground lamb

2 tbsp. fat-free dressing

2 tbsp. chopped parsley

2 oz. bulgur wheat

4 oz. light feta cheese

½ small chopped onion

8 oz. cherry tomatoes, halved

1 clove crushed garlic

½ cucumber, sliced and halved

½ tsp. cumin

½ tsp. ground coriander

1 ½ oz. craisins

Directions

Put the wheat into a skillet then cover with water and allow to boil. Cook for five minutes. The wheat needs to be tender then drain completely.

Combine garlic, lamb, onion, and wheat together. Mix the parsley, cumin, craisins, and coriander. Stir until all is incorporated. Divide the meat into 12 even portions.

Set your oven to broil or warm up a grill. Take one portion of the meat and press it around a skewer to form an oval. Continue with the remaining portions. Put them on a broiler pan or grill. Cook for about ten minutes. Turn about halfway through to brown both sides.

While the meat is cooking, combine parsley, cucumbers, mint, tomatoes, and feta. Toss in the dressing. Serve with the koftas.

Vegetable Chili

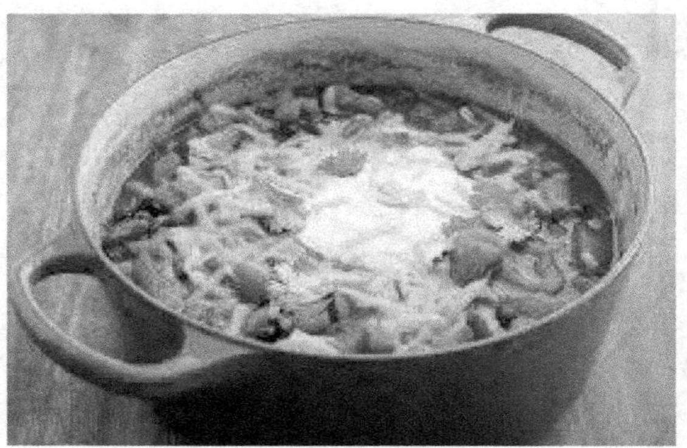

Serves: 3

Time: 20 minutes

Ingredients

1 tsp. chopped rosemary

7 oz. Romano peppers, seeded and sliced

1 red onion, sliced

Cilantro - garnish

14 oz. black beans, drained and rinsed

½ c strong low-fat grated cheese

12 oz. cherry tomato and basil sauce

2 tsp. chipotle paste

Cooking spray

Directions

Coat a pan generously with nonstick spray. Allow it to heat up and add the rosemary, peppers, and red onion. Cook for five minutes.

Add the chipotle paste, beans, and cherry tomato and basil sauce. Allow to simmer for about ten minutes. The peppers need to be tender.

Serve with some grated cheese and cilantro.

Enjoy.

Beef and Broccoli Stir-Fry

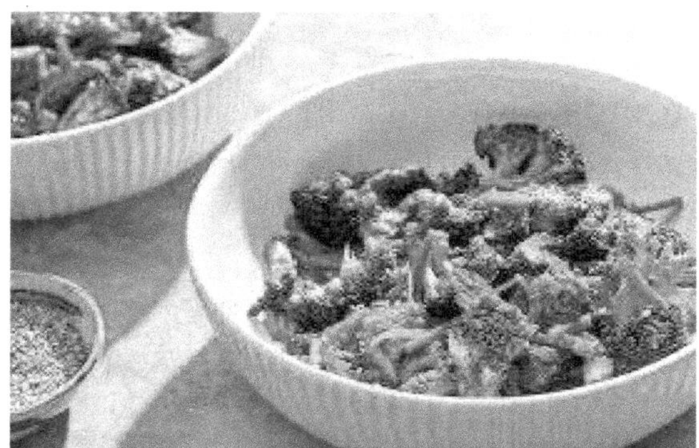

Serves: 4

Time: 50 minutes

Ingredients

1 tsp. rice vinegar

1 tsp. ginger, grated

4 scallions, shredded

4 tbsp. oyster sauce

12 oz. beef steak, cut into 1/2 -inch strips

2 red chilies, thinly sliced

Cooking spray

5 oz. shiitake mushrooms, sliced

1 tbsp. light soy sauce

1 red thickly sliced onion

8 oz. broccoli, cut in half

Directions

Combine the soy sauce and ginger and add the steak and coat well. Allow to sit for 15 minutes.

Use cooking spray to coat a wok then allow to heat up. When hot, place the steak mixture. Stir-fry the steak for five minutes until browned. Put the steak in a bowl for later use.

Put chili, broccoli, mushrooms, and onion in the wok and cook for about five minutes until veggies are tender. Add water or more cooking spray, so food doesn't burn.

Put the steak along with its juices back into the wok and add the rice vinegar and oyster sauce. Stir to combine. Cook a few minutes more until everything is heated through.

Garnish with scallions. Enjoy.

Spicy Peanut Vegetarian Chili

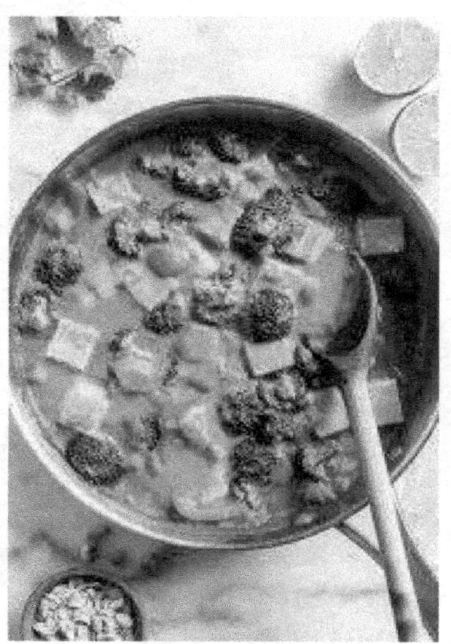

Serves: 4

Time: 50 minutes

Ingredients

2 c vegetable broth

¼ tsp. dried oregano

1 16 oz. can white beans, drained and rinsed

1 c chopped onion

1 15 oz. can tomato sauce

1 can black beans, drained and rinsed

2 tbsp. chili powder

1 28 oz. can diced tomatoes

2/3 c powdered peanuts

1 tsp. chipotle chili powder

1 tbsp. peanut oil

2 cloves minced garlic

Directions

Add oil to a Dutch oven and allow to heat up. Add the onion and garlic then sauté until tender and fragrant. Add the salt, chili powder, oregano, and pepper. Cook for another two minutes. Add the broth, beans, tomato sauce, corn, tomatoes, and powdered peanuts. Allow to boil then reduce the heat and simmer for 30 minutes.

Spoon into serving bowls and enjoy.

Chicken and Vegetables

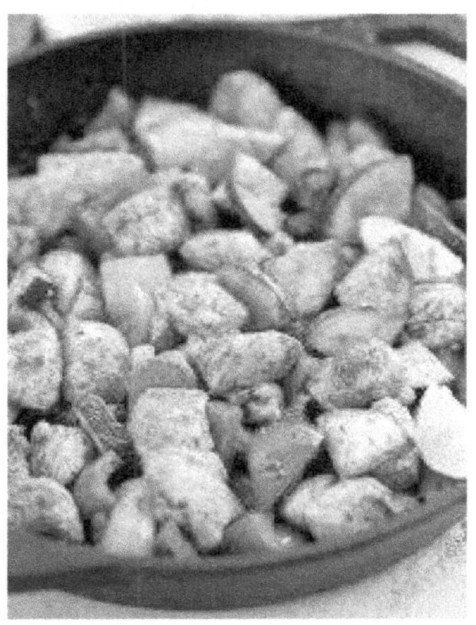

Serves: 6

Time: 50 minutes

Ingredients

4 yellow or red sliced bell peppers

3 to 4 cloves minced garlic

2 small diced Vidalia onions

1 8 oz. can tomato sauce

3 small zucchini, sliced

3 16 oz. cans diced tomatoes

8 oz. sliced mushrooms

3 lb. bag boneless skinless chicken breast

Directions

Cut the chicken into cubes. Put into a large pan along with the garlic and onion. Cook until almost done.

Add the tomato sauce, bell peppers, canned tomatoes, zucchini, and mushrooms. Cover and allow to cook for about 20 minutes. The vegetables need to be tender then taste to see if you need more pepper and salt

Serve over rice or as it is. Store leftovers in the refrigerator for one week or can be frozen to be eaten later.

Taco Chicken

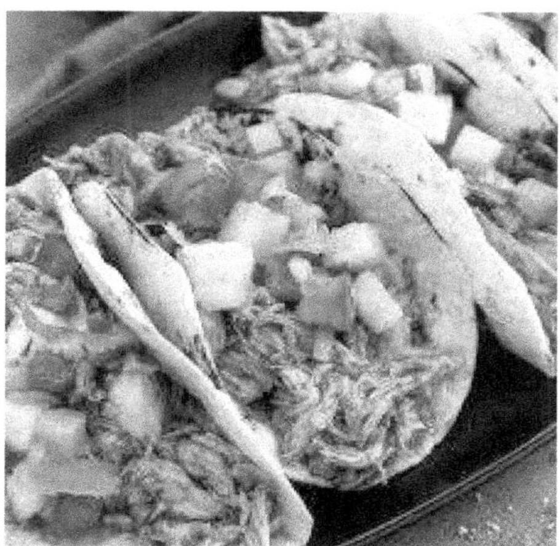

Serves: 2

Time: 40 minutes

Ingredients

1 c salsa

1 packet taco seasoning

¼ c nonfat sour cream

4 4 oz. chicken breast

Directions

Heat your oven to 375.

Put the taco seasoning in a reseal-able bag. Place the chicken and shake to coat. Place the chicken in a baking dish that is greased with nonstick spray. Bake for 30 minutes but take out of the oven at 25 minutes and top with salsa. Place back in the oven and bake for five more minutes. Remove from the oven and top with sour cream. Serve as it is or shred for tacos. Enjoy.

Vegetable Stir-Fry

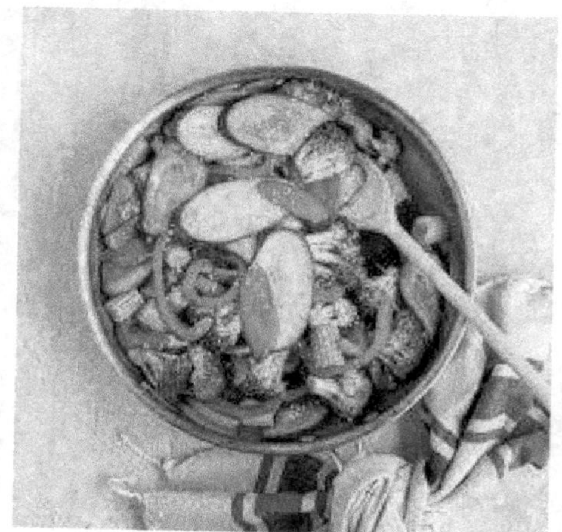

Serves: 5

Time: 25 minutes

Ingredients

1 chili, finely chopped

4 tbsp. soy sauce

2 red peppers, sliced and cored

1 onion, sliced

11 oz. baby corn, halved

1 lb. oriental mushrooms

2 tsp. sesame oil

2 cloves crushed garlic

1 lb. Chinese leaf lettuce, shredded

Cilantro for Garnish

Directions

Put oil in a wok and heat it.

Place the garlic and chili and let cook for 30 seconds.

Add the peppers, mushrooms, Chinese lettuce, and corn. Stir-fry for four minutes until they are tender-crisp.

Pour soy sauce over everything and toss to coat.

Serve garnished with cilantro.

Black Bean and Turkey Sloppy Joes

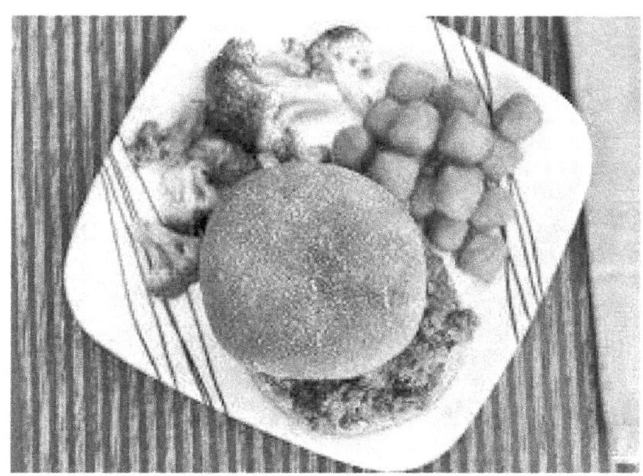

Serves: 4

Time: 70 minutes

Ingredients

1 14 oz. can diced tomatoes with green chilies

1 tsp. minced garlic

1 tsp. Mrs. Dash onion and herb blend

1 lb. ground turkey

1 6 oz. can tomato paste

1 14 oz. can black beans, drained and rinsed

1 ½ c low sodium tomato juice

1 tsp. paprika

1 tbsp. olive oil

1 medium chopped onion

2 tsp. chili powder

Directions

Put the turkey into a skillet and brown then drain any fat. Put all of the ingredients into the skillet and cook until the desired thickness.

Serve on buns or over toast.

Lemon Chicken Kebabs

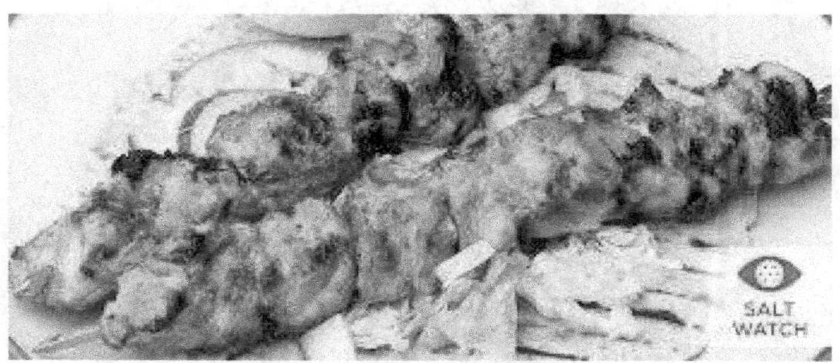

Serves: 4

Time: 55 minutes

Ingredients

2 tbsp. olive oil

Vegetables such as tomatoes and zucchini

2 lemons, juiced

1 tbsp. lemon zest

4 chicken breasts, cubed

Dipping Sauce:

2 cloves crushed garlic

Zest and juice of ½ lemon

3 tbsp. chopped basil

8 oz. plain goat cheese yogurt

Garnish:

2 tsp. basil

Directions

Put lemon juice, oil, pepper, salt, and lemon zest in a bowl and mix together well. Place the chicken and coat well. Cover the bowl and allow to marinate about 30 minutes.

While this marinates, combine the yogurt, pepper, garlic, lemon juice, salt, lemon zest, and basil in a bowl to make the dipping sauce. Put in the refrigerator until needed.

Thread the vegetables and the chicken onto eight to 12 skewers. Make sure you alternate them. Grill kebabs about five minutes per side. Turn them often, so they don't burn. As they cook, baste them with leftover marinade.

When chicken is done, serve with dipping sauce. Garnish with basil.

Enjoy.

Chapter 4: Veggies and Fruits

Black Bean and Rice Casserole

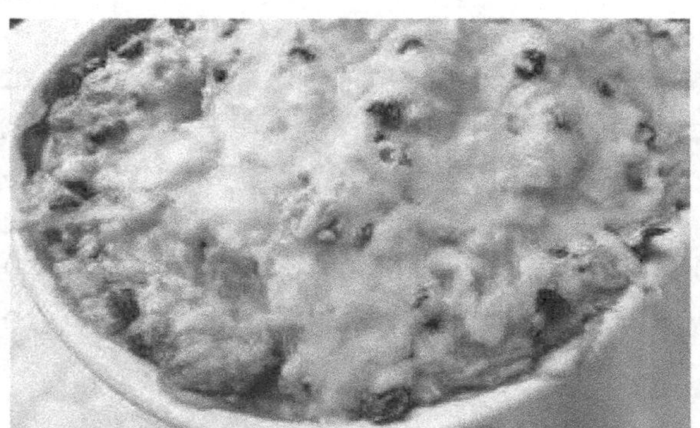

Serves: 8

Time: 90 minutes

Ingredients

1 cup vegetable broth

1/3 cup each:

Diced onion

Brown rice

1 tablespoon olive oil

1 lb. chopped chicken breast (no skin or bones)

1 medium thinly sliced zucchini

½ cup sliced mushrooms

¼ teaspoon cayenne pepper

½ teaspoon cumin

1/3 cup shredded carrots

1 can (4 ounces) diced green chilies

1 can (15 ounces) drained black beans

2 cups shredded Swiss cheese

Directions

Prepare a pot with the vegetable broth and rice, bringing it to a boil. Lower the heat setting and cook covered on low for 45 minutes.

Program the oven temperature to 350°F.

Spray a baking dish with some cooking spray.

Pour the oil in a pan over medium heat. Toss in the onion and cook until tender, and blend in the chicken, zucchini, mushrooms, and seasonings. Continue cooking until the chicken is heated and the zucchini is lightly browned.

In a large mixing dish, combine the onion, cooked rice, chicken, zucchini, beans, chilies, mushrooms, one cup of Swiss cheese, and the carrots.

Empty the ingredients into the casserole dish along with the remainder of the Swiss cheese as a topping. Cover and bake 30 minutes. Uncover, and continue cooking ten more minutes.

Broccoli Casserole

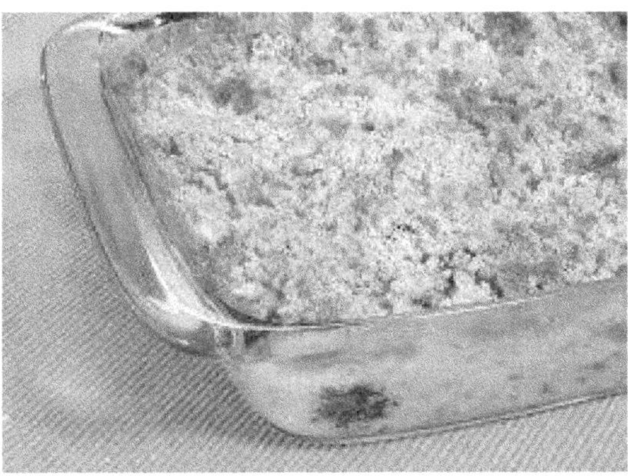

Serves: 12

Time: 50 minutes

Ingredients

4 cups cut up broccoli

1 sleeve Ritz crackers

2 cups cheddar cheese

Directions

Add the casserole ingredients into a Pyrex dish with the crumbled crackers on top.

Bake long enough to melt the cheese at 375°F.

Veggies with Grilled Pineapple

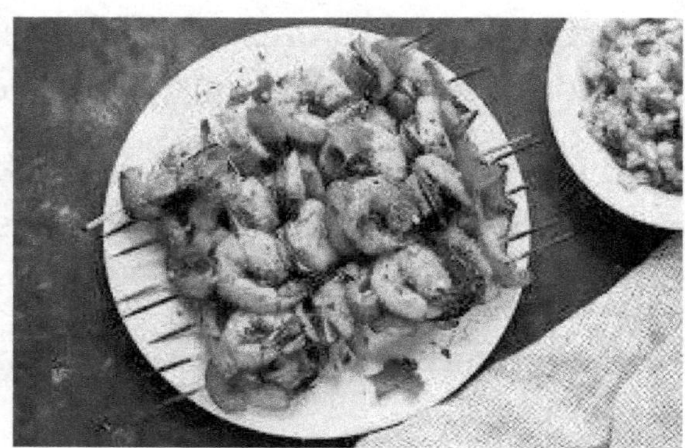

Serves: 6

Time: 40 minutes

Ingredients

1 cup of each:

Diced potatoes

Bell peppers

Raw mushrooms

1 cup cherry tomatoes

1 medium chopped onion

1 can of pineapple chunks – natural juices

2 teaspoons each:

Dill weed

Chopped garlic

1 teaspoon celery seed/salt

3 tablespoons olive oil

1 ½ teaspoons each: **Optional**:

Onion powder

Cayenne pepper

Garlic powder

Pepper and salt to taste

Directions

Chop the veggies

Option 1: Add the veggies on a piece of oil sprayed foil. Arrange the package on the grill using medium heat for 20-25 minutes (turning every five minutes).

Option 2: Place the veggies on wooden skewers that have been soaked in water. Cook on a med-high grill, turning every five minutes or so.

Oven: Bake at 400°F, checking every 10 minutes.

Vegetarian Frittata

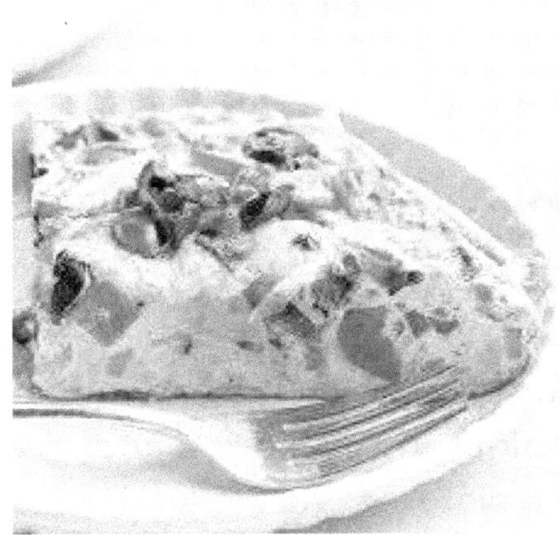

Serves: 6

Time: 60 minutes

Ingredients

6 ounces button mushrooms

1 pound asparagus

1 shallot

1 garlic clove

1 tablespoon olive oil

1 small zucchini

6 large eggs

1/3 cup 1% milk

¼ teaspoon of freshly ground black pepper

1 teaspoon salt

1 tablespoon chopped chives

Dash of nutmeg

2 medium/1 large tomato

¼ cup freshly grated parmesan cheese

Directions

Set the oven temperature to 350°F.

Prepare the Asparagus: Wash and trim cutting it into one-inch pieces. Blanche the cut asparagus for one to two minutes. Shock it by adding it to ice water. Drain and set to the side.

Wash and slice the mushrooms. Saute them in the oil for ten minutes using medium heat. Mince the shallots and garlic and add – cooking two more minutes. Transfer the mushrooms to a plate and set aside.

Slice the zucchini lengthwise and into half-moon shapes.

Whisk the eggs, milk, chives, pepper, salt, and nutmeg in a large mixing dish. Add the mushroom mixture, asparagus, and zucchini.

Spray a two-quart baking dish with cooking spray and add the egg/veggie mixture.

Arrange the thinly sliced tomatoes on top and sprinkle with the parmesan cheese.

Bake 30-35 minutes. You can place the frittata under the broiler for two to three minutes to brown the top.

Cool and serve at room temperature or straight from the fridge.

Chickpea and Feta Salad

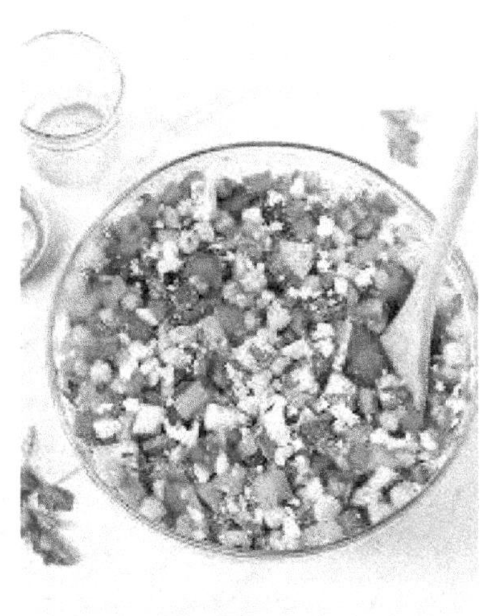

Serves: 1

Time: 55 minutes

Ingredients

¾ cup chopped raw vegetables

¼ cup each:

Can/fresh chickpeas

Crumbled feta cheese

1 tablespoon lemon juice

2 tablespoons olive oil

1 teaspoon dried oregano

Dash each of:

Pepper

Salt

Directions

Use your imagination for the chopped veggies. Include peppers, avocado, tomatoes, onions, and celery or your favorites.

Rinse and drain the chickpeas.

Combine all of the ingredients and chill in the fridge until ready to serve.

Cucumber and Onion Salad with Vinegar

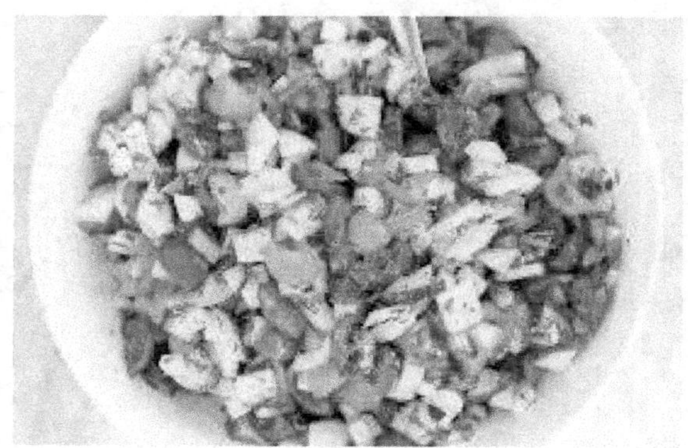

Serves: 6

Time: 70 minutes

Ingredients

Pinch of salt and pepper

1 red onion

3-5 cucumbers (peeled)

½ cup each:

White vinegar

Water

1/3 cup sugar

Directions

Slice the cucumbers and onions very thin and add to a salad dish.

Combine the water, vinegar, salt, pepper, and sugar and pour over the veggies.

Add a cover and marinate for a minimum of one hour.

Coleslaw

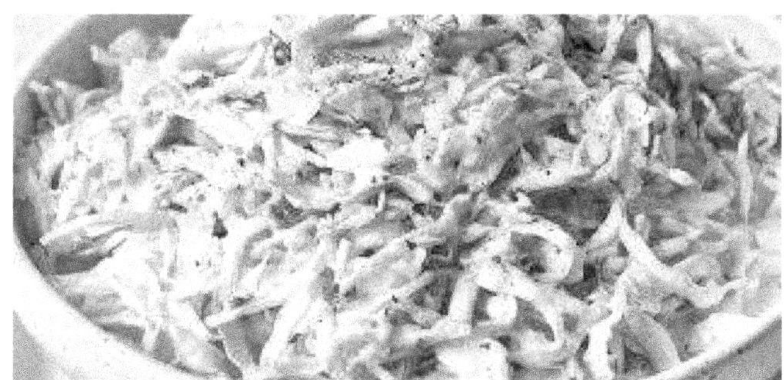

Serves: 6

Time: 35 minutes

Ingredients

1 small shredded carrot

3 cups green cabbage - shredded

¼ cup minced onion

1 tablespoon vinegar

1/3 cup mayonnaise

2 teaspoons sugar

½ teaspoon each:

Celery seed

Salt

Directions

Prepare the onion, carrots, and cabbage into a bowl.

Mix the dressing and pour over the slaw.

Lentil Vegetarian Loaf

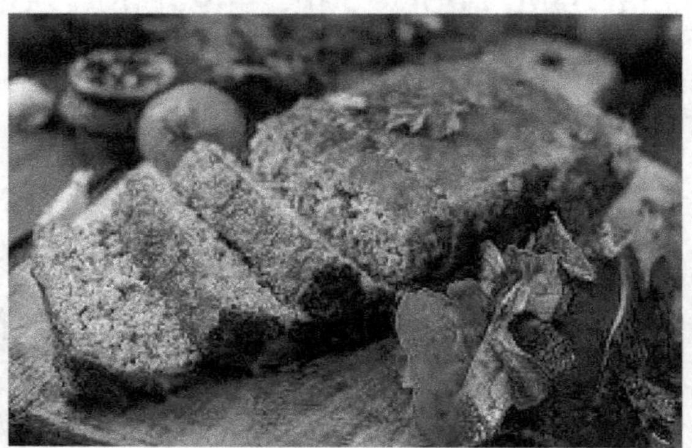

Serves: 10

Time: 2 hours 20 minutes

Ingredients

1 ½ cups rinsed - dried lentils

2 yellow onions

3 cups cooked brown rice

2 tablespoons canola/olive oil

½ cup ketchup

1 can tomato paste (6 ounces)

1 teaspoon each of:

Marjoram

Garlic powder

Sage

½ cup - quartered cherry tomatoes

¾ cup tomato/pasta sauce

To Taste:

Salt

More ketchup

Directions

Preheat the oven to 350°F.

Rinse and cook the lentils in 3 to 4 cups of water for approximately 30 minutes.

Drain and slightly mash the lentils.

Peel and chop the onions. Cook in the oil until golden.

Combine the onions, lentils, tomato paste, rice, tomatoes, sauce and spices into a large pot. Mix well.

Press the mixture into a well-greased baking dish with ½ cup of ketchup over the top.

Bake for one hour.

Baked Tomatoes

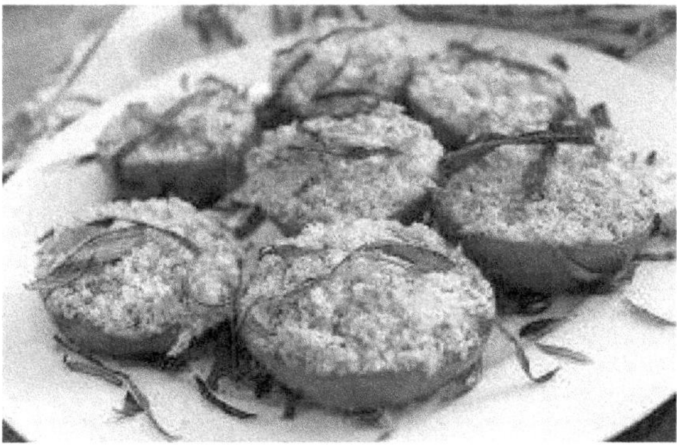

Serves: 6

Time: 60 minutes

Ingredients

Olive oil spray

5-6 large tomatoes

Greek seasoning

¼ cup low-fat parmesan cheese

Optional: ¼ cup pine nuts

Directions

Set the oven temperature in advance to 350°F. Spray a baking pan with the olive oil.

Slice the tomatoes lengthwise into halves and arrange them on the baking pan.

Sprinkle them with the cheese, nuts, and a bit of Greek seasoning as you desire.

Bake on the middle oven rack for 50 minutes.

Acorn Squash- Stuffed with Cheese

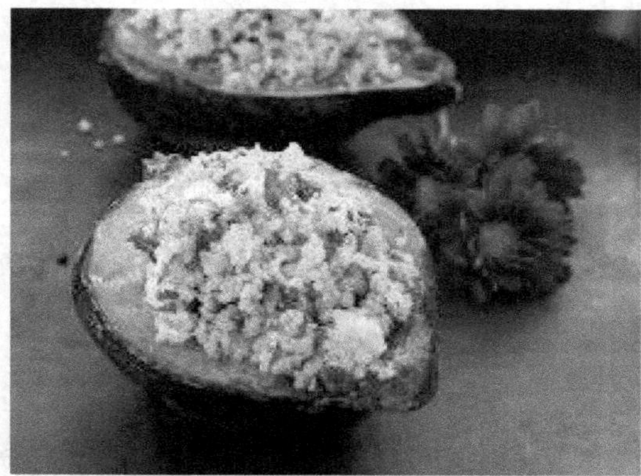

Serves: 4

Time: 60 minutes

Ingredients

1 pound ground turkey breast (extra-lean)

2 acorn squash

1 can (8 ounces) tomato sauce

1 cup each:

Sliced fresh mushrooms

Chopped onion

Diced celery

1 teaspoon each:

Garlic powder

Basil

Oregano

1 pinch black pepper

1/8 teaspoon salt

1 cup shredded cheddar cheese (reduced-fat)

Directions

Program the oven temperature to 350°F.

Slice the squash in half and remove the seeds. Arrange the squash, cut side down, in a dish and microwave on high for 20 minutes.

Brown the turkey in a skillet and add the onion and celery. Saute two to three minutes. Blend in the mushrooms, and add the sauce and seasonings. Divide into quarters and spoon into the squash.

Cover and bake for 15 minutes.

Garnish with the cheese and bake until the cheese has melted.

Spicy Sweet Potato Fries

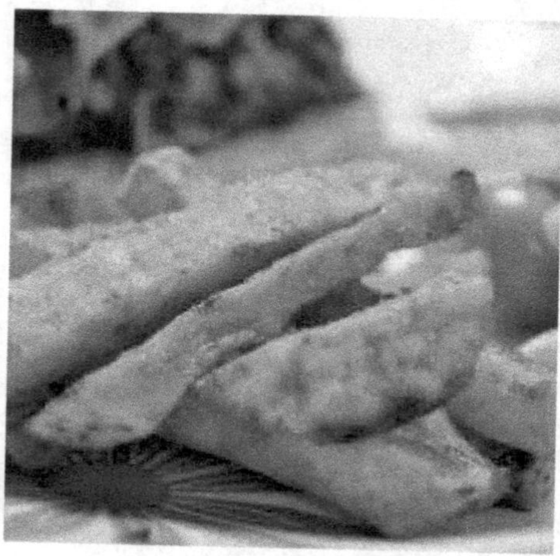

Serves: 4

Time: 40 minutes

Ingredients

1 ½ tablespoons olive oil

2 medium sweet potatoes

¼ teaspoon salt

1 teaspoon ground cumin

½ teaspoon each:

Onion powder

Chili powder

Directions

Program the oven setting to 450°F.

Wash and cut the potatoes lengthwise into fry strips. Combine all ingredients together in a dish and shake

Arrange them on a baking sheet on some parchment paper or foil.

Bake and turn every 5 to 6 minutes - for a total of 20 minutes cooking time.

Spinach Lasagna

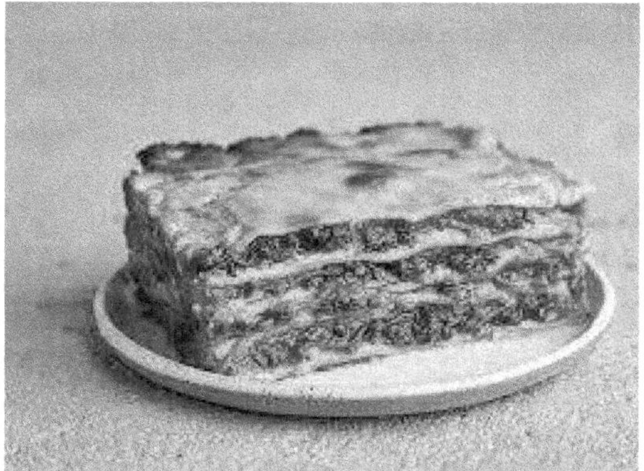

Serves: 8

Time: 2 hours

Ingredients

1 large egg

2 cups cottage cheese (1% milkfat)

2 cups part-skim mozzarella cheese

10 ounces baby spinach

1 jar spaghetti/marinara tomato sauce

1 cup water

9 lasagna noodles

1/8 teaspoon black pepper

Directions

Program the oven temperature to 350°F.

Combine the thawed, drained spinach, one cup of mozzarella, cottage cheese, egg, and the seasonings in a large mixing bowl.

Spray a 9x13x2-inch casserole dish with some cooking spray.

Layer ½ cup of the sauce, 3 noodles, and ½ of the cheese mixture. Repeat, and top with the noodles one cup of mozzarella. Pour water around the edges and toothpicks on top to place a piece of foil over the noodles.

Bake covered for one hour to 1 ½ hours. Let it rest 15 minutes.

Squash and Apple Bake

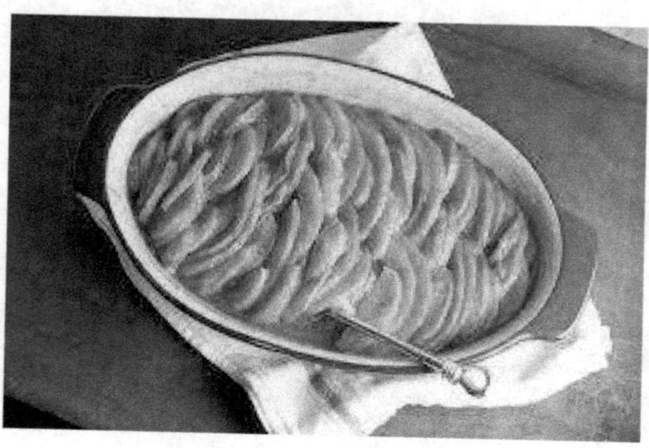

Serves: 6

Time: 70 minutes

Ingredients

2 medium apples

1 medium butternut squash

1 tablespoon each:

Splenda

All-purpose flour

½ teaspoon salt

¼ cup melted butter

2 teaspoons ground cinnamon

Directions

Program the oven temperature to 350°F.

Peel and core the apples and cut them into thin wedges. Peel and cut the squash into ¾-inch cubes.

Combine the squash and apples together in a baking dish.

Add the remainder of ingredients together and add to the top of the mixed apples and squash.

Bake for 50 to 60 minutes in a covered dish. For the last ten minutes, you can remove the top if you prefer the topping crispier.

Eggplant Pesto Mini Pizza

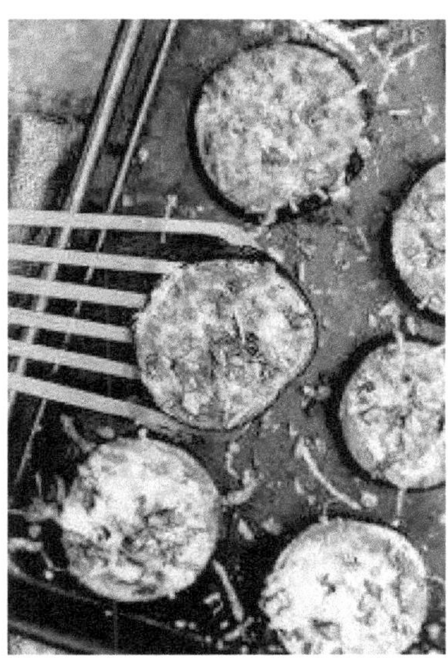

Serves: 4

Time: 55 minutes

Ingredients

1 each chopped:

Bell pepper

Tomato

Eggplant

1 medium sliced red onion

1/8 teaspoon salt

3 cloves of garlic

Pinch of oregano

¼ cup each:

Extra-virgin olive oil

Pesto sauce

Hummus

Vegan Parmesan cheese

Sandwich thins - Arnold Orowheat used

Optional: Pepper flakes

Directions

Set the oven to 400°F.

Chop the vegetables and combine the oil, pepper, salt, oregano, and pepper flakes if desired. Arrange on a baking tin and toast for approximately 30 to 45 minutes or until they are done the way you like them.

Toast the buns and spread the hummus on them, add the veggies, and a bit of pesto sauce. Sprinkle with the vegan cheese and enjoy.

Vegetarian Chili

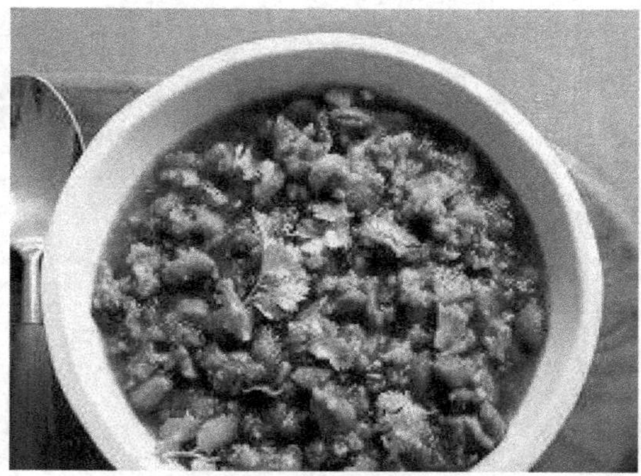

Serves: 8

Time: 15 minutes

Ingredients

1 can (15 ounces) each:

Dark red kidney beans

Pinto beans

Light red kidney beans

Black beans

2 cans (28 ounces) crushed tomatoes

1 can (28 ounces) diced tomatoes

3 cups celery

1 small diced each of bell peppers:

Yellow

Red

1 medium red onion

4 tablespoons chili powder

3 tablespoons garlic powder

2 tablespoons ground cumin

Directions

Drain and rinse all of the beans. Dice the veggies.

Lightly spray a large pan on the stovetop using medium heat and cook the veggies about six to seven minutes or until they are softened.

Combine the spices, beans, and tomatoes in a slow cooker or a Dutch oven.

Chapter 5: Fruit Salads

California Roll in a Bowl

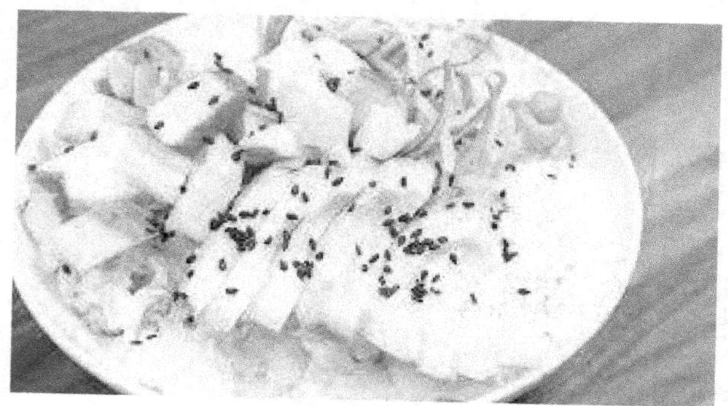

Serves: 4

Time: 15 minutes

Ingredients

1 head chopped lettuce

1 cup cooked brown rice

1 English cucumber – seedless – thinly sliced

1 (8 ounces) package cooked shrimp/crabmeat – chopped

1 grated carrot

1 ripe diced avocado

3 tablespoons pickled ginger

Ingredients for the Dressing

1 tablespoon light soy sauce

½ teaspoon wasabi powder – to taste

3 tablespoons rice wine vinegar

Garnishes:

1 large sheet seaweed/nori (toasted and in small bits)

1 tablespoon sesame seeds

Directions

Combine each of the fixings for the dressing in a mixing dish and whisk well.

Divide it into four sections and enjoy.

Note: You can locate the ginger in the Asian section of the supermarket.

Israeli Salad

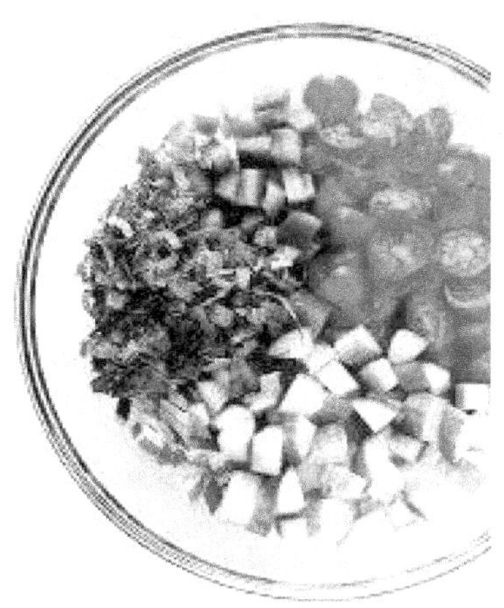

Serves: 8

Time: 5 minutes

Ingredients

1 medium peeled cucumber

3 medium tomatoes

1 yellow/green bell pepper

2 tbsp. lemon juice

3 tbsp. extra-virgin olive oil

1 tsp. of salt and fresh ground pepper

Directions

Chop all of the veggies into small bits.

Combine the rest of the ingredients and enjoy.

Grape Salad

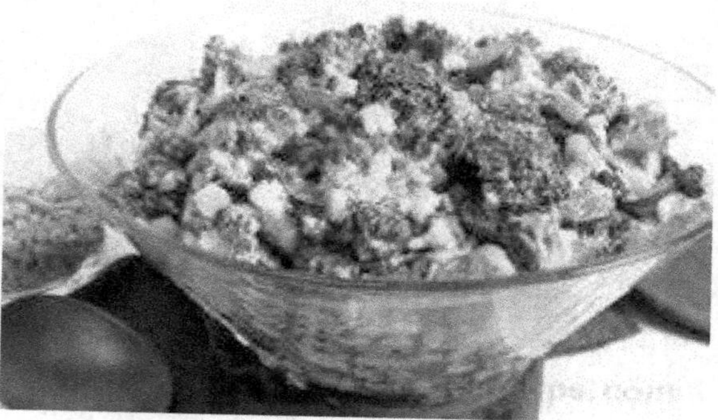

Serves: 16

Time: 65 minutes

Ingredients

2-4 pounds of grapes (green, red, or both)

1 package of fat-free– 8 ounces each:

Sour cream

Softened cream cheese

½ cup each:

Splenda/your choice

Walnuts/Pecans

¼ cup brown sugar

4 tablespoons vanilla extract

Directions

Wash and drain the grapes.

Combine the sour cream, cream cheese, vanilla, and sugar—blending well for about three to four minutes on high with a mixer.

Toss in the grapes and toss until covered.

Pour into a 9x13 cake pan. Sprinkle lightly with the brown sugar. Add the nuts.

Chill about one hour before serving.

Caramel Apple Salad

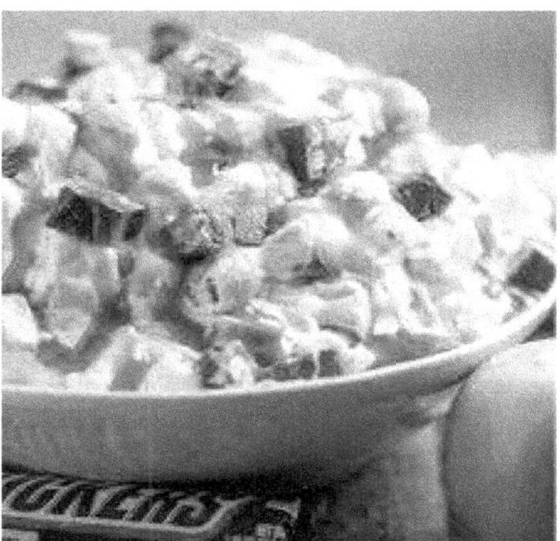

Serves: 16

Time: 30 minutes

Ingredients

1 tub (8 ounces) Cool Whip Free

1 box Instant Butter Scotch Pudding mix (sugar-free)

1 can (14 ounces) pineapple tidbits with the juice

4 large each:

Fuji apples/Red Delicious

Granny Smith apples

Directions

Mix the pineapple with its juice and the pudding mix in a large mixing container.

Dice the apples into small portions and fold in the Cool Whip.

Mix well, and chill in the refrigerator until ready to eat.

Caprese Salad

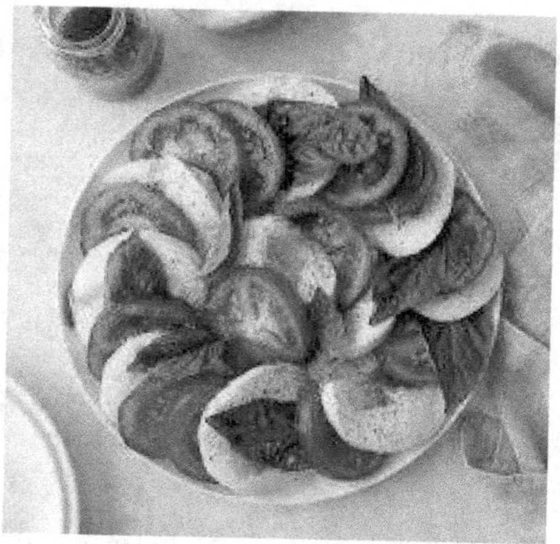

Serves: 2

Time: 10 minutes

Ingredients

6 ounces strawberries

1 ripe avocado

1 (7 ounces) sliced mozzarella ball

Small handful salad leaves

2-3 tablespoons balsamic dressing – your choice

Pepper and salt

Directions

Toss in the salad leaves, avocado, strawberries, and cheese into a serving dish.

Add the tasty dressing and sprinkle with the pepper and salt. Gently toss and enjoy.

Sunshine Fruit Salad

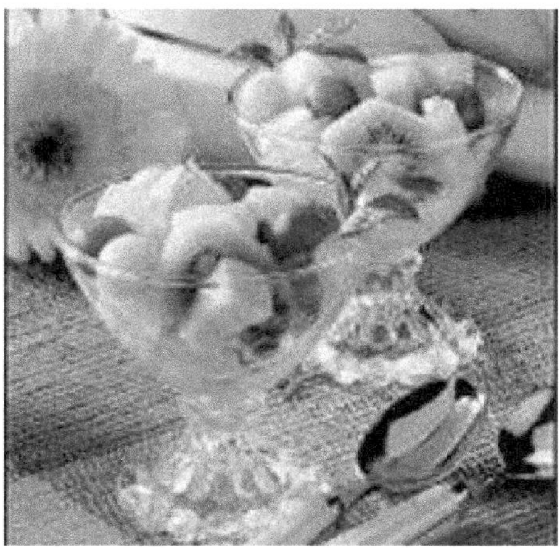

Serves: 10

Time: 65 minutes

Ingredients

2 cans (15 ounces each) mandarin oranges in light syrup

3 cans (20 ounces each) pineapple chunks in 100% juice

2 large bananas

3 medium kiwi fruits - bite-sized

Directions

Drain the oranges and pineapple. Reserve the pineapple juice.

Combine all of the fruit (omit the bananas).

Submerge the fruit with the juice and chill for a minimum of one hour.

Slice and stir in the bananas before serving.

Chapter 6: Snacks and Desserts

Mini Cheesecakes

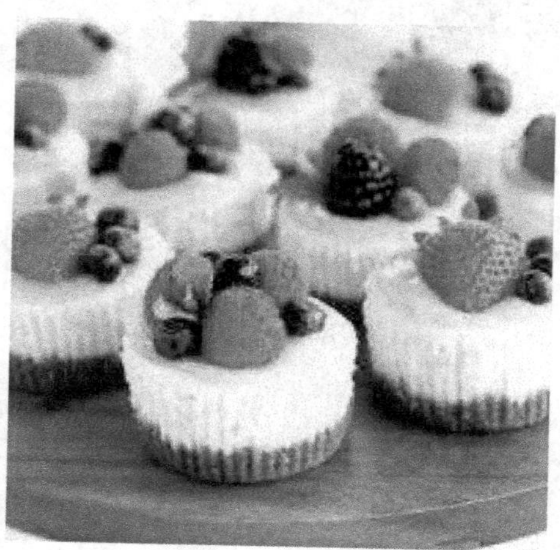

Serves: 20

Time: 2 hours 15 minutes

Ingredients

3 ounces cream cheese

12 ounces fat-free cream cheese

12 low-fat vanilla wafers

½ teaspoon vanilla

½ cup sugar

2 eggs

Cherry pie filling

Directions

Set the oven temperature to 350ºF.

Let the cream cheese sit out at room temperature.

Line 12 muffin tins with foil cake liners and add a wafer to each one.

Combine the regular and fat-free cheese until smooth. Blend in the sugar, vanilla, and eggs - beating until smooth.

Pour the batter into the tins and bake for 20 minutes.

Refrigerate for a minimum of two hours - preferably overnight.

Add the cherry filling to each one and serve.

Black Bean Brownies

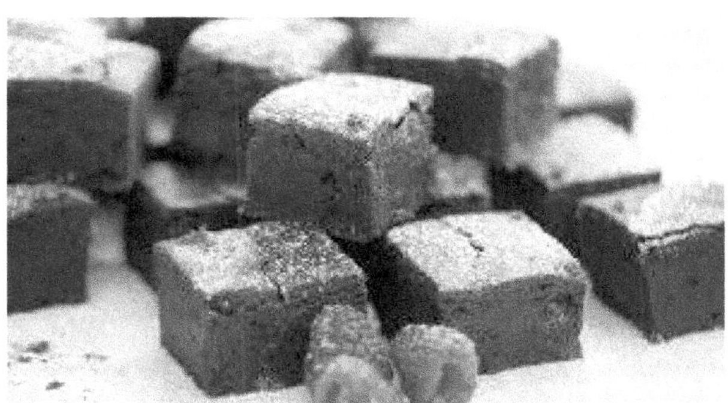

Serves: 16

Time: 40 minutes

Ingredients

4 large eggs

1 can (15 ounces) black beans

3 tablespoons cocoa powder

½ cup granulated Splenda

1 tablespoon instant coffee*

2 tablespoons olive/canola oil

1 teaspoon each:

Baking powder

Vanilla

Directions

Set the oven temperature to 350°F. Spray an 8x8 pan with some non-stick cooking spray.

*Dissolve the coffee in one tablespoon of hot water and mix with the rest of the ingredients. Drain and rinse the black beans, adding them last.

Bake 30 minutes, and perform the toothpick test for doneness.

Let cool before slicing into 2x2-inch brownies.

Coconut Meringue Cookies

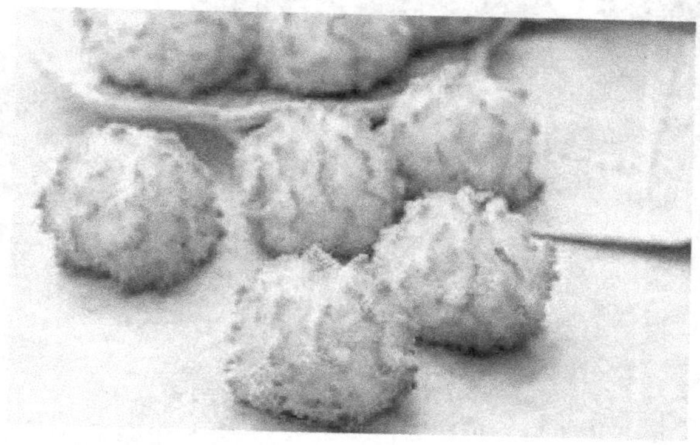

Serves: 20

Time: 30 minutes

Ingredients

2 egg whites

Dash of salt

1 ½ cups coconut sweetened shredded

2/3 cup granulated sugar

¼ teaspoon vanilla extract

Directions

Whip the eggs with a dash of salt to form stiff peaks. Stir in the sugar and fold in the coconut.

Bake 18 to20 minutes at 325°F.

Healthy Breakfast Cookie

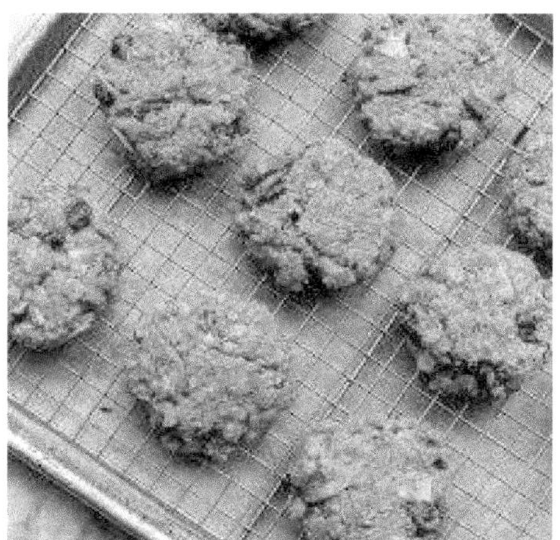

Serves: 30

Time: 20 minutes

Ingredients

2 large eggs

¼ cup butter

½ cup each:

Honey

Chopped - dried apricots

Raisins

1 cup each:

Grated carrots

Chopped walnuts

All-purpose flour

Rolled oats

1 ½ cups Cheerios

1 teaspoon each:

Cinnamon

Nutmeg

Directions

Mix the butter, honey, and egg in a mixing bowl. Combine the mixture with the apricots, walnuts, and raisins.

In a separate container, mix the cinnamon, nutmeg, flour, and oats.

Combine all components and mix well. Fold in the Cheerios.

Drop the dough onto a baking sheet about one inch apart.

Bake 15 minutes or until the cookie is firm.

Blueberry Muffin

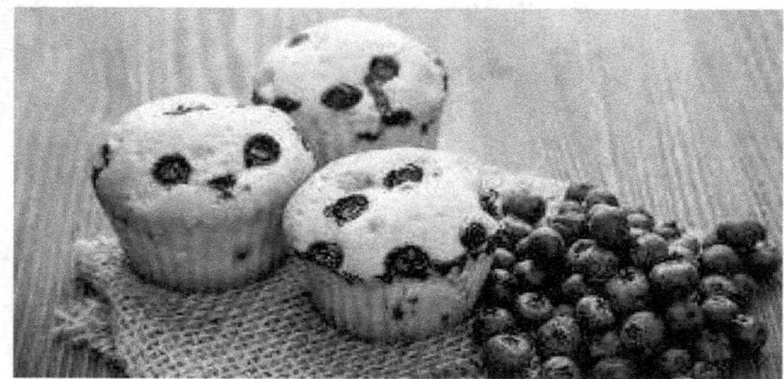

Serves: 12

Time: 35 minutes

Ingredients

1 cup of each:

Flour

Old-fashioned oats

1 tsp. each:

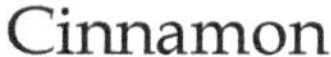

Cinnamon

Baking soda

½ tsp. of salt

½ cup each:

Unsweetened applesauce

Water

Sugar

2 egg whites

1 cup frozen blueberries

Directions

Prepare 12 muffin tins and program the oven to 350°F.

Combine the salt, soda, cinnamon, oats, and flour.

Add the egg whites, sugar, water, and applesauce.

Blend in the blueberries

Bake 20 to 25 minutes until lightly browned.

Pumpkin Muffins

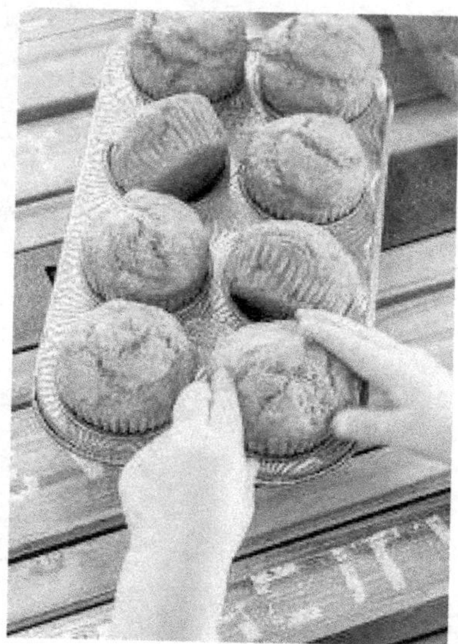

Serves: 18

Time: 40 minutes

Ingredients

1 can/1 pound pumpkin

½ cup flaxseed meal

1 box spice cake mix

Directions

Program the oven to 350°F.

Line a muffin tin with paper liners or cooking spray.

Combine all of the ingredients and bake 25 minutes.

Check for doneness with a toothpick in the center. If it comes out clean – it's done.

Enjoy when you just don't have time for the 'from scratch' recipe.

Carnivore diet Cookbook

Simple and easy recipes

Haile Banister

Table of Contents

Introduction

Are you looking for a protein-rich diet that will help you strengthen your muscles? Do you a dietary approach that is rich in protein but low in carbs? Then look no further, as we are about to introduce you to the carnivore diet, which is going to boost your protein intake up to many folds. The diet offers an all-meat meal plan with no use of plant-based products. But the carnivore diet does not recommend an unplanned and disorganized meat consumption; it suggests a three-stage formula to introduce this dietary regime into your lifestyle. And this cookbook brings you a complete account of the carnivore diet and how does it work. You will also learn a lot of interesting things about this diet that could make you change your mind about this diet. This three-stage carnivore diet is as follows:

Stage 1 (At first stage of the carnivore diet) – Full Carnivore Diet

"The full carnivore diet is the first stage of the carnivore diet in which all kinds of meat are consumed. This is the most crucial stage of this diet, as it helps get rid of the addiction to plants and persuades one to stick to this diet for the long run." Says Dr. Shawn Baker, a well-known carnivore diet proponent, who follows and recommends the carnivore diet for everyone who is looking for a healthier lifestyle. The full carnivore diet, in a nutshell, is as follows:

Steak and potatoes

Fish and vegetables

Bacon and eggs

Vegetable soup

Grilled chicken

Milk shake

Stage 2 (Second stage of the carnivore diet) – Reduced Carnivore Diet

The second stage of the carnivore diet is as follows:

Steak and eggs

Grilled chicken

Bacon and eggs

Chicken with vegetables

Milk shake

Vegetable soup

Stage 3 (Third stage of the carnivore diet) – Basic Recipes

The third stage of the carnivore diet is as follows:

Steak and rice

Stage 1, the full carnivore diet , is one of the most difficult stages of this diet to follow. It is advised to follow this stage for only two to three months.

Stage 2 is the most commonly used stage of the carnivore diet . It is a very easy stage to follow.

Stage 3 is still another stage that is often regarded as a difficult stage of this diet, but this is a myth.

The carnivore diet is explained in the most simple language. It can be followed by anyone who's ready to take the risks and responsibilities of this diet and wants to have a healthy lifestyle. It is a very effective way to reduce or stay away from any kind of health ailments as well as to get rid of the addiction to plants, which are plant foods that are a source of carbohydrates, proteins, fats as well as micronutrients.

How the Carnivore Diet Works

Most low-carb diets tend to restrict most plant-based options since carbohydrates come from plants. The most stringent low-carb meal plan the carnivore diet, emphasizes elimination of all plant-based foods, including seeds, nuts, and non-starchy veggies common on other similar diet plans such as paleo, keto, and Atkins. Carbohydrates are not a crucial nutrient despite the widespread belief, which means that we do not require them to function appropriately and survive.

Nevertheless, this does not imply that we are essentially meant to survive with no carbs.

Like the keto diet, this meal plan promotes a state of ketosis as you switch from sugars as the primary energy source for your body to fat (ketones). However, with this diet, the ketosis state is not required, and it is not as central as it is with the keto diet. Due to this, it is advisable to consume sufficient high-fat animal-based foods to keep your energy levels up.

Basic Principles of a Carnivore Diet:

Our metabolism always needs time to adjust to the new dietary regime, so try following some basic rules while introducing it into your lifestyle:

1. Start with Baby Steps:

Start with small targets and challenges, plan a carnivore diet only for 2 or 3 three weeks, and see how it turns out for then repeat the same routine for another two weeks or so.

2. Meat Based meals:

Instead of abruptly switching to an exclusive carnivore diet, start phasing into the diet by increase the proportion of meat only meals in your routine diet. Keep your refrigerator and freezer filled with a variety of meats- seafood, poultry, beef, lamb, and pork in different cuts like boneless, ground, chops, steaks, etc.

3. Stay Hydrated!

Eating a lot of meat can dehydrate the body because when protein breakdown, they release more uric acid, and it takes more water to get out of the body, which leaves the dieter dehydrated. So, drink lots of water as it will also keep your electrolyte levels balanced and your acidic load low

4. Prefer Grass-Fed, Pasture-Raised, and Organic Meat:

You can stay healthy on this diet by making the right choices and choosing organic and healthy meat over-processed and packaged meat.

Carnivore Diet Meal Plan

As mentioned earlier, it is recommended to ease into the carnivore diet using the 3-level strategy until you work your way to eating just beef. The meal plan below will steadily alter the selection of meat over the first 4 weeks until you reach the third level.

Week 1 Diet Plan

For your first week on the carnivore meal plan, you will notice a couple of dairy items that you can still enjoy. This helps you to not feel deprived.

Monday
Breakfast: 5 slices (about 4 ounces) of bacon and 1-2 (3 ounces) 100% pork sausages
Lunch: The grilled beef burger patty only (10 ounces) with a slice of cheese
Dinner: Four fresh racks of lamb (12 ounces)
Tuesday
Breakfast: 3 (5 ounces) grilled pork sausages, 3 slices (4 ounces) of bacon
Lunch: Roasted salmon cutlets on the bone (15 ounces) with butter **Dinner**: Grilled porterhouse steak (12 ounces) with butter
Wednesday
Breakfast: Grilled trout fillets (10 ounces) with butter
Lunch: Roasted pork belly (10 ounces)
Dinner: Slow roast topside of beef (12 ounces)
Thursday **Breakfast**: Ground beef burger patty- grilled with some cheese
Lunch: Roast salmon (15 ounces) with butter **Dinner**: Grilled porterhouse steak (12 ounces)
Friday **Breakfast**: 2 grilled chicken breasts with skin (8 ounces)
Lunch: Grilled trout fillets (16 ounces) **Dinner**: Slow roast topside of beef (12 ounces)
Saturday **Breakfast**: 3 (5 ounces) grilled 100% pork sausages, 3 slices (4

ounces) of bacon
Lunch: 4 lamb chops (12 ounces)
Dinner: Grilled ribeye steak (12 ounces)
Sunday
Breakfast: 2 (8 ounces) grilled chicken breasts with skin
Lunch: 4 (12 ounces) pork chops fried or grilled
Dinner: Grilled ribeye steak (12 ounces)
Week 1 Shopping List
Topside of beef: 24 ounces
Ribeye steak: 24 ounces
Porterhouse steak: 24 ounce
Beef (Grounded): 18 ounces
Salmon cutlets: 30 ounces (or other fatty fish)
Trout: 26 ounces
Lamb Chops: 24 ounces
100% pork sausages: 13 ounces
Pork belly: 10 ounces
Pork chops: 12 ounces
Bacon: 12 ounces
Cheese: 1/2 pounds
Butter: 1 pound Chicken breasts

Week 2 Diet Plan

In week 2 of your carnivore diet, we will eliminate most by products. You can still cook with some butter, though you should not use dairy products such as cheese. Also, during the second week, adjust to rarer meat cuts for your nutritional benefit. You can also introduce organ meats in this week.

Monday
Breakfast: 2 grilled chicken breasts (about 8 ounces)
Lunch: Slow roast topside of beef (12 ounces)
Dinner: 4 fresh lamb chops (12 ounces) Tuesday
Breakfast: Ground beef patty-grilled (8 ounces) **Lunch**: Roast salmon (around 15 ounces)
Dinner: Ribeye steak- grilled (8 ounces) +beef liver (roasted) (around 4 ounces)
Wednesday **Breakfast**: 5 slices (about 4 ounces) of bacon and 1-2 (3 ounces)

100% pork sausages
Lunch: Grilled porterhouse steak (12 ounces) with butter
Dinner: Slow roast topside of beef (12 ounces)
Thursday
Breakfast: Ribeye steak-grilled (12 ounces)
Lunch: 3 chicken breasts-grilled with skin (12 ounces)
Dinner: Ground beef burger patty- grilled (12 ounces)
Friday
Breakfast: Grilled steak (about 8 ounces) with some butter
Lunch: Slow roast beef (8 ounces) + roasted beef liver (4 ounces) **Dinner**: 4 grilled or fried pork chops (about 12 ounces)
Saturday
Breakfast: Grilled ground beef burger (8 ounces)
Lunch: 15 ounces of roast salmon with butter
Dinner: Grilled sirloin steak (12 ounces) Sunday
Breakfast: Grilled steak (8 ounces) **Lunch**: Slow roast beef (12 ounces)
Dinner: 3 (12 ounces) grilled chicken breasts with skin + 4 ounces of roasted beef liver

Week 3 Diet Plan

During week 3, you need to remove all by-products of milk, and then shift towards eating more beef. You will also eat less of fish and poultry and more of beef. You will also eat more of organ meat.

Monday
Breakfast: 8 ounces of grilled beef burger patty
Lunch: 8 ounces of Slow roast beef + 4 ounces of roast beef liver **Dinner**: 15 ounces of Roasted salmon (or any fatty fish) cutlets on the bone
Tuesday
Breakfast: 5 slices (about 4 ounces) of bacon and 1-2 (3 ounces) pork sausages
Lunch: Grilled beef burger patty (12 ounces)
Dinner: Grilled porterhouse steak (about 12 ounces)
Wednesday
Breakfast: Grilled ribeye steak (8 ounces)
Lunch: 12 ounces of Grilled beef burger patty
Dinner: 4 pork chops grilled or fried (12 ounces) Thursday
Breakfast: Grilled porterhouse steak (8 ounces) **Lunch**: 3 grilled chicken

breasts with skin (12 ounces)
Dinner: 8 ounces of Slow roast topside of beef + 4 ounces of slowcooked beef Kidney
Friday **Breakfast**: Grilled ground beef burger patty (8 ounces)
Lunch: Grilled ribeye steak (8 ounces) + roasted beef liver (4 ounces) **Dinner**: Grilled porterhouse steak (12 ounces)
Saturday **Breakfast**: 3 fresh lamb chops (8 ounces)
Lunch: 12 ounces of Grilled ground beef burger patty
Dinner: 12 ounces of Slow roast topside of beef Sunday
Breakfast: 8 ounces of Grilled ribeye steak **Lunch**: 12 ounces of Grilled ground beef burger patty
Dinner: 8 ounces of Slow roast topside of beef + 4 ounces of slowcooked beef Kidney

Recipes

1. Carnivore Pancake Patties

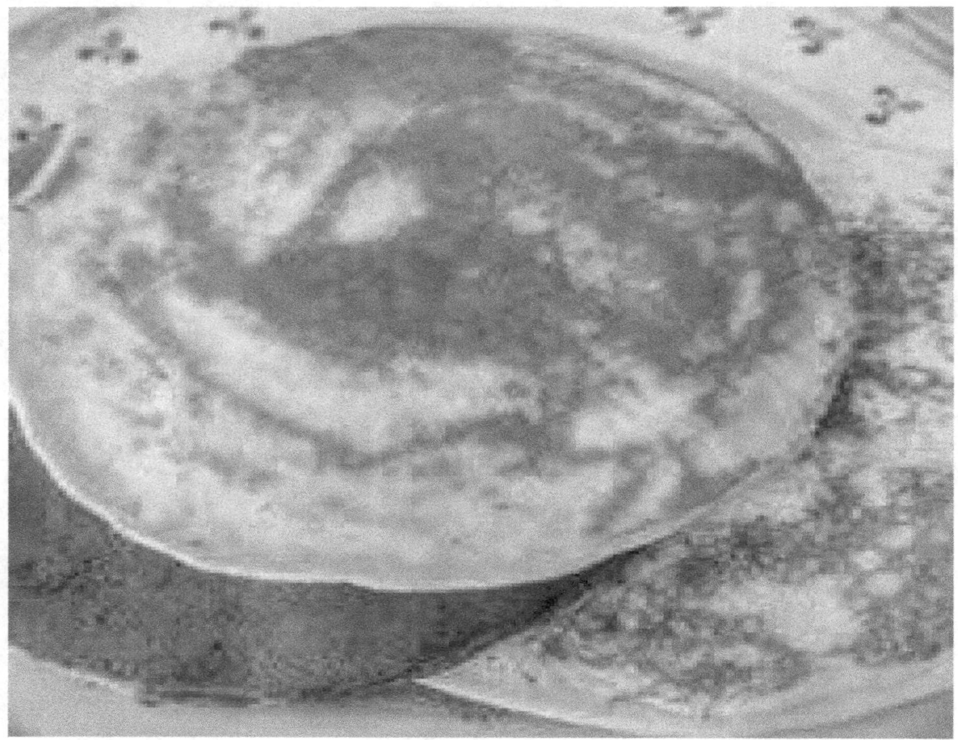

Prep Time: 20 min

Cooking Time: 30 min

Number of Servings: 6

Ingredients:

- 4 eggs
- 12 oz. pasture-raised sausages
- 2½ oz. pork rinds

Directions:

1. **Foreheat the oven to 375 degrees F and line a baking pan with aluminum foil.**
2. **Put the pork rinds in the food processor and process until smooth.**
3. **Combine sausages with the eggs and pork rinds in a bowl.**

4. **Form thick patties out of this mixture and arrange on the baking pan.**
5. Bake for about 30 minutes and dish out to serve in a platter.

Nutritional Values (Per Serving):

Calories: 302

Fat: 23.2g

Saturated Fat: 7.8g

Carbohydrates: 0.2g

Fiber: 0g

Sodium: 694mg

Protein: 22.3g

2. Beef Liver and Bacon Muffins

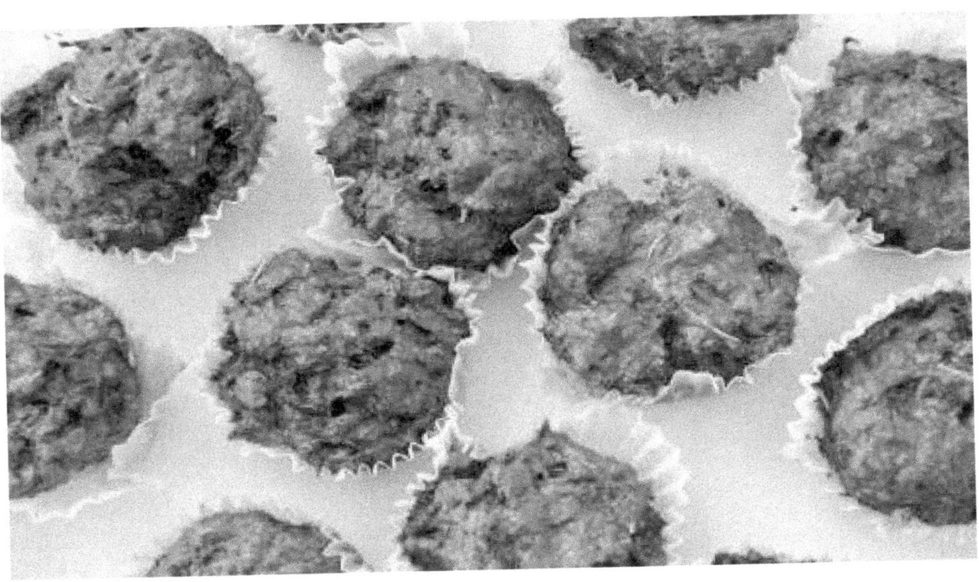

Prep Time: 10 min

Cooking Time: 30 min

Number of Servings: 8

Ingredients:

- 12 oz. beef liver
- ¼ cup bone broth
- 12 oz. ground beef, grass-fed
- 12 oz. bacon, cooked
- 1 teaspoon oregano
- 1 teaspoon rosemary
- 1 teaspoon thyme
- 1 tablespoon salt

Directions:

1. **Foreheat the oven to 350 degrees F and grease a muffin pan lightly.**
2. **Blend the liver with cooked bacon and place in a bowl.**
3. **Stir in the ground beef, bone broth, and spices. Mix well.**
4. **Transfer into the muffin pan and place in the oven.**
5. Bake for about 30 minutes and dish out to serve hot.

Nutritional Values (Per Serving):

Calories: 388

Fat: 22.5g

Saturated Fat: 7.5g

Carbohydrates: 3.1g

Fiber: 0.2g

Sodium: 1920mg

Protein: 40.6g

3. Carnivore Waffles

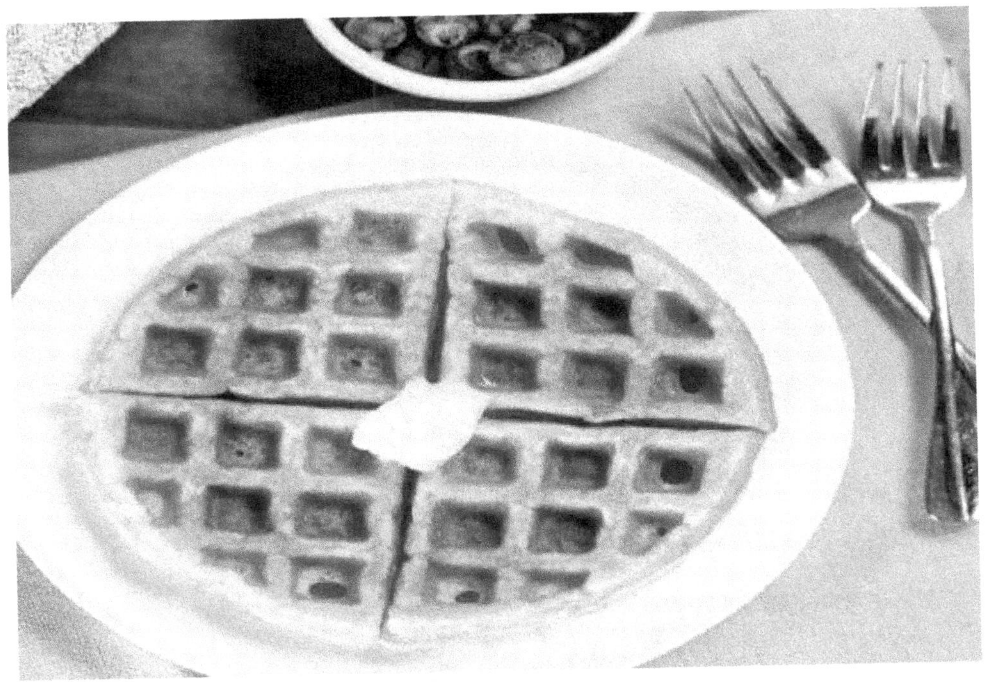

Prep Time: 5 min

Cooking Time: 4 min

Number of Servings: 1

Ingredients:

- ¼ cup raw breakfast sausage, chopped
- 2 eggs, whisked
- Coconut oil spray

Directions:

1. **Combine the whisked eggs with the sausage in a bowl.**
2. **Spray coconut oil spray on the waffle iron and pour it in the egg-sausage mixture.**
3. **Cook for about 4 minutes and remove from the waffle iron.**
4. Dish out in a platter and serve warm.

Nutritional Values (Per Serving):

Calories: 266

Fat: 20.7g

Saturated Fat: 6.9g

Carbohydrates: 0.7g

Fiber: 0g

Sodium: 423mg

Protein: 18.8g

4. Carnivore Breakfast Sandwich

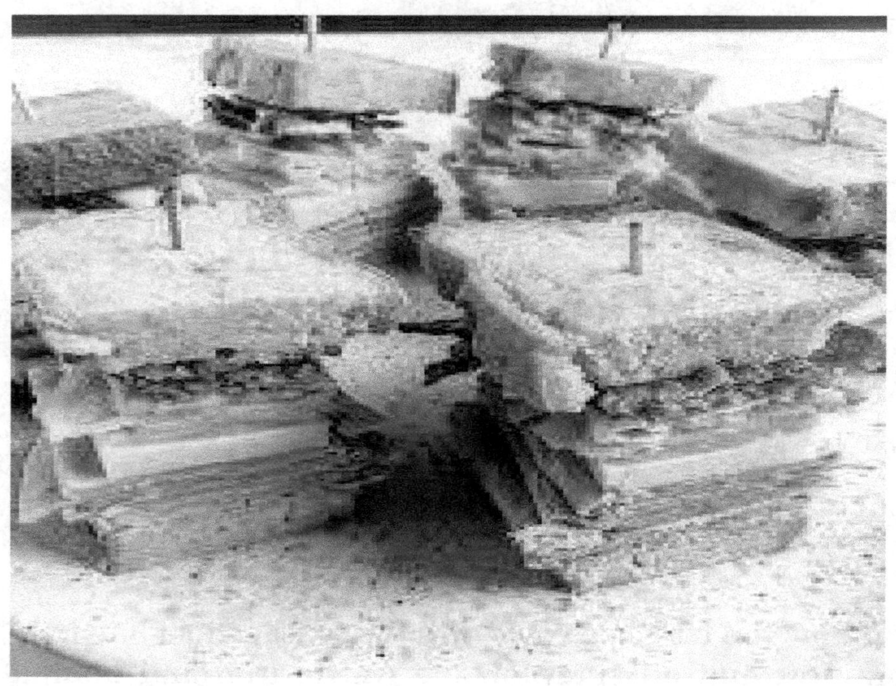

Prep Time: 5 min

Cooking Time: 8 min

Number of Servings: 1

Ingredients:

- 1 egg
- 2 beef sausage patties
- 1-ounce cheddar cheese
- 1 teaspoon butter

Directions:

1. **Put butter and beef sausage patties in a skillet over medium heat.**
2. **Cook for about 6 minutes on both sides and transfer into a plate.**
3. **Crack an egg in the same skillet and fry it for 2 minutes.**
4. **Place the fried egg on one sausage patty and top with cheese.**
5. Cover with the second sausage patty and serve immediately.

Nutritional Values (Per Serving):

Calories: 448

Fat: 36g

Saturated Fat: 15g

Carbohydrates: 1g

Fiber: 0g

Sodium: 288mg

Protein: 33

5. Ham and Egg Breakfast Cups

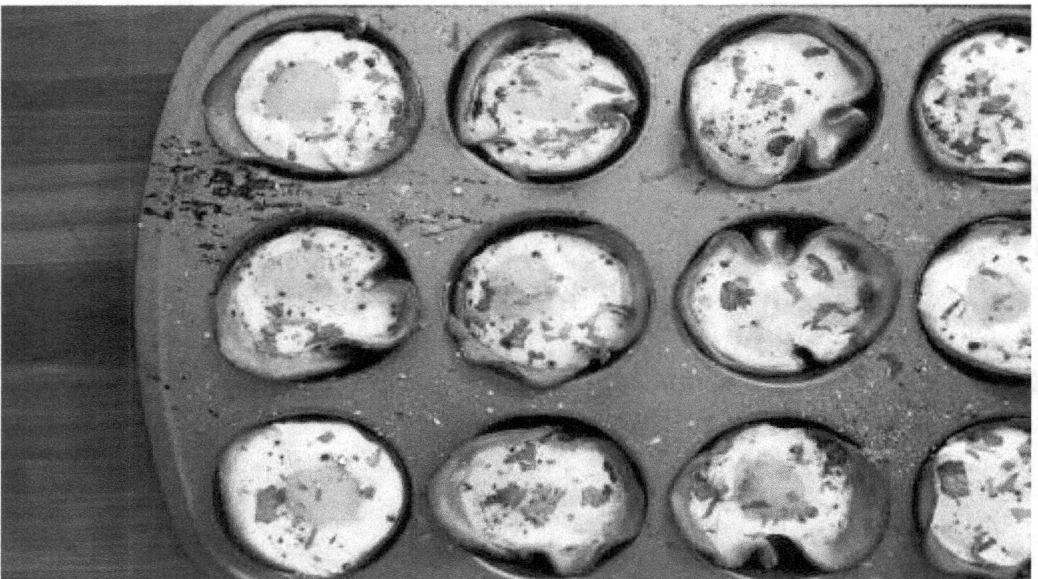

Prep Time: 10 min

Cooking Time: 20 min

Number of Servings: 6

Ingredients:

- 6 tablespoons cheddar cheese, grated
- 6 thin ham slices
- 6 eggs
- Cooking oil spray
- 1 tablespoon milk

Directions:

1. **Foreheat the oven to 350 degrees F and grease a muffin pan lightly.**
2. **Line the tins in the muffin pan with ham slices and put 1 tablespoon of cheddar cheese over each ham slice.**
3. **Whisk the eggs with milk and pour evenly into the muffin tins.**
4. **Transfer the muffin tray into the oven and bake for about 20 minutes.**
5. Dish out in a platter and serve warm.

Nutritional Values (Per Serving):

Calories: 139

Fat: 9.3g

Saturated Fat: 3.7g

Carbohydrates: 1.6g

Fiber: 0.4g

Sodium: 472mg

Protein: 12g

6. Homemade Pork Breakfast Sausage

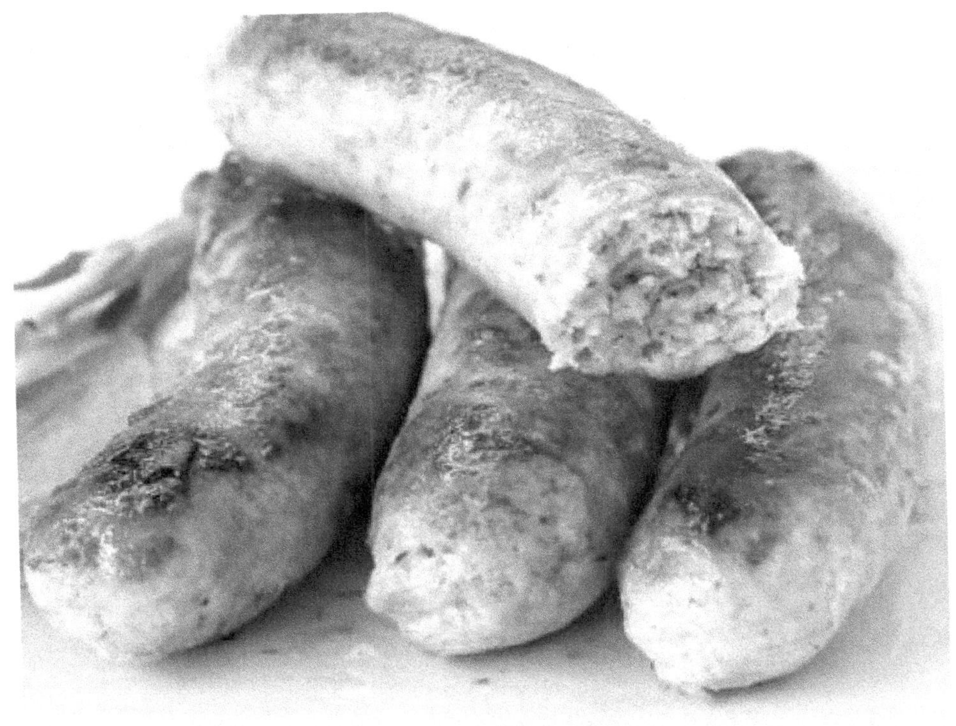

Prep Time: 15 min

Cooking Time: 20 min

Number of Servings: 3

Ingredients:

- ½ teaspoon kosher salt
- 1 pound lean ground pork
- ½ teaspoon ground thyme
- ¼ teaspoon ground allspice
- ½ teaspoon fresh ground black pepper
- ½ teaspoon dried rubbed sage
- 1/8 teaspoon cayenne pepper
- Cooking spray

Directions:

1. **Combine the ground pork with the rest of the ingredients in a bowl.**
2. **Form 8 patties out of the ground pork mixture.**
3. **Sprinkle a pan with cooking spray and fry half of the patties for about 10 minutes.**
4. Fry the remaining patties for about 10 minutes and serve on a platter.

Nutritional Values (Per Serving):

Calories: 311

Fat: 22.9g

Saturated Fat: 0g

Carbohydrates: 0.6g

Fiber: 0.2g

Sodium: 388mg

Protein: 25.8g

7. Baked Chicken Thighs

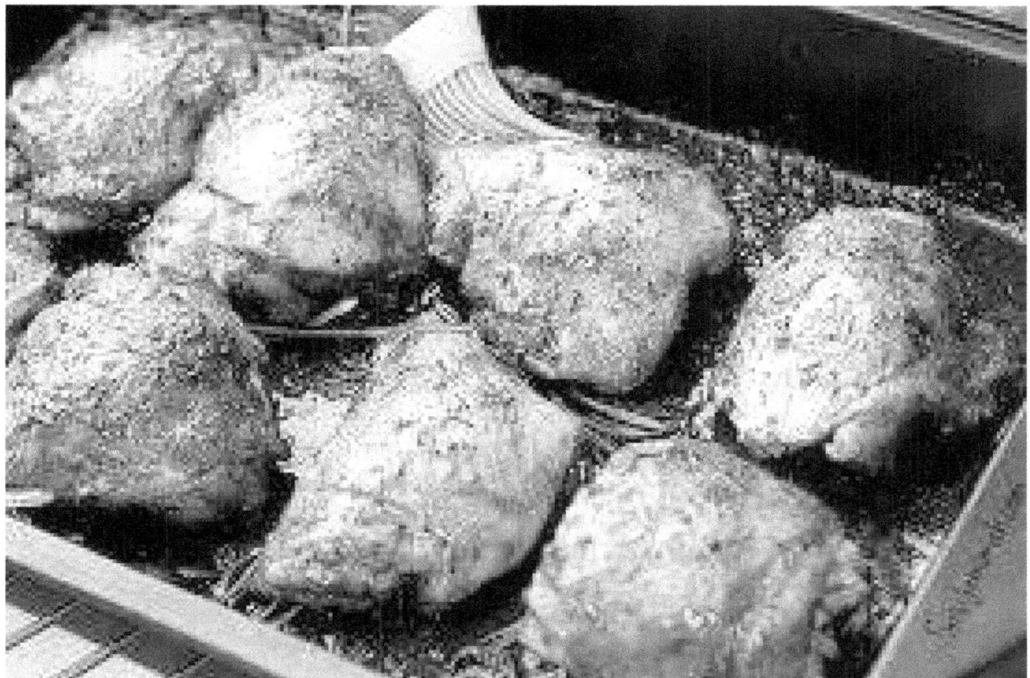

Prep Time: 10 mins

Cooking Time: 16 mins

Number of Servings: 4

Ingredients:

- Salt
- 2 tablespoons butter, divided
- ground black pepper
- 2 teaspoons dried oregano
- 1 tablespoon fresh lemon juice
- 1 tablespoon lemon zest, grated
- 1 teaspoon dried thyme

- 1½ pounds bone-in chicken thighs

Directions:

1. Preheat the oven to 420 degrees F.
2. In a large mixing bowl, add 1 tablespoon of the butter, lemon juice, lemon zest, dried herbs, salt, and black pepper and mix well.
3. Add the chicken thighs and coat with the mixture generously.
4. Refrigerate to marinate for at least 20 minutes.
5. In an oven-proof skillet, melt the remaining butter over medium-high heat and sear the chicken thighs for about 2-3 minutes per side.
6. Remove from the heat and immediately transfer the skillet into the oven.
7. Bake for about 10 minutes.
8. Remove from the oven and set aside for about 2-3 minutes.
9. **Serve hot.**

Nutritional Values (Per Serving):

Calories: 338

Fat: 19.7g

Saturated Fat: 4.5g

Trans Fat: 15.2g

Carbohydrates: 1g

Fiber: 0.5g

Sodium: 186mg

Protein: 49.4g

8. Grilled Duck Breast

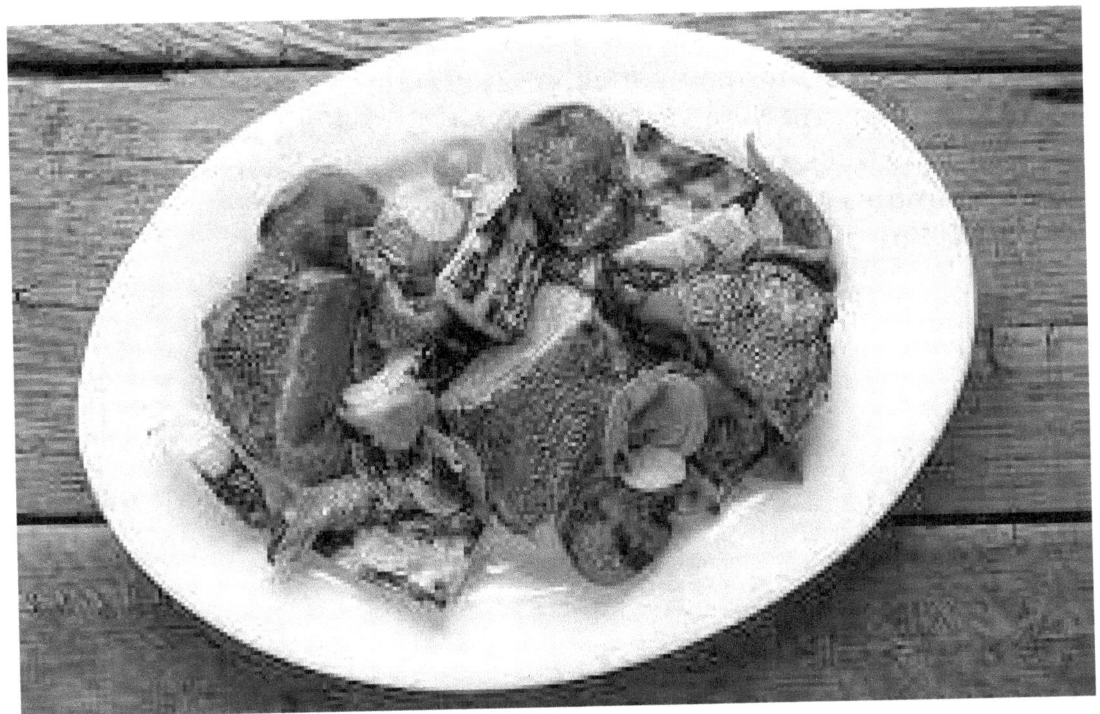

Prep Time: 10 mins

Cooking Time: 16 mins

Number of Servings: 2

Ingredients:

- 2 shallots, sliced thinly
- 1 tablespoon fresh ginger, minced
- 2 tablespoons fresh thyme, chopped
- Salt and freshly ground black pepper, to taste
- 2 duck breasts

Directions:

1. In a large bowl, place the shallots, ginger, thyme, salt and black pepper and mix well.
2. Add the duck breasts and coat with marinade evenly.
3. Refrigerate to marinate for about 2–12 hours.
4. Preheat the grill to medium-high heat. Grease the grill grate.
5. Place the duck breast onto the grill, skin-side down, and cook for about 6–8 minutes per side.
6. **Serve hot.**

Nutritional Values (Per Serving):

Calories: 337

Fat: 10.1g

Saturated Fat: 0g

Trans Fat: 10.1g

Carbohydrates: 3.4g

Fiber: 0g

Sodium: 80mg

Protein: 55.5g

9. Pan-Seared Pork Chops

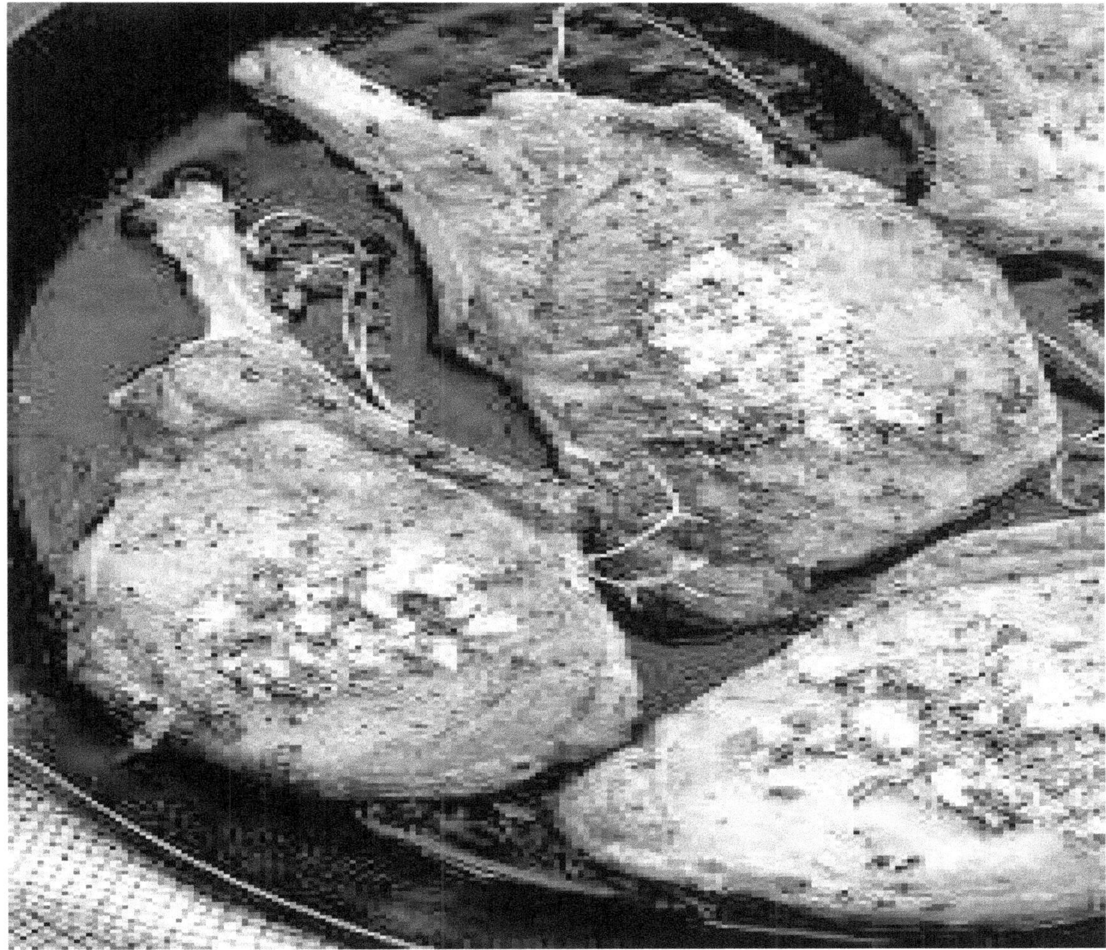

Prep Time: 10 mins

Cooking Time: 12 mins

Number of Servings: 4

Ingredients:

- 2 tablespoons butter, melted
- 1 tablespoon Worcestershire sauce
- 1 teaspoon fresh lemon juice

- ½ teaspoon garlic paste
- Salt and freshly ground black pepper, to taste
- 4 (6-ounce) (½-inch thick) boneless pork chops

Directions:

1. In a large bowl, add all the ingredients except for pork chops and mix well.
2. Add the pork chops and coat with the mixture generously.
3. Cover the bowl and set aside at room temperature for about 10-15 minutes.
4. Heat a greased skillet over medium-high heat and cook the pork chops for about 5 minutes, gently shaking the skillet occasionally.
5. Flip the pork chops and reduce heat to low.
6. Cook for about 1-2 minutes.
7. **Serve hot**

Nutritional Values (Per Serving):

Calories: 308

Fat: 13g

Saturated Fat: 3.1g

Trans Fat: 9.9g

Carbohydrates: 0.9g

Fiber: 0g

Sodium: 177mg

Protein: 44.6g

10. Grilled Lamb Chops

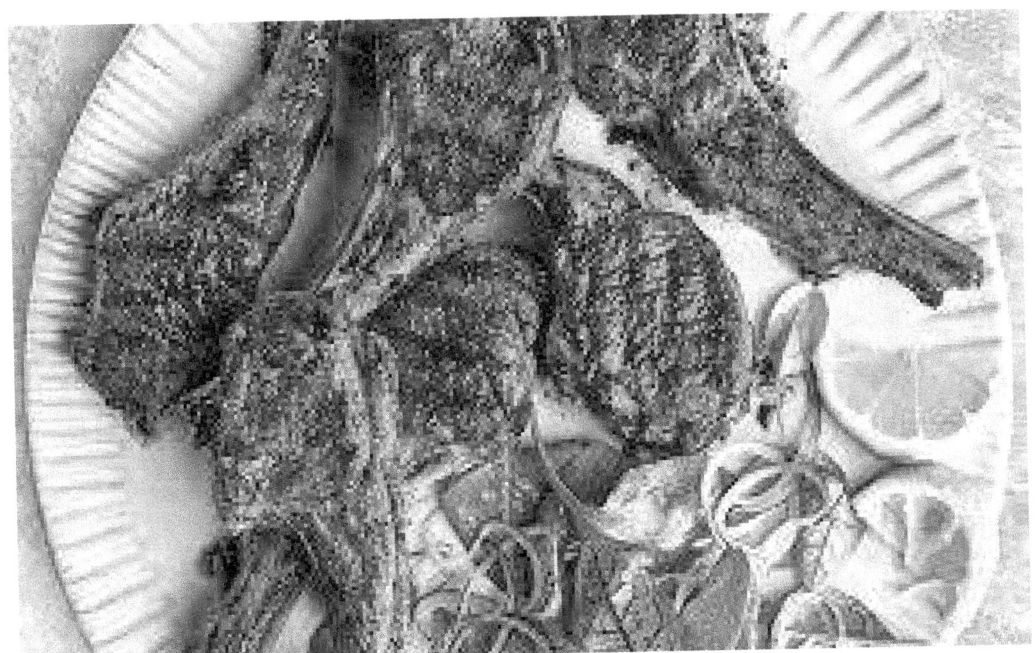

Prep Time: 10 mins

Cooking Time: 9 mins

Number of Servings: 4

Ingredients:

- ¼ cup butter, melted
- 2 tablespoons fresh oregano, chopped
- 1 teaspoon garlic, minced
- Salt and freshly ground black pepper
- 4 (8-ounce) (½-inch-thick) lamb shoulder blade chops
- 2 tablespoons fresh lemon juice

Directions:

1. Mix the ingredients
2. Place the chops and marinade into a large sealable plastic bag.
3. Seal the bag and shake vigorously to coat evenly.
4. Set aside at room temperature for about 1 hour.
5. Remove the lamb chops from the bag and discard the marinade.
6. With paper towels, pat dry the lamb chops.
7. Season the lamb chops with a little salt.
8. Preheat a large cast-iron grill pan over medium-high heat and cook 2 lamb chops for about 3 minutes.
9. Move the lamb chops and cook for about 3 more minutes.
10. Now, flip the lamb chops to their sides and adjust the heat to medium-low.
11. Cook for about 2-3 minutes.
12. Repeat with the remaining lamb chops.
13. Remove the lamb chops from heat and set aside for about 5 minutes before serving.

Nutritional Values (Per Serving):

Calories: 459

Fat: 31g

Saturated Fat: 7.9g

Trans Fat: 23.1g

Carbohydrates: 1.8g

Fiber: 1g

Sodium: 201mg

Protein: 44.5g

Conclusion

All bariatric surgeries can have some potential risks and side effects, and as we have already briefly discussed, gastric sleeve surgery is no exception. However, in comparison to other forms of bariatric surgery, gastric sleeve is by far more safe. It's one of the reasons why it's rapidly becoming one of the more popular weight loss surgeries.

In order to give you the most well rounded view of gastric sleeve surgery possible, we'll discuss the possible risks and side effects here.

Moderate Side Effects

- Moderate side effects can be expected to happen in the days immediately following surgery, but these also go away very quickly and are not dangerous at all. Examples of moderate side effects include pain, bleeding, and swelling.

Severe Side Effects

- Severe side effects are far less common for gastric sleeve surgery. Some potential complications include stomach acid leaking, inflammation in the stomach, or even bloating in the abdomen. Longer term severe side effects would include infections and pneumonia.

- While it is a severe side effects, blood clots are extremely rare in patients who undergo gastric sleeve surgery. In fact, less than one percent of all gastric sleeve patients will ever develop blood clots.

- Remember to take these potential side effects into consideration when you consider any type of bariatric surgery. Also remember that no two patients will ever experience the same combination or same level of risks at the same time. Next, we'll discuss some long term risks of the aftermath of gastric sleeve surgery that can possibly happen overtime.

Risks

- The first risk that you can take with gastric sleeve surgery is possibly having an allergic reaction to the anesthesia or other medication.

- Most of the other risks of gastric sleeve surgery would happen in the aftermath, mainly during the two week long recovery period. Examples can include developing infections in the incision area or in the bladder and kidneys, suffer from blood loss, damage to the intestines or organs in the stomach area, sutures becoming rejected, or the intestines becoming blocked.

One thing you have to be aware with gastric sleeve surgery risks is that the risks can develop over the course of several months following the surgery. The good news is that most of these risks can be prevented by simply following your surgeon's Directions, following your dieting regimen, and getting the necessary exercise.

The greatest possible risk of gastric sleeve surgery would be the stomach expanding. If you eat too much food, it can cause your stomach to expand and increase capacity. Remember that your stomach has been reduced by as much as eighty percent, so expanding your stomach beyond the twenty percent it would be after surgery can lead to some potential complications, such as developing malnutrition, lower vitamin levels, kidney stones, or gastritis.

All in all though, don't let these potential risks and side effects dishearten you from undergoing gastric sleeve surgery at all. The chance of you developing any of these risks during or following surgery are very minimal if you follow your doctor's Directions, and gastric sleeve surgery is regarded overall as being one of the safest weight loss surgeries available.

Last but not least, we'll discuss the new diet you'll have to embark on before and after surgery.

Dieting Before Surgery

- Your stomach and liver are located very closely to one another. When the surgeon will get to your stomach to perform the surgery, they will need to retract your liver with a device to move it out of the way. The overwhelming majority of individuals who are obese will also have fatty liver disease, which is where fat cells will gather around the liver cells, and causes it to function improperly…not to mention increasing the size of it.

- When the liver expands, it makes it much more difficult for the surgeon to get out of the way, which in turn makes it significantly more difficult for the actual operation and can lead to complications. Therefore, the goal of your diet before gastric sleeve surgery should be to lower the size of the liver via your diet as much as possible.

- As a large liver will only increase your surgical risk, embarking on a healthy diet before surgery is very important to ensure that the operation proceeds as smoothly as it should. You'd be surprised to know that your liver will decrease in size very quickly if you can adhere to a strict diet in just two weeks before the date of the surgery.

- Your doctor may recommend a different two week diet than the one we're going to discuss here, but this diet should serve as a golden rule (if you will call it that) for all pre-weight loss surgery diets. Begin by increasing your protein consumption by eating more lean meats, and lower your carbohydrate consumption. This means avoiding bread, pasta and rice. Finally, you'll need to eliminate all sugary foods completely. Candy, juice, soda, cake, you name it.

- For breakfast, try consuming more protein shakes such as from a supplement store. The only thing to watch out for in these shakes is to make sure that there are no sugars in them. For lunch and dinner alike, focus on eating more vegetables and lean meats.

- You can eat snacks throughout the day, but only ones that are healthy and low in carbs. Examples of this clued veggies, berries, nuts, and salads. It's also important that you stay hydrated throughout the days, so drinking plenty of water is critically important. An added benefit of water is that it will control the hunger you feel. Plus, it's common knowledge that water is good for you.

- In the three days before surgery, you will have to adhere to a strict liquid diet and stop drinking all beverages that are carbonated and/or have caffeine in them.Clear liquids that you can drink include protein shakes (though less shakes than you were consuming before), water, popsicles (provided they are sugar free), Jell-O, and broth.

- All in all, if you can adhere to this kind of strict surgery, the size of your liver should drastically decrease in the weeks before your surgery and the risk of developing any potential complications during surgery will dramatically decrease.

Dieting After Surgery

- At this point, you have completed the surgery and you may already be home following your stay in the hospital. However, now is no time to return to your previous eating habits. Whereas the previous diet you embarked on was designed to prevent complications from happening during your surgery by reducing the size of your liver, the new diet that you will embark on is focused on preventing the risk of complications after the surgery.

At times, this new diet may seem far more extreme than the previous diet, and even if you find yourself second guessing your decision to have gastric sleeve surgery, just know that this diet is essential to bringing your weight down and preventing the onset of risks. We'll go over what specific foods you can and cannot have for the weeks following your surgery and then beyond that.

- For the first week, you'll have to adhere to clear liquids only. Whereas before you spent two to three days with only clear liquids, you're now going to have to add seven days to that. Fortunately, the ghrelin hormone will be nearly eliminated at this point, so your desire to eat high amounts of 'normal foods' will be nearly eliminated as well. Foods you can eat during this time, provided they are all sugar free, include water, un-carbonated drinks, broth, decaf tea and coffee, jell-o, and popsicles. Specific foods that you should avoid include carbonated drinks, sweet drinks, non-decaf caffeine, and sugar.

- For the second week after surgery, you'll still have to adhere a liquid diet, but with less limitations than the clear liquid diet. For this week, you'll want to add more proteins to the mix. Examples of foods that you can eat during this time include protein powders mixed with liquid, sugar free ice cream, oatmeal, sugarless juices, creamy soups, non fat yogurts, soupy noodles, and sugar free pudding. While this diet definitely has less limitations than before, you can't get too overconfident at this point and eat foods you shouldn't be eating.

- Good news! For the third week after surgery, you'll be able to add some real foods to your diet instead of strictly liquids. However, you should still keep your intake of fats and sugars down if not avoiding them completely. For this week, focus on taking smaller bites and eating the individual bites more slowly, only trying one new food per meal (meaning you should not have two or more kinds of foods at the same meal), and continue to get plenty of protein. This is because you must give your body the time it needs to react to these 'new' foods; remember that's gone well over a month by now without the foods it is used to in taking and digesting. It will need more time to adjust fully.

- There are specific new foods that you can now add to your diet, as well as a few others that you should continue to avoid. New foods that you can add are protein shakes mixed with yogurt and non-fat milk, hummus, low fat cheese, mashed fruit, canned tuna or salmon, mayonnaise, steamed fish (as long as you chew well), scrambled eggs, soup, grounded beef, grounded chicken, soft cereals (tip: allow your cereal to sit in the milk to become soft), soft vegetables, soft cheese, almond milk, and coconut milk. None of these foods should be crunchy and you should remember to chew slowly with all of them.

Foods that you should continue to avoid in the third week are sugars, pasta, rice, bread, fibrous vegetables, and smoothies with high sugar levels.

- For the fourth week, you can continue to introduce more real foods that you're accustomed to. Remember though, your stomach is still very sensitive, and you aren't yet at the point where you can eat anything you want however you want. You still have to eat slowly, eat soft foods whenever possible, and only introduce one new food per meal.

During this time, you should continue consuming protein shakes, as they are one of your best sources of protein throughout this dieting process. You can introduce more fish, fruits, softened vegetables, chicken and beef. All of these foods should be as softened as much as possible and chewed thoroughly. You can also re-introduce potatoes to your diet (mashed, baked and sweetened alike) and cereal. You can also re-introduced caffeine products to your diet, but not to the point that it becomes a regular part of your diet. Be very discretionary as you add caffeine to your diet.

For the fourth week, you should focus primarily on eating three small meals throughout the day and getting plenty of water. But as long as your surgeon approves it, you should also be able to add snacks to your diet at this point. Examples of snacks that you can add include fresh fruit, small portions of baked or sweetened potatoes, small portions of oatmeal, one egg, a small portion of baby carrots, or a small portion of crackers.

Some foods you will have to continue to avoid. Most sodas, fried food, fibrous vegetables, candy and sugar, desserts, pasta, pizzas, whole milk, dairy in general, and nuts will all have to continue to be avoided in the fourth week of your diet.

- For the fifth week, your body will be able to tolerate more foods, but you could still feel an upset stomach at times. Continue to eat three small meals and remain fully hydrated throughout the day. Continue to take your prescribed medication and vitamins, and focus mainly on getting enough protein into your system (sixty grams at the least). Again, protein shakes are an excellent way to get plenty of protein in your system. You should also try to exercise more now, and your body should start to lose weight at a faster rate. Continue to adhere to a strict dieting plan, and when you do eat snacks, only eat from small portions.

CPSIA information can be obtained
at www.ICGtesting.com
Printed in the USA
BVHW060734210721
612420BV00004B/832

9 781803 570457